# Handbook of Laboratory Animal Management and Welfare

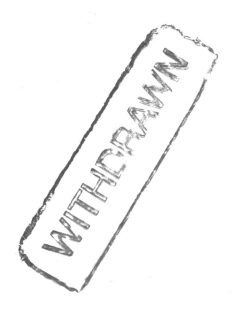

# Handbook of Laboratory Animal Management and Welfare

## Third edition

**Sarah Wolfensohn**

BSc, MA, VetMB, Cert LAS, CBiol, FIBiol, Dip ECLAM, MRCVS
*Head of Department, Veterinary Services, University of Oxford*

and

**Maggie Lloyd**

MA, VetMB, CertLAS, DipHE, MRCVS
*Home Office*

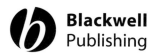

**Blackwell**
Publishing

© 2003 by Blackwell Publishing Ltd

Editorial Offices:
Blackwell Publishing Ltd, 9600 Garsington Road, Oxford OX4 2DQ, UK
  Tel: +44 (0)1865 776868
Blackwell Publishing Professional, 2121 State Avenue, Ames, Iowa 50014-8300, USA
  Tel: +1 515 292 0140
Blackwell Publishing Asia, 550 Swanston Street, Carlton, Victoria 3053, Australia
  Tel: +61 (0)3 8359 1011

First published 1994 by Oxford University Press
Second edition published 1998 by Blackwell Science
Third edition published 2003 by Blackwell Publishing Ltd
3   2006

ISBN-13: 978-1-4051-1159-1
ISBN-10: 1-4051-1159-3

Library of Congress Cataloging-in-Publication Data
Wolfensohn, Sarah.
   Handbook of laboratory animal management and welfare/Sarah Wolfensohn, Maggie Lloyd.– 3rd ed.
     p. cm.
Includes bibliographical references (p.   ) and index.
   ISBN 1-4051-1159-3 (pbk. : alk. paper)
   1.  Laboratory animals – Handbooks, manuals, etc.   2.  Animal welfare – Handbooks, manuals, etc.   3.  Animal experimentation – Handbooks, manuals, etc.
   I. Lloyd, Maggie.   II. Title.

   SF406.W64 2003
   636.088′5 – dc22

                                                                    2003015192

A catalogue record for this title is available from the British Library

Set in Times
Printed and bound in Great Britain
by TJ International Ltd, Padstow, Cornwall

The publisher's policy is to use permanent paper from mills that operate a sustainable forestry policy, and which has been manufactured from pulp processed using acid-free and elementary chlorine-free practices. Furthermore, the publisher ensures that the text paper and cover board used have met acceptable environmental accreditation standards.

For further information on Blackwell Publishing, visit our website:
www.blackwellpublishing.com

*This book is dedicated to our families,*
*Simon, Rebecca and Joseph, Andrew, Michael and Elizabeth*
*in recognition of the unfailing support they have given us*

# Contents

## SECTION 2: SPECIES

**For each species covers:**

Behaviour                   Handling
Housing                     Pain and stress recognition
Feeding                     Common diseases and health monitoring
Water                       Biological data and useful reference data
Environment                 Drug doses for anaesthesia
Breeding                    Drug doses for analgesia
Growth

# Acknowledgements

Mr Chris Trower made a significant contribution to Chapter 16 for which we are very grateful. Mr Roger Francis made helpful comments on birds and exotic species and provided photographs. Thanks are also due to our colleagues both at Oxford University Veterinary Services and the Home Office for their advice and comments, particularly Dr Manuel Berdoy, Mr Paul Finnemore and Dr Paul Honess.

# Section 1
# General

# Chapter 1
# Education and training for the licence holder

## INTRODUCTION

The Animals (Scientific Procedures) Act 1986 (ASPA) covers procedures carried out on certain types of animals (protected animals) for a scientific purpose, which may have the effect of causing pain, suffering, distress or lasting harm (regulated procedures) (see Chapter 2). The Act places clear responsibilities on people with specific roles under the Act. In order to fulfil their responsibilities effectively, it follows that appropriate education and training will be required, depending on the role of the person. In addition, the European Commission (EC) Directive for the Protection of Vertebrate Animals used for Experimental and other Scientific Purposes (86/609/EEC) specifies that those carrying out experiments shall have appropriate education and training. Education involves the acquisition of relevant knowledge and development of a suitable attitude towards experimental work using live animals including an understanding of alternative methods and the ethical issues, whereas training involves the acquisition of manual skills. Both of these are important: an increased awareness of the practical and ethical issues by the scientific community will assist in the implementation of the legislation, which would be ineffective if it were forced upon a research community that was insensitive to the requirements of the law.

## ATTITUDES

At first glance, the 3 million or so animals used for science annually in the UK compares favourably with the hundreds of millions used for food or killed by cats (Woods *et al.*, 2003). It might be considered, therefore, in terms of animal welfare, that the use of animals for science is less problematic. Yet, it is the basis of heated, and sometimes violent, debate. There may be several reasons for this. First, while anybody can have a direct effect on the number of animals used for food or killed by cats by changing their own behaviour, it is difficult to have a direct influence on the number of animals used for research. Secondly, there is the issue of suffering, since scientific procedures may have the potential to incur pain, suffering, distress or lasting harm (which is why they are regulated). Many people would argue that this is a form of torture. It is indeed worth noting that the ASPA is an enabling Act, protecting the researcher from other pieces of animal legislation (e.g. 1911 Protection of Animals Act), which would otherwise prevent such potentially harmful scientific investigations using animals.

Society is, therefore, faced with a moral dilemma:

1. we have dominion over animals
2. animals suffer
3. the use of animals (including for food) can involve suffering.

What should society allow, and how?

This book is more concerned with ethical behaviour (i.e. about ways of eliminating or minimising suffering) than moral philosophy, but it is worth being aware of the two major schools of thoughts that have fed ethical thinking: the consequentialist and the non-consequentialist approaches. Pro- and anti-vivisectionists are found in both camps; and to some extent (albeit with large shades of grey), the positions adopted by lobby groups also reflect these two approaches.

The *consequentialist* attitude encompasses a number of ethical traditions, including utilitarianism. This approach is essentially based on a cost–benefit calculation that aims to maximise overall pleasure (benefit) and minimise pain (cost). This is a powerful approach, although not one without problems, particularly where the costs and benefits are in different currencies. How does one weigh the pleasures/pain of animals against those of humans? The attitude of some philosophers and animal welfare groups can be placed in this category: they would like to see an end to animal experimentation, but they agree that it is not yet possible (e.g. Singer, 1976). However, they highlight that much needs to be done in understanding the true costs, which they view as being currently underestimated.

The *non-consequentialist* arguments are based on the inherent value of life and the principle of rights (e.g. Regan, 1983). It argues that, whatever the benefits, there are things that should not be done: the use of sentient animals for one's own ends is viewed as ethically unjustifiable. If aliens invaded us, would we have a right not to be experimented on? This is a position often adopted by the generally smaller 'Animal Rights' groups. Unlike welfare groups who take a more pragmatic, gradualist approach to reform, animal rights groups tend to have a more extreme abolitionist view (not larger cages but empty cages).

Where does the Act stand? This section has deliberately asked more questions than it has answered in trying to illustrate that animal ethics is about more than just our emotional reactions to animals. The rest of the book is concerned with practical ethics; but before reading further, you might consider where you stand in this spectrum of views; and indeed, where you think that the legislation, which is covered in the next chapter, should stand.

## TRAINING

Personal licensees bear primary responsibility for the care and welfare of animals on which they have carried out regulated procedures; therefore, they must be appropriately qualified to take on this responsibility. This will involve acquiring knowledge of the legal framework and needs of the relevant species as well as practical skills relating to the handling of animals and conduct of regulated procedures.

Project licence holders take responsibility for the direction of a programme of work, and must be able to manage such a programme taking all opportunities for reduction, refinement and replacement.

Holders of certificates of designation have responsibility for maintaining the fabric of the establishment and for appropriate staffing, and for ensuring that management systems are in place for prevention of unauthorised procedures. It is also the certificate holder who is obliged to ensure that appropriate training facilities are available not only for licence applicants, but also for those people carrying out humane methods of killing, as listed in Schedule 1 to the Act, and for people carrying out non-regulated procedures using live animals. These people also need to be aware of the ethical issues surrounding the use of animals in scientific procedures.

Applicants for personal licences since 1994 have been required to complete an accredited training programme. The purpose of accreditation is to achieve common and high standards for licensee training, which will facilitate free movement of licensees within the UK and Europe as well as ensuring high standards in the use of animals in scientific procedures. The accreditation schemes operated by the Institute of Biology and the Universities Accreditation Scheme are currently recognised by the Home Office for this purpose. The contents of the programmes are laid down by the Home Office and divided into individual modules as described below.

## Module 1: Legislation

1.  Historical background.
2.  Introduction to ethical aspects of the use of animals in experimental procedures.
3.  The ASPA.
4.  Other legislation relevant to the use of animals.

## Module 2: Principles of animal care

1.  Recognition of well-being, pain, suffering and distress in relevant species.
2.  Handling and restraint of relevant species.
3.  Humane methods of killing.
4.  Local procedures for security, administration, supply and disposal of animals.
5.  Health and safety.

## Module 3: Principles of animal use

1.  Biology and husbandry of relevant species.
2.  Common diseases in the relevant species.
3.  Health monitoring, and disease prevention and control.
4.  Introduction to anaesthesia and analgesia.
5.  Conduct of minor procedures.

## Module 4: Surgery

1.  Surgical anaesthesia and analgesia.
2.  Conduct of surgical procedures.

## Module 5: Project management

1. Further ethical considerations.
2. Analysis of the scientific literature.
3. Alternatives to using animals – the three Rs.
4. Project design.
5. Project licence management.
6. European and international legislation.

The syllabus is inexhaustive and course organisers are encouraged to include other topics that they may consider relevant. Training can be achieved through lectures, tutorials, discussions, videos and reading, but the importance of practical experience must be emphasised. There must be an assessment at the conclusion of the formal training programme, since it is the acquisition of knowledge that is required, not simply the attendance at a course. The aim of this book is to supplement other training methods and to bring useful information together in one volume, particularly for Modules 1–4 for the *personal* licensee, but the reader is encouraged to observe others and gain as much experience as possible.

In general, people applying for licences or certificates should complete modules as shown in Table 1.1. Exemptions from training requirements will be considered for those with relevant experience, such as overseas researchers or veterinarians with particular expertise in a species. Requests for exemption from training requirements should be discussed with the local Home Office Inspector.

**Table 1.1**   Training modules for licence applicants.

| Target audience | Modules | | | | |
|---|---|---|---|---|---|
| | 1 | 2 | 3 | 4 | 5 |
| *Those not applying for licence* | | | | | |
| Personnel with administrative responsibility only | + | | | | |
| Non-licensed animal users: those killing by a Schedule 1 method | + | + | | | |
| *Licence applicants* | | | | | |
| Undergraduates applying for limited licences to work personally under close supervision | + | + | | | |
| Personal licence applicants who will be performing minor non-surgical procedures; brief terminal procedures under anaesthesia | + | + | + | | |
| Personal licence applicants who will be performing major surgical procedures under terminal or recovery anaesthesia | + | + | + | + | |
| Project licence applicants | + | + | Individual needs may vary | + | |

## CORE COMPETENCIES OF PERSONAL LICENCE HOLDERS

A personal licence holder bears the primary responsibilities for animals on which they have performed regulated procedures. As such, he or she must possess the appropriate knowledge, skills and attitudes to carry this out effectively. The list below indicates the minimum standards, which might be expected of an experienced licence holder.

## Module 1: Legislation

In order to fulfil their responsibilities, a new personal licence holder should be able to perform the following:

- Relate the main requirements of the legislation controlling the use of animals in the UK, including not only the ASPA, but also other relevant legislation (see Chapter 2).
- Relate the responsibilities of personal licence holders under ASPA.
- Relate the responsibilities of other key personnel under ASPA.
- Discuss the arguments put forward by both sides in the debate on the ethics and morals of using animals in experiments.

## Module 2: Principles of animal care

A new personal licence holder should be able to perform the following:

- Handle and manipulate the commonly used laboratory species or any other species named in the licence application (Chapter 6 and Section 2).
- Identify the sex and age of the animals to be used (Chapter 6 and Section 2).
- Recognise when the animal is deviating from normal behaviour and showing signs of ill health or distress, and describe what action to take to prevent pain or suffering (see Chapters 4, 6 and 8 and Section 2).
- Relate the local rules in the institution relating to health and safety, security, supply and disposal of animals (see Chapter 3).
- Describe humane methods of killing listed in Schedule 1 for the species and stage of development they will be working with (see Chapter 5).

## Module 3: Principles of animal use

A new personal licence holder should be able to perform the following:

- Describe the normal husbandry and nutritional requirements of the animals, together with their social, behavioural and environmental needs (Chapter 6 and Section 2).
- Relate the importance of disease prevention in the animals and discuss how diseases are monitored (Chapter 6 and Section 2).
- Describe the general principles of general anaesthesia and relate acceptable methods of anaesthesia and analgesia for the species used and procedures to be carried out (see Chapters 7 and 8).
- Dose and take samples from the species involved with due regard for volumes and sites and different methods for different species (Chapter 9 and Section 2).

## Module 4: Surgery

A new personal licence holder should be able to perform the following:

- Describe the methods of anaesthesia and analgesia suitable for recovery surgery (see Chapters 7 and 8).
- Relate the principles of aseptic surgery and how this may be achieved (see Chapter 10).
- Perform incisions, deep dissection and haemostasis competently (see Chapter 10).
- Relate the differences between different types of suture materials, indicating when each might be appropriate (see Chapter 10).
- Describe and perform different types of suture patterns suitable for different tissues and animals (see Chapter 10).
- Discuss the care of the recovering animal (see Chapters 4 and 8).

It is unexpected that a new personal licence holder will be able to demonstrate all these competencies to a high level. The object of mandatory-training courses is to establish a sound foundation on which competence can be effectively built. Mandatory-training courses usually only cover general principles, and provide limited opportunities to acquire manual skills. Therefore, in the UK, there is emphasis on 'on-the-job' training under the supervision of those already expert in the field, and a supervision condition is usually added to new personal licences.

Training is an ongoing process, and there should be available a mechanism for updating licensees on a regular basis on developments in, for example, laboratory animal science, animal welfare, anaesthesia, the law and ethics. Methods of reduction, refinement and replacement must also be regularly addressed. Thus, there is a need to maintain quality training and guidance after the issue of a licence. The project licence holder is responsible for ensuring that personal licensees receive adequate supervision until they are competent in the techniques to be applied (see Chapter 11).

## FURTHER INFORMATION

You must read the *Guidance on the Operation of the Animals (Scientific Procedures) Act 1986* (HMSO 2000: HC 321, ISBN 00-1-556706-X) before applying for a licence.

*The Home Office Code of Practice for the Housing and Care of Animals used in Scientific Procedures*. ISBN 0-10-210789-0.

*The Home Office Code of Practice for the Housing and Care of Animals in Designated Breeding and Supplying Establishments*. ISBN 0-10-212595-3.

HMSO (1992). *Education and Training of Personnel under the Animals (Scientific Procedures) Act 1986*. Report of the APC for 1992.

Laboratory Animal Science Association. *Directory of Animal Research Training Courses*. Published annually. PO Box 3993, Tamworth, Staffordshire, B78 3QU.

National Research Council (1991). *Education and Training in the Care and Use of Laboratory Animals: A Guide for Developing Institutional Programs*. National Academy Press. ISBN 0-309-04382-4.

Regan, T. (1983). *The Case for Animal Rights*. Berkeley: University of California.

Reports of FELASA Working Groups (2001). FELASA recommendations for the education and training of persons involved in animal experiments. Reprinted from *Laboratory Animals*. Categories A and C: 29 (1995), pp. 121–31; Category B: 43 (2000), pp. 229–35; Category D: 33 (1999), pp. 1–15.

Singer, P. (1976). *Animal Liberation* (2nd edn). Jonathan Cape, London.
Smith, M.W. (ed.) (1984). Report of the working party on courses for animal licensees. *Laboratory Animals* 18, 209–20.
www.homeoffice.gov.uk/animalsinsp/index.htm, Home Office website.
Woods, M., McDonald, R.A. and Harris, S. (2003). Predation of wildlife by domestic cats *Felis catus* in Great Britain. *Mammal Review* 33, 174–88.

## Journals

*Animal Welfare.* Universities Federation for Animal Welfare, Potters Bar, Herts. ISSN 0962-7286.
*ILAR News.* Institute of Laboratory Animal Resources, National Research Council, Washington. ISSN 0018-9960.
*Lab Animal.* Nature Publishing Co., New York. ISSN 0093-7355.
*Lab Animal Europe.* PO Box 24, Hull.
*Laboratory Animals.* Royal Society of Medicine Services, London. ISSN 0-023-6772.
*Animal Technology.* The Journal of the Institute of Animal Technology. ISSN 0264-4754.
*Comparative Medicine.* The Journal of the American Association for Laboratory Animal Science. ISSN 023-6764.

## Videos and audio-visual programmes

*Animals in Science Teaching* (1988). British Universities Film and Video Council and Universities Federation for Animal Welfare.
Association of British Pharmaceutical Industries, Interactive videos: *Animal Care Training –* 1. Health and Safety; 2. Animal Handling; 3. Principles of Anaesthesia; 4. Principles of Surgery; 5. Post Operative Care; 6. Euthanasia and Carotid Cannulation.

## General textbooks

Fowler, M. and Miller, R.E. (eds) (1999). *Zoo and Wild Animal Medicine.* Saunders.
*Guide for the Care and Use of Laboratory Animals* (1996). National Research Council. National Academy Press. ISBN 0-309-05377-3.
*Guide to Care and Use of Experimental Animals*, Vol. 1 (1980). Canadian Council on Animal Care, Ottawa, Ontario. ISBN 0-919087-00-0.
*Guide to Care and Use of Experimental Animals*, Vol. 2 (1984). Canadian Council on Animal Care, Ottawa, Ontario. ISBN 0-919087-08-6 (or set of two volumes ISBN 0-919087-10-8).
*Guidelines on the Care of Laboratory Animals and Their Use for Scientific Purposes:* Vol. 1 (1987), *Housing and Care*; Vol. II (1989). *Pain, Analgesia and Anaesthesia*; Vol. III (1989), *Surgical procedures*; Vol. IV (1990). *Planning and design of experiments*; Laboratory Animal Science Association, London and Universities Federation for Animal Welfare, Potters Bar, Herts.
Harkness, J.E. and Wagner, J.E. (1983). *The Biology and Medicine of Rabbits and Rodents* (2nd edn). Lea and Febiger, Philadelphia.
Hau, J. and van Hoosier, G.L. (2002). *Handbook of Laboratory Animal Science* (2nd edn). Vol. 1. Essential Principles and Practices. CRC Press.
Hau, J., van Hoosier, G.L. and Ardehali, A. (2002). *Handbook of Laboratory Animal Science* (2nd edn) Vol. 2. Animal Models. CRC Press.
Inglis, J.K. (1980). *Introduction to Laboratory Animal Science and Technology.* Pergamon Press, Oxford.
Moore, M. (ed.) (1999). *Manual of Veterinary Nursing.* British Small Animal Veterinary Association. ISBN 0-9052-1450-1.

Nevalainen, T., Hau, J. and Sarviharju, M. (eds.) (1995). *Frontiers in Laboratory Animal Science.* Kandrup. ISSN 0901-3393.

Poole, T.B. (ed.) (1999). *The UFAW Handbook on the Care and Management of Laboratory Animals* (7th edn). Longman, London.

Tuffery, A.A. (ed.) (1994). *Laboratory Animals. An Introduction for New Experimenters* (2nd edn). John Wiley and Sons Ltd.

van Zutphen, L.F.M., Baumans, V. and Beynen, A.C. (eds.) (1993). *Principles of Laboratory Animal Science.* Elsevier.

## WEBSITES

Useful websites are given in the table opposite.

Useful websites.

| Organisation | Website address | Comments |
|---|---|---|
| *Organisations* | | |
| American Association of Laboratory Animal Science | http://www.aalas.org/ | |
| American Society of Mammalogists | http://www.mammalsociety.org | Useful information about field methods, etc. |
| Animal Procedures Committee | http://www.apc.gov.uk | |
| Arkanimals | http://www.arkanimals.com | Environmental enrichment magazine, aimed at zoo animals |
| Biomed Net | http://biomednet.com/hmsbeagle | News magazine, with features and articles relevant for biomedical research, includes medline |
| BVA Animal Welfare Foundation | http://www.bva-awf.org.uk/ | |
| Centers for Disease Control (US) | http://www.cdc.gov | Information about the CDC, including its journal, *Emerging Infectious Diseases* |
| Convention on International Trade in Endangered Species | http://www.cites.org | |
| European Society for Laboratory Animal Veterinarians | http://www.eslav.org | |
| Farm Animal Welfare Council | http://www.fawc.org.uk/ | |
| Food and Drug Administration | http://www.fda.gov | |
| Federation of European Laboratory Animal Science Associations | http://www.felasa.org | |
| Home Office: Guidance on ASPA 86 | http://www.archive.official-documents.co.uk/document/hoc/321/321.htm | |
| Home Office: Schedule 1 Methods | http://www.homeoffice.gov.uk/si3278.htm | |
| Home Office: Forms | http://www.homeoffice.gov.uk/comrace/animals/index.html | |
| Humane Society of the United States | http://www.hsus.org | |
| Institute of Biology | http://www.iob.org | |

*(Continued)*

(*Continued*).

| Organisation | Website address | Comments |
|---|---|---|
| Institute of Laboratory Animal Resources (ILAR) | http://dels.nas.edu/ilar | Contains links to journals and other useful sites |
| Lab Animal | http://www.labanimal.com | Web page for Lab Animal magazine |
| Laboratory Animals | http://www.lal.org.uk | Laboratory animals: journal home page |
| Laboratory Animals internet links | http://www.lal.org.uk/links-menu.html | A list of useful websites, with links to mailing lists and journals, and details of meetings and relevant legislation worldwide |
| National Library of Medicine | http://www.nlm.nih.gov | National Library of Medicine at the National Institute for Health, Bethesda Maryland; includes access to free medline, human gene map and visible human project |
| Research Defence Society | http://www.rds-online.org.uk | Promoting the understanding of animal research in medicine |
| *Animals and animal services* | | |
| B & K Universal Ltd | http://www.bku.com | |
| Charles River UK Ltd | http://www.criver.com | |
| Database of Gene Knockouts | http://www.bioscience.org/knockout/knochome.htm | |
| Ellegaard Gottingen Mini pigs | http://www.minipigs.dk | |
| Harlan UK Ltd | http://www.harlan.com | |
| Mouse Genome Informatics | http://www.informatics.jax.org | |
| Pathology of Laboratory Animals | http://www.afip.org/vetpath/polatab.html | Notes and references on pathology of laboratory animals |
| Rat Life | http://www.ratlife.org | Natural behaviour of rats |
| Taconic | http://www.taconic.com | A US supplier; much useful information about strains of laboratory rodents, including growth curves |
| The Jackson Laboratory | http://www.jax.org/ | The Jackson laboratory; includes access to the mouse genome database |

*Equipment*

| | | |
|---|---|---|
| Allentown Caging Equipment Company | http://www.acecaging.com | Caging |
| Animalcare Ltd | http://www.animalcare.co.uk | Surgical equipment |
| Arnolds Veterinary Products Ltd | http://www.arnolds.co.uk | Surgical equipment |
| Arrowmight Ltd | http://www.arrowmight.com | Caging |
| Bell Isolation Systems | http://www.bell-isolation-systems.com | Containment systems |
| Biozone Ltd | http://www.biozoneglobal.com/ | Containment systems |
| Brookwick Ward & Co Ltd | http://www.brookwickward.com | Surgical equipment |
| Burge Equipment | http://www.burge.co.uk | Cage washers, etc. |
| Burtons of Maidstone Ltd | http://www.burtons.uk.com | Anaesthetic equipment |
| Carl Zeiss Ltd | http://www.zeiss.com | Ophthalmic equipment |
| Cook UK Ltd | http://www.cookincorporated.com | Catheters, etc. |
| Cox (Surgical) Ltd | http://www.coxagri.com | Surgical equipment |
| Datesand Ltd | http://www.datesand.com | Environmental enrichment |
| Ellman International (UK) Ltd | http://www.ellman.com | Surgical equipment |
| Ethicon Ltd | http://www.ethicon.com | Sutures |
| Ferno UK Ltd | http://www.ferno.co.uk | Heating pads |
| Kruuse UK Ltd | http://www.kruuse.com | Anaesthetic equipment |
| Lab Animal Buyers Guide | http://guide.labanimal.com/guide/ | List of suppliers of animals, equipment, etc. |
| Labtrac | http://www.stoeltingco.com | Animal identification |
| Lomir Biomedical Inc | http://www.lomir.com | Surgical instruments |
| Moredun Isolators | http://moredun.mri.sari.ac.uk | Isolators |
| PLEXX bv | http://www.plexx.nl | Bedding materials |
| PMI Lab diet | http://www.labdiet.com | Diets |
| Prima Tec management | http://www.PrimaTec.co.uk | Management systems |
| Rocket of London Ltd | http://www.rocketmedical.com | Surgical equipment |
| Scanbur A/S | http://www.scanbur.com | Caging |
| Shor-Line Ltd | http://www.shor-line.com | Caging |
| Steris Ltd | http://www.steris.com | Washing equipment |
| Swann Morton Ltd | http://www.swann-morton.com | Surgical equipment |
| Taconic | http://www.taconic.com | Cryopreservaiton |

*(Continued)*

(*Continued*).

| Organisation | Website address | Comments |
|---|---|---|
| Tecniplast Ltd | http://www.tecniplast.it | Caging |
| Thames Medical | http://www.thamesmedical.com | Anaesthetic equipment |
| Thoren Caging Systems Inc | http://www.thoren.com | Ventilated cages |
| Uno Roestvastastaal BV | http://www.unobv.com | Caging |
| *Alternatives* | | |
| European Centre for the Validation of Alternative Methods | http://ecvam-sis.jrc.it | |
| Netherlands Centre for Alternatives to Animal Use (NCA) | http://www.nca-nl.org | Much information on alternatives to animals in biomedical research |
| Norwegian College of Veterinary Medicine | http://oslovet.veths.no/NORINA | Gives access to the NORINA database of training materials |

# Chapter 2
# The regulatory framework

*The little I have hitherto learned is almost nothing in comparison with that of which I am ignorant.*

Descartes

## A BRIEF HISTORY OF THE USE OF ANIMALS IN RESEARCH

From ancient times people have strived to understand the workings of nature and the universe. Experiments with animals date back to at least the fifth century BC, and experiments performed in the second century AD formed the basis of medicine for many centuries to come. However, scientific investigation into the natural world, including animal-based research, vanished in the Middle Ages with the rise of Christianity, as such scientific studies were perceived as a challenge to the authority of the church.

Roger Bacon published *Opus Majus*, in 1265, in which he noted the causes of error – authority, custom, popular prejudice and the concealment of ignorance with the pretence of knowledge. He pointed out that the two methods of acquiring knowledge are argument and experience. Bacon asserted that argument alone is not enough, for 'the strongest argument proves nothing so long as the conclusions are unverified by experience.' Bacon's insistence on the gathering of data is one of the central tenets of modern science.

The birth of modern science dates to 1543 and the publication of Copernicus' *De Revolutionibus Orbium Coelestium* (*On the Revolutions of the Heavenly Spheres*) and Vesalius' *De Humani Corporis Fabrica* (*On the Fabric of the Human Body*), which challenged systems of belief dating back to the second century. Previously, medicine had been largely based on the teachings of Galen, whose knowledge of human anatomy was largely deduced from animal dissections (the dissection of human bodies was generally unacceptable in ancient times), and whose treatment of disease was based on the doctrine of the four bodily humours. Vesalius performed detailed dissections of the human body, and spotted inaccuracies in Galen's descriptions. In challenging them, he destroyed the foundation of medieval medical practice, which, like astronomy, was based on ancient tradition and inherited knowledge.

William Harvey discovered the circulation of the blood and published his book *On the Motion of the Heart and Blood* in 1628. He made his discovery using both dead and live animals, and is considered the inventor of modern laboratory science. Harvey's discovery of the circulation led to a more extensive use of vivisection in Europe. In the nineteenth century, French physiologist Claude Bernard published *An Introduction to the Study of Experimental Medicine*. This book provided a sound rationale for scientific medicine, which greatly accelerated its development. By the early twentieth century, the knowledge accruing from the increasing use of animals in scientific research was testimony to the success of the method.

As the use of animals in research increased, so too did opposition to vivisection. In 1789, utilitarian philosopher Jeremy Bentham wrote of animals 'the question is not, can they reason, nor can they talk, but can they suffer?' opening the debate on the ethics of animal use in experiments. A Society for the Prevention of Cruelty to Animals was founded in 1824. Princess Victoria extended her patronage to the society in 1835, and it became the Royal Society for the Prevention of Cruelty to Animals (RSPCA). In August 1874, the use of two dogs in an experimental demonstration of epilepsy created uproar at a meeting of the British Medical Association in Norwich. At the meeting there were vociferous protests against the experiments, which were performed by the French physiologist Eugene Magnan. At one stage, the President of the Royal College of Surgeons of Ireland cut the bindings holding one of the dogs and released it. The RSPCA later took Magnan and the three Norwich doctors who had arranged the demonstration to court, accusing them of unnecessary cruelty to the animals. In this first prosecution against the use of animals in experiments, the Norwich men were found not guilty because they did not perform the demonstration, and Magnan had returned to France. Nevertheless, the magistrates granted that the RSPCA was justified in bringing the action, and declined to award defence costs.

The first anti-vivisection societies originated in 1875, and the best known of these was probably the Society for the Protection of Animals Liable to Vivisection, founded by Frances Power Cobbe, which later became the Victoria Street Society (VSS) and then the National Anti-Vivisection Society (NAVS), which survives today. Miss Cobbe served as Honorary Secretary for 18 years, before deciding to leave NAVS due to differences in opinion with other members. On 14 June 1898, she founded the British Union for the Abolition of Vivisection, which remains very active, campaigning in schools, via the media, and in the political arena for a ban on the use of animals in research.

The VSS presented the first anti-vivisection bill in history to the House of Lords in 1875. The scientific community were obliged to present a bill themselves in opposition to this, and following these bills and the Norwich prosecution a Royal Commission was set up to study the issues. The result of this was the Cruelty to Animals Act 1876, the first law written specifically to regulate animal experimentation.

In 1926, Charles Hume founded the University of London Animal Welfare Society (now the Universities Federation for Animal Welfare) to try to get people to think rationally about their attitude to animals. He published the first edition of the UFAW *Handbook on the Care and Management of Laboratory Animals* in 1947 (now in its seventh edition). He also commissioned Russell and Burch to write *The Principles of Humane Experimental Technique* in 1959, which brought out the concept of the three Rs – replacement, reduction and refinement. This provided a sound basis for humane experimentation, and this basis was formally instituted in the current piece of legislation, the Animals (Scientific Procedures) Act 1986 (ASPA).

## LEGISLATION AND ANIMAL USE

Legislation governing the protection of animals has been in existence for many centuries. In the UK, laws were passed against cruelty to animals late in the seventeenth century. In 1822, Martin's Act (after its sponsor Richard Martin) was passed that primarily protected cattle and horses (it did not include cats, dogs or birds), and was amended in 1835 to protect all domestic animals.

In 1831, British physiologists attempted self-regulation with the publication of Marshall Hall's five principles, which are as follows:

- An experiment should never be performed, if the necessary information could be obtained by observations.
- No experiment should be performed without a defined, obtainable, objective.
- Scientists should be well informed about the work of their predecessors and peers in order to avoid unnecessary repetition of an experiment.
- Justifiable experiments should be carried out with the least possible infliction of suffering (often through the use of lower, less sentient animals).
- Every experiment should be performed under circumstances that would provide the clearest possible results, thereby diminishing the need for repetition of experiments.

Hall also proposed that results should be made available for public scrutiny. These principles bear a great deal of similarity to the three Rs, published 128 years later, and to the current piece of legislation.

A moral Code of Practice (CoP) for work with experimental animals was drawn up by the Committee of the British Association for the Advancement of Science, which published guidelines in 1871.

The Cruelty to Animals Act, which related to experiments calculated to cause pain to living animals, was passed in 1876, and set up a system of licensing and certification. The central purpose of the law was to reconcile the needs of science with the just claims of humanity and this principle is implicit in all the various laws, conventions and directives which have been passed since. The main differences from the present legislation were that 'experiment' was not clearly defined and that initially the main concern was only over surgical procedures. However, there was increasing concern over the wide variety of types of non-surgical work being performed. Pain was not clearly defined in the 1876 Act and there was little control over the purposes for which techniques could be used once permission had been given. There was no explicit justification required in order to limit the suffering caused in pursuit of relatively trivial purposes. There was no control over the scientific design of the experiment, the number of animals or the species used or the competence of licensees. The law only applied while the animal was under experiment, there was no control over the animals' care and welfare outside this time, and no control over the breeding and supply of experimental animals.

Despite its limitations, the 1876 Act stood for 110 years, but by the 1960s a strong case for updating the legislation was made and the Littlewood Committee reported that the provisions of the Act 'had not matched up with modern scientific and technological requirements'. Certain administrative changes were made including strengthening the Inspectorate (the government body responsible for overseeing the implementation of the legislation) and setting up an independent Advisory Committee. Pressure for change continued into the 1970s and in 1976, coinciding with 'Animal Welfare Year' and the Centenary of the 1876 Act, the Committee for Reform of Animal Experimentation (CRAE) was formed. Lord Halsbury brought a Private Members' Bill before Parliament in 1979, and in 1980 the Home Office Advisory Committee was asked to make recommendations for reform. In 1983 CRAE, the British Veterinary Association (BVA) and the Fund for Replacement of Animals in Medical Experimentation (FRAME) joined forces to negotiate the White Papers and the ASPA was passed in 1986.

## THE ANIMALS (SCIENTIFIC PROCEDURES) ACT 1986

The ASPA is an enabling Act: it allows people to carry out actions that would otherwise be prevented by other legislation. It provides protection for animals used in experimental or other scientific procedures. It aims to ensure that any research using animals is original, properly justified, and has no less severe or non-animal alternative.

The types of animals covered by the provisions of the Act (protected animals) are living vertebrates other than man, and *Octopus vulgaris*. Death is defined as the point where there is permanent cessation of the circulation, or destruction of the brain. Fetal, larval and embryonic forms are covered from specific stages in development: for mammals, birds and reptiles, this is the mid-point of gestation or incubation, and for other species the point at which they become capable of independent feeding.

The types of experimental or scientific procedures (regulated procedures) that are covered by the Act are those that may have the effect of causing the animal pain, suffering, distress or lasting harm. The use of anaesthesia or analgesia is disregarded when making the judgement whether there may be any harm, hence procedures carried out on anaesthetised or decerebrated animals are still regulated under the Act (see Box 2.1). A procedure is also regulated if:

- it is part of a series of treatments which cause no harm individually but which may cause pain, suffering, distress or lasting harm when applied together
- it is applied to an animal before the stage of development where it becomes a protected animal, but the animal survives to become a protected animal
- it results in the birth or hatching of a protected animal which may cause pain, suffering, distress or lasting harm, hence the breeding of harmful mutant animals or genetically modified animals (see Chapter 13) is also a regulated procedure under the Act.

Certain procedures are exempted from regulation under the Act. Ringing, tagging or marking an animal solely for identification purposes are not regulated provided it causes no more than momentary or transient pain and no lasting harm. Killing an animal by an approved method listed in Schedule 1 to the Act (see page 75) is not a regulated procedure. Recognised veterinary, agricultural or husbandry practices are also not regulated under the Act, although these are covered by other legislation (see Table 2.1). Similarly, testing medicines as part of a test under the Medicines Act is not regulated under ASPA.

---

**Box 2.1**

Regulated procedures under the ASPA:

- *protected animals* are used
- for a *scientific purpose*
- and there may be *pain, suffering, distress or lasting harm.*

---

**Table 2.1**    Legislation relevant to animal use in the UK.

*Protection of animals*
- *Animals (Scientific Procedures) Act 1986*
  Provides protection for animals used for scientific purposes.
- *Protection of Animals Acts 1911–1988*
  Provides protection for captive animals which may not be covered by other legislation, for example stock animals.
- *Wildlife and Countryside Act 1981 (amended 1991)*
  Provides protection for wild animals and plants. This Act makes it an offence to kill, injure, trade in or take a listed species from the wild, to possess a scheduled species or to damage, destroy or obstruct access to their habitat.
- *Wild Mammals Protection Act 1996*
  Protects wild mammals from acts of wilful cruelty, such as beating, stabbing, burning or drowning.
- *Protection of Badgers Act 1992*
  Protects badgers from being taken, injured, sold, killed or treated cruelly. It also protects their setts.
- *Veterinary Surgeons Act 1966*
  Defines procedures which may only be carried out by registered veterinary surgeons, for example, acts of veterinary surgery and prescription of veterinary medicines.

*Control of animal diseases/zoonoses*
- *The Animal Health Act 1981*
  Seeks to safeguard the health of animals by controlling movement and import of animals and animal products. Orders made under this Act include:
  – Rabies Control Order 1974 and the Rabies (Importation of Dogs, Cats and Other Mammals) Order 1974 .
  Describe the action to be taken in an outbreak of rabies, and lay down requirements for importation of rabies susceptible animals, including quarantine.
  – The Movement of Animals (Records) (Amendment) Order 1960
  – The Movement of Animals (Records) (Amendment) Order 1989
  – Movement and Sale of Pigs Order 1975
  – The Movement and Sale of Pigs (Amendment) Order 1987
  – The Pigs (Records, Identification and Movement) Order 1995
  – Bovine Animals (Identification, Marking and Breeding Records) (Amendment) Order 1993.
  These require records to be kept of the movement of animals in order to facilitate control of diseases.

*Wild animals and species*
- *Convention on International Trade in Endangered Species (CITES)*
  CITES (of Wild Fauna and Flora) is an international agreement between governments. Its aim is to ensure that international trade in specimens of wild animals and plants does not threaten their survival.
- *Endangered Species (Import and Export) Act 1976*
  This law implements the CITES into UK legislation. This controls the movement of endangered species, live or dead, part or whole organism, across international borders.
- *The Dangerous Wild Animals Act 1976*
  Dangerous animals listed under this Act can only be kept under licence from the local authority. The Act includes some venomous snakes, wolves and elephants.

*(Continued)*

**Table 2.1**    (*Continued*).

*Transport of animals*
- *Welfare of Animals (Transport) Order 1997 (Animal Health Act 1981)*
  Lays down requirements to safeguard the welfare of animals being transported.
- *International Air Transport Association (IATA) Live Animals Regulations*
  These guidelines describe appropriate methods for transportation of different species.

*Control of dangerous drugs and firearms*
- *The Medicines Act 1968*
  Controls the manufacture, distribution and marketing of medicines. This defines POMs, which may only be given to animals under the direction of a veterinary surgeon.
- *The Misuse of Drugs Act 1971*
  Controls the use of 'dangerous or otherwise harmful' drugs (controlled drugs), such as those which may be addictive or drugs of abuse.
- *The Poisons Act 1972*
  Controls the use of non-medicinal poisons.
- *Firearms Regulations*
  Several Acts and sets of regulations control the supply and use of firearms.

*Health and Safety*
- *Health and Safety at Work Act 1974*
  Requires employers to take reasonable steps to ensure the health, safety and welfare of their employees at work.
- *Control of Substances Hazardous to Health (COSHH) Regulations 1999*
  Requires employers to weigh up the risks to the health of their employees arising from exposure to hazardous substances and to prevent, or where this is not reasonably practicable, adequately control exposure.

---

> **Box 2.2**
>
> Regulated procedures may only be carried out, if authorised
>
> - by the personal licence (ASPA Section 3a)
> - by the project licence (ASPA Section 3b)
> - the place is specified in both licences (ASPA Section 3c).

Section 3 of the ASPA describes the system of control laid down by the Act to regulate the use of animals in scientific procedures. The Act places controls at three levels, namely the person, the programme of work and the place where the work is done (see Box 2.2).

## The personal licence

A personal licence is granted by the Secretary of State and qualifies the holder to perform specific regulated procedures, on specified types of animals, at specified places. A personal licence is the endorsement of the Secretary of State that a person is competent and suitable to perform the procedures, that is, it is concerned with practical competence. It is personal to the holder, not to the programme of work the person

---

**Box 2.3**    Main responsibilities of the personal licence holder.

*The personal licensee bears primary responsibility for the health and welfare of animals on which they have carried out scientific procedures.*

- Checking the welfare of experimental animals daily.
- Taking precautions as required to control severity.
- Notifying the project licence holder of breaches of the severity limit.
- Seeking veterinary advice as required.
- Making suitable arrangements for periods of absence.
- Humane killing of protected animals at the end of procedures, if they are in severe pain or if requested by a Home Office Inspector.
- Labelling of cages or pens.
- Ensuring they have appropriate personal and project licence authorities.
- Record keeping.

---

may be working under, and a personal licence holder may work under several different project licences. However, it does not authorise the performance of any procedures that are not also authorised by a project licence. Project licence holders should hold a list of personal licensees working on their projects.

Personal licences may only be granted to people over the age of 18 years who have appropriate education and training and who are competent to perform the procedures. Before applying for a personal licence, the applicant must first have completed an appropriate training course, such as those described in Chapter 1, or provide evidence that they already have adequate knowledge of the subject. The application must be endorsed by a sponsor, who must be a personal licence holder, and who can vouch for the biological knowledge and character of the applicant. A personal licence continues in force until revoked, but they must be reviewed at intervals of not more than 5 years. It may initially be issued with an additional *supervisory condition*, requiring the holder to be supervised when carrying out procedures until they are judged to be competent.

## The personal licence holder

*The personal licensee bears primary responsibility for the health and welfare of animals on which they have carried out scientific procedures.*

There are a number of standard conditions attached to all personal licences, which define the responsibilities of the holder (see Box 2.3). There may also be other additional conditions as requested by the Secretary of State. These conditions require the holder to ensure that they have the necessary authority on personal and project licences and that the place is specified in both, forbid the performance of procedures in public, place restrictions on the use of neuromuscular blocking agents, and prevent unauthorised re-use or release of animals. They also require the licensee to label cages or pens such that it is possible to identify the project, the regulated procedures that have been performed, and the responsible personal licensee. The personal licensee should keep records of the procedures they have carried out, and indicate whether they were supervised or not. They must check their animals daily and make suitable arrangements for any period of absence. They must be familiar with the severity limit and the constraints on adverse effects contained within the project licence, and notify the project licence holder in the event of any likely breach of these. They must also take effective precautions to prevent or alleviate any suffering caused, and to seek veterinary advice and treatment if required. There is also a condition requiring that all procedures are carried out under local or general anaesthetic, unless this would be more traumatic to the animal than the procedure, or would not be compatible with the aims of the procedure.

The personal licensee must humanely kill an animal immediately in three circumstances:

1. at the end of the series of regulated procedures, if the animal is suffering or likely to suffer adverse effects from those procedures
2. an Inspector from the Home Office requests it for humane reasons
3. an animal is suffering severe pain which is not temporary and which cannot be alleviated.

This applies regardless of how important the animal is for the experiment. The welfare of the animal comes first.

## The personal licence application form

An application for a personal licence should be completed carefully, and submitted to the Home Office only when it is complete and when all supporting documentation is available. Unsigned or incomplete applications will be returned. It is an offence under the ASPA to provide false or misleading information in support of an application. Notes to assist in completion of the form are available on the Home Office website. The numbers in the text refer to sections of the personal licence application form.

*7.* Full details of educational qualifications and relevant experience should be given: applicants should normally possess the equivalent of at least five GCSEs, or have received appropriate formal vocational training. Foreign researchers should be able to demonstrate competence in English to the level of TOEFL 550 or an equivalent, such as level 6 of IELTS. A personal licence is concerned with the competence of the holder, so any information pertinent to this needs to be included on the application form.

*9.* Applicants for personal licences are required to have successfully completed an accredited training programme comprising the subjects described in Modules 1–4. Exemptions from these requirements may be considered by the Home Office (see Chapter 1). Former personal licensees who are applying for reinstatement of their licences should discuss training requirements with their local Home Office Inspector. In general, anyone applying for a licence more than 5 years after relinquishing the previous licence should expect to undergo the full training programme.

*11.* Most new personal licensees will be subject to a condition of supervision by an experienced personal licence holder who works closely with them. This is done to ensure the attainment of competence, and in the case of scientists from abroad, to enable them to be given guidance about the requirements of the Act. The level of supervision required will vary between licensees: initially the supervisor may need to observe a licensee throughout the performance of a technique or procedure.

As technical competence is gained, the level of supervision may reduce to monitoring and discussing the work. A supervised licensee should at all times know who their supervisor is.

Regardless of whether or not they are under a supervision condition, all personal licensees should obtain guidance from the project licence holder about the way in which techniques and procedures forming part of the project are to be carried out. A supervision condition does not lessen the individual responsibility of the personal licensee to comply with the provisions of the Act and the terms and conditions of the licence.

*14.* All places at which it is intended to perform procedures should be listed, including non-designated places if appropriate. If after a licence has been issued there is a need to work at a place not specified on it, the licence will require amendment.

*15.* Column (a) lists the techniques for which authority is sought. This section should cover all of the techniques and species it is intended to use, as it will define the entire extent of personal authority. Reference to the details on the project licence will aid in describing the techniques in this section. However, since a personal licence is only concerned with personal competence, the purpose of the techniques should not be described, and care should be taken to make sure the techniques are worded in a sufficiently flexible manner to avoid inadvertent infringements. A technique is a technical act or omission, for example, dosing, bleeding, laparotomy, withholding food or water. For the administration of substances or removal of body fluids, each method and route should be specified, and abbreviations should not be used. More complex techniques, and those requiring a surgical approach, should be specified separately. The administration of an anaesthetic is a regulated procedure in its own right. Associated surgical techniques, such as tracheostomy, should be listed separately. Killing an animal for a scientific purpose at a designated establishment is a regulated procedure unless an appropriate method from Schedule 1 to the Act is used. Such methods should, therefore, be listed. The code 'S' should be used to indicate surgical techniques and 'NS' to indicate non-surgical techniques. Figure 2.1 gives some examples of personal licence techniques.

Column (b) lists the animal species for which authority is sought, and the stage of development, for example mature forms, or embryonic, larval or fetal forms. Column

| (a) Technique | (b) Animal | (c) Anaesthesia |
|---|---|---|
| 1. Administration of substances by admixture with food or water, by gavage or injection by the following routes: subcutaneous, intramuscular, intravenous............. (specify) (NS) | Mouse Rat Rabbit | AA |
| 2. Withdrawal of blood from a superficial blood vessel or via cannulae implanted under separate authority (NS) | Rat | AA/AB(L or G) |
| 3. Induction and maintenance of general anaesthesia by a route and method appropriate for the species and duration and nature of the procedure (NS) | Rat Rabbit | AA/AB(G)/AC |
| 4. Implantation of a cannula into a superficial blood vessel (S) | Rat | AB(G) |
| 5. Laparotomy followed by cannulation of the intestine (S) | Rat | AB(G) |

**Figure 2.1**  Personal licence techniques.

(c) lists the type of anaesthesia to be used for the techniques. The following codes should be used:

- AA: No anaesthesia throughout the technique.
- AB: Anaesthesia with recovery. This may be local (ABL) regional (ABR) or general (ABG).
- AC: Anaesthesia without subsequent recovery.
- AD: Use of neuromuscular blocking agents. This must be used in conjunction with an anaesthetic agent.

If anaesthesia is to be used in some kinds of animal but not in others, make this clear. Also, if another licensee will be administering the anaesthetic agent this should be made clear.

*16.* Some non-technical procedures, which do not require technical knowledge, may be delegated to non-licensed assistants. Examples of these procedures can be found in the *Guidance on the Operation of the Animals (Scientific Procedures) Act 1986*. These include tasks such as the filling of food hoppers with previously mixed diets, pairing or grouping of animals for breeding purposes, or the placing of animals in some previously set up altered environments. If this is deemed appropriate, an additional condition will be added to the licence to permit delegation. The personal licensee *must be within reach for assistance or advice if required*. Some tasks may be delegated in decerebrated or terminally anaesthetised animals provided the responsible personal licensee is present.

*Part 2.* In most cases the application should be signed by a sponsor. The Secretary of State seeks the sponsor's assurance, where necessary, that the applicant is competent, of suitable character and understands his duty under the law. The sponsor also provides assurance that the applicant has a sufficient command of English to be able to fulfil these duties. The sponsor must hold a personal licence. However, the duty to comply with the law remains with the licence applicant, not the sponsor.

## The project licence

A project licence specifies a programme of work covering a single theme or purpose, and authorises a series of regulated procedures to be applied to specified animals at a specified place or places to achieve the particular purpose set out in the programme of work. Project licences are issued to someone who can take overall responsibility for the work, usually a senior researcher. Licences may only be issued for work in certain categories, known as permissible purposes. These are as follows:

(a) the prevention, diagnosis or treatment of disease in man, animals or plants
(b) the assessment, detection, regulation or modification of physiological conditions in man, animals or plants
(c) the protection of the natural environment in the interests of the health or welfare of man or animals
(d) the advancement of knowledge in biological or behavioural sciences
(e) education or training other than in primary or secondary schools

(f) forensic enquiries

(g) the breeding of animals for experimental or other scientific use.

Sections 5(4) and 5(5) of the ASPA state the requirements for project licences. A project licence will only be granted if:

- the likely adverse effects on the animals (the costs) have been weighed against the benefits likely to accrue from the programme of work specified in the licence
- the purpose of the programme of work cannot be achieved by any other means not using protected animals
- the procedures use the minimum number of animals, involve animals with the lowest neurophysiological sensitivity, cause the least pain, suffering, distress and lasting harm, and are most likely to succeed.

That is, the project must take into account the three Rs, namely, reduction, refinement and replacement. Particular justification is required for projects which propose to use cats, dogs, non-human primates or equidae. Although many programmes of work continue for decades, project licences are issued for a maximum period of 5 years. After this time, a new application must be prepared. See Chapter 11 for more details on project licences. The application must explain the background, objectives and potential benefits of the work (Section 17 of the licence application), and demonstrate clearly how the objectives are to be achieved in the plan of work (Section 18). Section 19 of the project licence consists of protocol sheets, which set out exactly what is to be done to the animals. Section 19b(vi) covers the likely adverse effects of the procedures, and what steps will be taken to minimise these, including the use of analgesics and humane end points. Each protocol has a severity limit (either mild, moderate or substantial), which reflects the likely maximum severity that might be encountered. Procedures conducted entirely under terminal anaesthesia are listed as unclassified. The severity limits are not discrete entities but form a spectrum across a wide range of adverse effects. It is necessary to consider not only the immediate effects on the animal, but the longer-term effects as well, in order to gauge the overall effects of the procedure. For example, establishing a ruminal fistula has a high adverse effect initially but low adverse effect long term, whereas the effects of injecting a carcinogenic drug may be mild initially but very severe in the longer term. Also, if corrective action is taken to prevent suffering at an early stage, the severity limit may be kept down. For instance, by monitoring closely and humanely killing any animal that begins to exhibit more than mild adverse effects, it may be possible to place an otherwise moderate procedure into the mild severity band. This is the concept of *the humane end point*, which refines the experimental technique in order to reduce the overall suffering. A predetermined level of adverse effects is set down and if an animal starts to exceed this, it is killed (see Chapter 4, for further details on Humane end points).

In addition to the protocol severity limits, each project has an overall severity band, which reflects the average severity likely to be experienced and takes into account the individual protocol severity limits and the likely incidence of their occurrence. By limiting the occurrence of severe adverse effects to a small percentage of the animals involved, it may be possible to keep the overall severity band mild or moderate, even if the individual protocols have substantial severity limits (see Box 2.4).

> **Box 2.4**    Severity limits and bands
>
> - May be *unclassified*, *mild*, *moderate* or *substantial*.
> - Protocol *severity limit* – reflects the likely *maximum* severity for the individual protocol.
> - Project *severity band* – reflects the *average* severity over the whole project.

> **Box 2.5**    Main responsibilities of the project licence holder
>
> - Overall management of the programme of work.
> - Directing, supervising, training and managing personal licences working on the project.
> - Ensuring compliance with the terms and conditions of the licence.
> - Ensuring implementation of controls on severity.
> - Record keeping.
> - Preparing annual returns.

## *The project licence holder*

The project licence holder takes overall responsibility for a programme of work. He or she must ensure compliance with the terms and conditions of the licence and direct, train, manage and supervise any personal licence holders working on the project. The project licence holder is responsible for ensuring that the programme of work specified in the licence is adhered to, that controls on the severity of procedures are effectively implemented, and that only the estimated numbers of authorised species are used.

The project licence holder must keep full records of procedures performed under the licence. Project licence holders must submit an annual return detailing the regulated procedures which have been carried out during the year, produce lists of publications which have arisen during the lifetime of a project licence and may be asked to submit other reports on request.

There are a number of standard conditions attached to a project licence, and there may also be other additional conditions as requested by the Secretary of State. The standard conditions require the project licence holder to ensure that personal licensees working under the project only perform procedures authorised by the programme of work and by their personal licences, and at places specified in the licence. The project licence holder must also ensure that personal licensees are appropriately supervised, and are aware of the terms and conditions of the licence. The conditions also place controls on the use of neuromuscular blocking agents, use of anaesthesia, supply of animals and re-use of animals. They also detail the requirements for determining the fate of the animals at the end of the procedure.

## Designated establishments

In general, any place where scientific procedures are to be performed must be a designated scientific procedure establishment. These are inspected and approved by the Home Office, before a Certificate of Designation is issued to a person of seniority and authority at the establishment (the Certificate Holder or PCDh). The schedule to the

Certificate of Designation lists all the rooms where animals may be held or procedures performed, and what type of animal/procedure may be held/performed there. Procedures may not be performed in any room unless authorised on the schedule. Rooms are classified according to:

- LTH: long-term holding
- STH: short-term holding (less than 48 h)
- NSEP: non-sterile experimental procedure
- SEP: sterile experimental procedure
- SF: service facility
- SA: small animal
- PRI: primate
- CAT: cat
- DOG: dog
- LA: large animal.

## *The Certificate Holder (PCDh)*

The PCDh has overall legal responsibility for all the animal facilities and for all the procedures carried out in an institute. The responsibilities of PCDh fall into eight categories.

### *1. Ethical review process*

The PCDh is responsible for overseeing the ethical review process (ERP) (see pages 36–37 for more information) and for signing applications for project licences and amendments to certify that they have completed the local ERP at the establishment.

### *2. Prevention of unauthorised procedures*

It is the PCDh who has to ensure that all procedures carried out in the establishment are authorised by project and personal licences. He or she must put in place systems of management that ensure compliance with the requirements of the Act and the terms and conditions of the Certificate of Designation and licences issued under the Act.

### *3. Animal care and accommodation*

The PCDh is responsible for ensuring that the fabric of the buildings in which experimental or breeding animals are kept are maintained to a satisfactory standard to meet the Codes of Practice (CoPs) issued by the Home Office, and that the accommodation provides adequately for the animals' needs, including quarantine and acclimatisation. He must ensure that the physical environment and the well-being and state of health of animals are checked daily by a competent person. All animals must be provided at all times with adequate care and accommodation appropriate to their type or species, and any restrictions on the extent to which the animal can satisfy its physiological and ethological needs must be kept to the absolute minimum. There must be adequate fire and security provisions.

## 4. Staffing

The PCDh must ensure that there are sufficient staff at the establishment to maintain a high standard of animal care, and ensure that suitable arrangements are made to cover the absence of the named animal care and welfare officer (NACWO) or named veterinary surgeon (NVS). He or she must ensure that staff have appropriate education and training, and that there is access to appropriate education and training, and continuing professional development for licensees and others involved with animals as is required for them to meet their obligations.

## 5. Identification of animals

Each cage or confinement area should be properly labelled with the identity of the animals within to enable records to be kept as below. The PCDh must also ensure that personal licensees label cages as required by personal licence standard conditions. Dogs, cats and primates kept at the establishment must be individually and permanently identified. Equidae, other farm animals and adult birds should also be identified.

## 6. Record keeping

The PCDh is responsible for keeping daily records of the environmental conditions in enclosed animal areas, and of the source, use and final disposal of animals held and used at the establishment, including those animals killed by a Schedule 1 method. He or she is also responsible for keeping health records, which are prepared under the supervision of the NVS.

## 7. Source of animals

The PCDh must ensure that Schedule 2 animals are appropriately sourced, or that exemption from the requirement is obtained from the Secretary of State.

## 8. Disposal of animals

The PCDh is responsible for animals kept alive at the completion of regulated procedures. These may remain at the establishment under the supervision of the NVS provided that authority has been obtained from the Secretary of State and that a veterinary surgeon has determined that the animal is not suffering or likely to suffer adverse effects as a result of the procedure. Animals may be moved from the establishment if authority has been received from the Secretary of State and a veterinary surgeon has certified that they will not suffer if they cease to be kept at a designated establishment. Unauthorised re-use of animals must be prevented by appropriate systems of management.

   The PCDh must ensure that killing of any surplus stock must be done competently by a method listed in Schedule 1 or other method authorised by an additional condition on the certificate. A register of people competent to kill animals using a Schedule 1 method must be maintained, and someone must be available to perform humane killing at all times (see Box 2.6).

---

**Box 2.6**    Main responsibilities of the PCDh

- Maintenance of animal care and accommodation.
- Ensuring adequate staffing.
- Prevention of unauthorised procedures.
- Overseeing the ERP.
- Record keeping (including health records).
- Identification of animals.
- Sourcing of Schedule 2 animals.
- Disposal of animals (re-use and Schedule 1 killing).

---

**Box 2.7**    Responsibilities of the NACWO

- Provision of day-to-day care for protected animals.*
- Notification of the personal licence holder and/or NVS, or provision of care for animals whose health gives cause for concern.*
- Maintaining animal husbandry to CoP standards.
- Knowledge of Schedule 1 methods of humane killing.
- Ensuring protected animals are checked daily by a competent person.
- Recording of environmental conditions.
- Participation in ERP.

* Statutory responsibility.

---

## The named animal care and welfare officer

The Certificate of Designation names a person responsible for the day-to-day care of the protected animals held (the NACWO). The NACWO has responsibilities laid down in the Act (statutory responsibilities), and other additional responsibilities. Their statutory responsibilities require that the NACWO should contact the responsible personal licensee or arrange for the care or destruction of an animal if the health or welfare of that animal gives rise to concern. They may also notify the NVS (see below) in such circumstances. The responsibilities of NACWO extend to animals undergoing regulated procedures at the establishment, not just those held as stock. The Institute of Animal Technology has issued guidelines for NACWOs and provides opportunities for their continuing professional development. The NACWO reports to the PCDh.

The NACWO is usually a senior animal technician within a unit, and should have expert knowledge and relevant experience of animal technology. They must ensure that husbandry and care of animals are practised to the highest standards and ensure that the standards described in the relevant CoPs are met. They should be familiar with Schedule 1 methods of killing, and be able to apply them or know how to contact a suitably competent person if required. They should be familiar with the schedule to the Certificate of Designation that lists which rooms are suitable for which purpose. The NACWO is responsible for ensuring that all the animals are checked daily by a competent person and that the environmental conditions are recorded. The NACWO should be familiar with the project licences in use and participate in the local ERP (see Box 2.7).

## The named veterinary surgeon

The certificate also names a veterinary surgeon to advise on the health and welfare of the animals (the NVS). The NVS also has statutory responsibilities under the Act, and other additional responsibilities required by the Royal College of Veterinary Surgeons (RCVS) and Home Office. The RCVS has issued a CoP, currently under review, which sets out the duties and responsibilities of the NVS. Those wishing to become NVSs must undertake specific training, and there is an ongoing requirement for continuing professional development. The requirements of the RCVS are strict, and non-adherence can lead to disciplinary proceedings. This includes transgressions made by the NVS and also by others carrying out duties delegated by the NVS.

The statutory responsibilities require that the NVS should provide advice on the health and welfare of the animals, and contact the responsible personal licensee or arrange for the care or destruction of an animal if the health or welfare of that animal gives rise to concern. The NVS reports to the PCDh.

In addition, the NVS should visit all parts of the establishment frequently enough to be able to monitor the health and welfare of animals kept at the establishment. They must be able to diagnose and treat diseases in the protected animals, and advise on health screening and husbandry requirements. They should maintain health records in a format acceptable to the Home Office, be familiar with Schedule 1 methods of humane killing, and perform health certification of animals for fitness to travel or on discharge from the controls of the Act. The NVS should be familiar with the project licences in use, and be able to provide advice to licensees regarding refinement of techniques, non-animal alternatives, and selection of animal models. The NVS is expected to be familiar with the project licences in use and is often involved in the performance of techniques, training of licensees, and the drafting of new applications and amendments. They should take an active role in the ERP. The NVS is responsible for directing the use of controlled and prescription only medicines (POMs) in the animals (see Chapter 7) and should ensure that appropriate veterinary cover is provided at all times. Several veterinary surgeons may be involved with the care and welfare of animals at a designated establishment, but only one will be named on the Certificate of Designation (see Box 2.8).

---

**Box 2.8**   Main responsibilities of the NVS

- Provision of advice on the health and welfare of protected animals.*
- Notification of the personal licence holder or provision of care for animals whose health gives cause for concern.*
- Provision of advice to licensees on the three Rs.
- Direction of the use of POMs.
- Provision of veterinary care to protected animals.
- Maintenance of health records.
- Certification of fitness for travel or discharge.
- Participation in the ERP.

*Statutory responsibility.

## *Designated breeding and supplying establishments and Schedule 2*

Some types of protected animals may only be bred at or supplied from establishments which are themselves designated under the Act as designated breeding establishments (DBEs). Some animals may be bred at a non-designated establishment, for example, in holdings abroad, and then supplied from an establishment designated as a supplying establishment (DSE). These animals are listed in Schedule 2 to the ASPA. Currently this includes: mouse, rat, hamster, gerbil, guinea pig, rabbit, cat, dog, ferret, primate, European Quail (*Coturnix coturnix*), sheep (if genetically modified) and pig (if genetically modified).

Dogs and cats, however, may only be used in projects authorised by the Act if they have been bred at *and* obtained from a DBE. DBEs and DSEs are subject to many of the same requirements as scientific procedure establishments, in that they must have a PCDh, an NACWO and an NVS, and must be maintained to an appropriate standard. There must be records of the source, use, disposal and health of the animals; dogs, cats and primates must be permanently marked for identification purposes, and there must be suitable arrangements in the absence of the NACWO or NVS. There must be adequate security and fire precautions, and facilities for acclimatisation and quarantine. It is a condition of the certificate that all animals are provided at all times with adequate care and accommodation appropriate to their type or species, and that any restrictions on the extent to which the animal can satisfy its physiological and ethological needs are kept to the absolute minimum.

## Places other than designated establishments

Sometimes, it may be necessary to carry out scientific procedures away from designated establishments, for example on wild animals, on farms or on free-living fish in rivers. In these cases, the controls of the Act are more difficult to apply, since there is no responsible PCDh, NACWO or NVS. The need for using the PODE must be justified in the project licence, and the place must be specified on both personal and project licences. In practice, most project and personal licences with PODE availability have primary availability at a designated scientific procedure establishment, and the PODE work is considered by the ERP at the establishment.

## Additional controls

The Act provides for a number of other restrictions on the use of animals.

## *Re-use*

If, at the conclusion of a series of regulated procedures, an animal is used again in further scientific procedures *and a naive animal would have sufficed*, this constitutes re-use. Section 14 describes the regulations relating to the re-use of animals. No animal may be re-used unless authorised by the Secretary of State. Re-use will not be permitted if the animal has experienced severe pain. If the animal has been given a general anaesthetic with recovery, re-use will not be permitted unless the first use was essential preparation for the subsequent use, the anaesthetic was administered solely for immobilisation, or all further procedures are carried out under terminal anaesthesia.

If animals are subjected to several series of regulated procedures one after the other as a matter of scientific necessity, this constitutes *continued use* and is not subject to the same restrictions under Section 14 as re-use. Examples include surgical preparation of an animal model for subsequent applied studies, breeding transgenic or harmful mutants for use in other projects, or repeated blood sampling for the purpose of studying the time course of an infection or for pharmacokinetic studies.

## Schedule 2A

Schedule 2A requires that all experiments be carried out under local or general anaesthesia. This does not apply if the administration of an anaesthetic would be more traumatic to the animal than the experiment itself, or if anaesthesia is incompatible with the aims of the experiment. This is reiterated in the standard conditions of project and personal licences.

## Endangered species, wild animals and Great Apes

There are restrictions on the use of endangered species, wild animals and Great Apes. No endangered species may be used unless the research is aimed at conservation of the species itself, or for essential biomedical research where the species exceptionally proves to be the only one suitable for the purpose. Wild animals may only be used if no other animals suitable for the purpose are available, and they may only be released into the wild again provided they have been properly cared for, their state of health allows them to be set free, and they will not pose a danger to public health or the environment on release.

The Government stated in November 1997 that it would no longer issue licences for the use of Great Apes in scientific procedures. In fact, no Great Apes have been used in scientific procedures in the UK since the 1986 Act was introduced. Project licences for the testing of cosmetic or tobacco products will not be issued either.

## Schedule 1

Schedule 1 to the Act describes methods of humane killing. Killing a protected animal at a designated establishment using one of the methods described in Schedule 1 is not considered to be a regulated procedure, and no licence authorities are required. However, personnel who carry out killing by a Schedule 1 method must be competent to do so, and listed in a register maintained by the PCDh. Using a method not listed on Schedule 1, or a Schedule 1 method on an animal for which it is not deemed appropriate, constitutes a regulated procedure, and must be licensed by both project and personal licences (see Chapter 5).

## Administration of the Act

The Act is administered by the Secretary of State at the Home Office, who takes advice from a number of sources as to whether and on what terms to grant a licence or certificate under the Act. The main source of advice is a network of Home Office Inspectors. These are usually registered veterinary or medical practitioners with higher academic or clinical qualifications, who visit research establishments and study all applications for licences to work on animals to ensure the work is justified and meets the criteria laid down in the Act. Inspectors also visit establishments and conduct periodic reviews of licences and certificates in order to assess compliance with their terms and conditions. Any non-compliance is reported to the Secretary of State, who may revoke certificates or licences, impose retraining requirements, or formally admonish the licensee or PCDh. Offences under the Act may result in a prison sentence or a fine, or both. The Home Office issues CoPs in which the optimum environmental conditions and minimum cage sizes for protected animals are laid down. The Home Secretary also takes advice regarding project licence applications from the Animal Procedures Committee (APC). This is a panel of senior researchers, legal, veterinary and medical personnel, and representatives of welfare groups. They automatically study all applications for work of substantial severity on primates, any work on wild caught primates, work involving cosmetic or tobacco testing, or licences for training in microsurgical techniques. The Annual Report of the APC covers a wide range of issues to do with animal experimentation from ERPs to training of licensees and details of infringements.

## COMMUNICATION

Within a designated establishment, many people are involved in caring for and maintaining the welfare of protected animals. The Act describes five people with particular responsibilities towards animals, the PCDh, project licence holder, personal licence holder, NVS, and NACWO. Often, particularly in small establishments, it is necessary to combine some of these roles, for example the project licence holder may also hold a personal licence, the NVS may also be the NACWO, or the PCDh may hold a project licence. It is envisaged, however, that there should be at least three different individuals fulfilling these five roles. Open communication between these people is vital if everyone is to carry out their responsibilities effectively and if animal welfare is to be maintained. The animals cannot speak for themselves: they rely on personnel to attend to their needs. Figure 2.2 shows the lines of communication that must function effectively in order to maintain animal welfare.

## THE ETHICS OF USING ANIMALS IN EXPERIMENTS

The word 'ethics' is used in many contexts, often incorrectly, leaving the reader confused as to its meaning. For the purposes of this book, it is an examination of the acceptability of the motives that drive the behaviour of people (Dolan, 1999), whether they are scientists who use animals, or people who stand up for animal rights. This

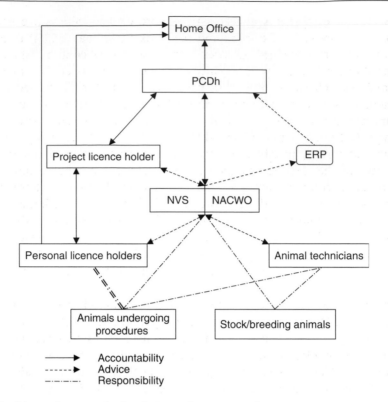

**Figure 2.2**   Lines of communication between key personnel.

section is not intended to provide a comprehensive guide to the ethics of using animals, and its brevity should not be taken to indicate that such considerations should be treated lightly. This book is intended as a practical handbook and the reader is urged to consult the list of further reading and to examine the texts for a more detailed consideration of the ethics of animal usage.

All use of animals for human benefit creates a dilemma. There is a spectrum of opinion on whether there is justification for using animals for our own ends: some people believe that animals have rights and it is wrong to use them, whether for food, in research, as beasts of burden, as pets, or to kill them as vermin. Another group believes it is acceptable for humans to use animals in any way we think fit. Most people fall somewhere in between.

The justification for using animals in biomedical research depends on them being different from humans, with a reduced capacity to suffer (this in itself is the subject of much debate), while the validity of the results obtained depends on their physiological similarity to humans. The debate about animal experimentation started over 130 years ago. It has waxed and waned over the decades but it has never gone away, and some aspects of the debate are essentially unchanged from those used a century ago. An important factual point is whether animal experimentation has been essential in the development of important medical advances or not. Many abolitionist groups claim that animal research has never resulted in any medical benefits, that it has misled scientists, or that it is unnecessary because we have alternative non-animal techniques. However, most doctors and scientists agree that animal research has played a major part in medical advances in the past and will continue to do so. Most researchers would like to see alternatives to animals developed, but most believe that animal research will continue to be necessary, at least for the foreseeable future. Other campaigners claim that animal research is cruel. There is no doubt that over 100 years ago it was cruel, before the advent of modern anaesthetic and analgesic drugs. But today things are very different: advances in veterinary science have made painless surgery possible, and everyone involved in animal research is very much aware of the need to maintain animal welfare. The regulations governing animal research contain many provisions to safeguard animal welfare. Research using animals can only be authorised provided the benefits outweigh the costs to the animals under a utilitarian framework (the end justifies the means), with some additional restrictions. For example, work on developing cosmetic or tobacco products is not considered acceptable; however, much 'benefit' can be derived from the work. Similarly, work on Great Apes will not be authorised in the UK, for whatever purpose.

For the most part, society accepts that the use of animals is necessary for medical progress, provided there are assurances over the purpose for which the work is carried out and the degree of suffering inflicted. Surveys have shown that people will accept a greater degree of suffering to animals in the pursuit of cures for devastating illnesses such as childhood leukaemia than for minor problems or for toxicity testing (see Aldhous et al., 1999). However, there is a significant sector in society which believes that however high the anticipated benefit, no animal should undergo more than transient suffering, which may be at odds with the interests of science and industry. A majority of people seems to support the use of mice in fundamental biomedical research if they come to no harm, but begins to show disapproval as soon as pain, surgery or illness became involved. If animal suffering cannot be ruled out, it may be hard to convince the public of the worth of such fundamental biological research. However, much research of this type is relatively benign, and so might win public support if measures to limit suffering were implemented effectively and described in detail. It is up to the scientist, therefore, to fully explain the nature of the work he or she is undertaking, and to put it in context, such that the public can understand the motives for the work and gain a greater understanding of research.

Regulated procedures using animals involve inflicting potential harm on them. The motive for this is usually to derive some benefit to man or other animals. For research to be conducted in an ethical manner, the researcher should analyse the motives behind the research – is it being done for a good enough reason, and could it be done any other way? Therefore, it is important to consider the following questions before embarking on an experiment involving animals.

## 1. Why are you doing it?

Can you justify what you are doing: is the potential benefit to be derived from the result significant enough to outweigh the likely costs to the animal?

## 2. Does what you propose to do raise ethical issues?

Is the planned experiment going to cause the animal any pain or any other form of suffering, such as isolation or confinement?

## 3. Is replacement possible?

Is it possible to achieve the same benefit by replacing all or part of the experiment with an *in vitro* experiment, a mathematical model or a human subject, or could a different animal species lower in the phylogenetic scale be used?

## 4. Is reduction possible?

Can you use fewer animals by improving the design of the experiment (e.g. factorial designs), collaborating with colleagues to use as many tissues as possible from each animal, or using 'spare' breeding animals or excess young? Can you get Home Office approval for re-use of some animals?

## 5. Is refinement possible?

Can you alter your experimental method in some way to decrease the potential for suffering, for example, by an improvement in surgical technique (e.g. using laparoscopy instead of a laparotomy), modifications to housing or bedding, or reducing the volume or frequency in a drug dosing regime?

   At all times throughout the experiment, consider what could be done to decrease the potential for suffering inflicted on the animals, and to maximise the likely benefit to be derived.

## The local ethical review process

Since 1 April 1999, all designated establishments have been required to implement a local ERP. The aims of the process are to provide independent ethical advice to the PCDh, to provide support to the named people, and to use ethical analysis to increase awareness of animal welfare issues and develop initiatives to lead to the widest possible application of the three Rs. This makes sure that all use of animals at the establishment is carefully considered, that all possibilities for reduction, refinement or replacement are taken account of, and that high standards of accommodation and care are achieved. The structure of the ERP should be designed to suit the size and nature of the establishment, and may consist of committees, e-mail discussion groups, project refinement groups or other formats, all of which should encourage local consideration of ethical issues. In general, as many people as possible should be involved in the ERP, to widen the debate as much as possible. The NACWO, NVS and representatives of the users should also be included. The ERP should include people who do not use animals, and lay people from outside the institution may also be appropriate members.

   The local ERP provides a mechanism to help PCDhs to meet their responsibilities and encourage wider local involvement in addressing issues surrounding animal use.

The inclusion of lay people from the local community among the membership when debating the issues may go some way towards satisfying the demand for public accountability of what research should be allowed to be performed on animals in the name of the public interest. The Holder of the Certificate of Designation has to decide not whether the proposed work can be done, but whether it should be done.

## STATISTICS OF ANIMAL USAGE

Project licence holders are required to submit detailed returns each year, from which it is possible to compile an accurate picture of the use of animals in regulated procedures in the UK. People working with experimental animals should be aware of some of the facts concerning their use.

> On 31.12.01 there were 248 designated Scientific Procedure establishments in the UK, with 3,309 project licences and 14,553 personal licensees covering the work that was done.
>
> (Home Office, 2002).

In 2001, 2,567,688 animals, of which 86% were rodents, were used in 2,622,589 regulated procedures, compared with 2,714,700 procedures in 2000. A total of 3,342 primates (Old World and New World) and 8,273 dogs, cats, ferrets and other carnivores were used. Primates and carnivores accounted for 0.45% of the total number of animals. Farm animals (pigs, sheep, goats, cattle and other ruminants) accounted for 0.75% of animals used. Transgenic animals or those with a potentially harmful genetic defect accounted for 33%, and this area of work is increasing. Medical, veterinary or biological research, development and production accounted for 62% of animals used. More than 30% of animals used were for breeding animals with harmful genetic defects or transgenic animals.

These figures should be considered in the light of other forms of animal usage. For example, more than 650 million poultry and 50 million cattle, pigs and sheep are slaughtered for food each year in the UK. To put this another way, for every 25 people in the UK, one animal is used in research and 300 are slaughtered for food each year.

## LEGISLATION CONTROLLING USE OF ANIMALS IN EXPERIMENTS IN OTHER COUNTRIES

### Europe

In Europe there are two documents which control the use of animals in experiments. In 1985, the 26 countries of the Council of Europe reached an agreement on the use of animals in research and published the *Convention for the Protection of Vertebrate Animals Used for Experimental and Other Scientific Purposes* (ETS 123). This has no legislative force, but countries which ratify the Convention agree to implement its provisions through their national laws. The European Union (EU) ratified the Convention in 1998, therefore EU member states must implement its provisions. The implementation tool is the EU Directive for the Protection of Vertebrate Animals used for Experimental and other Scientific Purposes (86/609/EEC). All EU members are compelled to implement its provisions as minimum standards via their national laws. The requirements of EU Directive 86/609 (and, therefore, European Convention ETS 123) are reflected in the ASPA in the UK.

## The USA

In the USA, the primary federal law concerning the protection of laboratory animals is the Animal Welfare Act (AWA). The aim of the AWA is 'to insure that animals intended for use in research facilities or for exhibition purposes or for use as pets are provided humane care and treatment'. The AWA is enforced by the US Department of Agriculture, Animal and Plant Health Inspection Service (APHIS). In the AWA, the term 'animal' includes any live or dead dog, cat, monkey, guinea pig, hamster, rabbit, or such other warm-blooded animal, used, or intended for use in research, testing, experimentation, or exhibition purposes or as a pet. However, it specifically excludes rats (*Rattus* spp.), mice (*Mus* spp.) and birds used in research, horses unused for research purposes and farm animals used or intended for use as food, or livestock or poultry used or intended for improving animal nutrition, breeding, management, production or food quality. The Act lays down standards for facilities and operations, health and husbandry systems, and transportation. It is the responsibility of the research facility to ensure that all scientists, research technicians, animal technicians and other personnel involved in animal care, treatment and use are qualified to perform their duties, and ensure that adequate training is available for personnel. Each research facility must have an attending veterinarian to provide veterinary care to the facility's animals. The facility must appoint an Institutional Animal Care and Use Committee (IACUC). The people on this committee must be qualified through experience and expertise to assess the establishment's animal programme, facilities and procedures, according to the requirements of the Association for the Accreditation and Assessment of Laboratory Animal Care (AAALAC, see Chapter 6). An IACUC consists of at least three members, including a chairman, a veterinary surgeon with training or experience in laboratory animal science and medicine with responsibility for animals at the research facility, and a non-affiliated member to provide representation for the general public. The IACUC is required to review the establishment's programme for humane care and use of animals, and inspect all of the animal facilities for compliance with the required standards, at least once in every 6 months. Their findings are reported to the head of the facility. If any deficiencies are noted, the reports must contain a reasonable and specific plan and schedule with dates for correcting each deficiency. Any failure to adhere to the plan and schedule that results in a significant deficiency remaining uncorrected must be reported to APHIS. The IACUC may also make recommendations regarding any aspect of the research facility's animal programme, facilities or personnel training.

If a researcher proposes to conduct research where there is a potential for pain, harm or distress to the animals, the principal investigator must do a search for alternatives. The IACUC must approve any proposed research and significant changes in ongoing research to assure compliance with the AWA.

# OTHER RELEVANT LEGISLATION IN THE UK

There are many other pieces of legislation, regulations and guidelines which may be relevant to certain areas of laboratory animal use. Failure to comply with the requirements of these may result in prosecution under both the ASPA and other legislation. Many of these are summarised in Table 2.1. The list is not exhaustive, so for further information, consult the list of further reading.

# FURTHER INFORMATION

Aldhous, P., Coghlan, A. and Copley, J. (1999). Let the people speak. *New Scientist* May 1999.

Australian Council for the Care of Animals in Research and Teaching (1992). *Animal Pain: Ethical and Scientific Perspectives*. (eds. T.R. Kuchel, M. Ros, J. Barrell) Obtainable from UFAW.

Bateson, P. (1986). When to experiment on animals. *New Scientist* 20 February 1986.

Bunyan, J. (1991). *Handbook for the Animal Licence Holder* (2nd edn). Institute of Biology, London. ISBN 0 900 490 276.

Carruthers, P. (1992). *The Animals Issue – Moral Theory in Practice*. Cambridge University Press.

CITES Convention on International Trade in Endangered Species of Wild Fauna and Flora: www.cites.org

Council of Europe (1986). *European Convention for the Protection of Vertebrate Animals Used for Experimental and Other Scientific Purposes*. Council of Europe, Strasbourg. Obtainable HMSO, London.

Cooper, M.E. (1987). *Introduction to Animal Law*. Academic Press.

Dawkins, M. and Gosling, M. (1992). *Ethics in Research on Animal Behaviour*. Academic Press.

Dawkins, M.S. (1980). *Animal Suffering, the Science of Animal Welfare*. Chapman and Hall.

Dolan, K (1999). *Ethics, Animals and Science*. Oxford, Blackwell Science.

European Union: List of Animal Welfare Legislation: http://europa.eu.int/comm/food/fs/aw/aw_references_en.html

Hampson, J. (1985). *Laboratory Animal Protection Laws in Europe and N. America*. RSPCA, Horsham, W. Sussex.

Hollands, C. The Animals (Scientific Procedures) Act 1986. *The Lancet* 5 July 1986. 32–33.

Home Office (1998). *The Ethical Review Process*.

Home Office (2000). *Guidance on the Operation of the Animals (Scientific Procedures) Act 1986*. London: The Stationery Office.

Home Office (2002). *Statistics of Scientific Procedures on Living Animals*, Great Britain 2001. The Stationery Office, London.

Hughes, T.I. (ed.) (1990). Bio-ethics 1989. A report of the *Proceedings of an International Symposium on the Control of the Use of Animals in Scientific Research. Animal Welfare Foundation of Canada*, Ontario, Canada.

Institute of Animal Technology (1998). Guidance notes on the role of the Named Animal Care and Welfare Officer in establishments designated under the Animals (Scientific Procedures) Act 1986.

Jasper, J.M. and Nelkin, D. (1992). *The Animals Rights Crusade: The Growth of Moral Protest*. The Free Press, New York.

Johns Hopkins University Center for Alternatives to Animal Testing:http://caat.jhsph.edu/

Langley, G. (ed.) (1989). *Animal Experimentation: The Consensus Changes*. Macmillan Press.

Leahy, M.P.T. (1991). *Against Liberation: Putting Animals in Perspective*. Routledge, London.

Littlewood, Sir S. (1965). *Report of the Departmental Committee on Experiments on Animals*. Cmnd 2641. HMSO, London.

MRC (2000). *Mice and Medicine.* MRC, London.

O'Donoghue (ed.) (1998). The ethics of animal experimentation. *Proceedings of the EBRA/FELASA European Congress*, 17–18 December 1996. EBRA, London.

Paton, W. (1984). *Man and Mouse: Animals in Medical Research.* Oxford University Press.

Paterson, D. and Palmer, M. (eds.) (1989). *The Status of Animals, Ethics, Education and Welfare.* CAB International.

Philips, M.T. and Sechzer, J.A. (1989). *Animal Research and Ethical Conflict.* Springer-Verlag. ISBN 0387 969357.

Rachels, J. (1990). *Created from Animals. The Moral Implications of Darwinism.* Oxford University Press.

Regan, T. and Singer P. (eds.) (1976). *Animal Rights and Human Obligations.* Prentice-Hall, Englewood Cliffs.

Research Defence Society: http://www.rds-online.org.uk

*Responsibility in the Use of Animals in Medical Research* (1993). MRC Ethics Series.

Rhodes, P. (1985). *An Outline History of Medicine.* Butterworths.

Rollin, B.E. (1990). *The Unheeded Cry. Animal Consciousness, Animal Pain and Science.* Routledge, London.

Rowan, A.N. (1989). *Of Mice, Models and Men. A Critical Evaluation of Animal Research.* State University of New York Press.

Royal College of Veterinary Surgeons (1992). *Code of Practice for Named Veterinary Surgeons.*

Royal College of Veterinary Surgeons. *Legislation Affecting the Veterinary Profession in the United Kingdom.* Available from the RCVS: www.rcvs.org.uk.

Rupke, N.A. (ed.) (1987). *Vivisection in Historical Perspective.* Croom Helm Ltd.

Russell, W.M.S. and Birch, R.L. (1959). *The Principles of Humane Experimental Technique.* Special Edition UFAW 1992.

Silverman, J., Suckow, M.A. and Murthy, S. (eds) (2000). *The IACUC Handbook.* CRC Press.

Singer, P. (1976). *Animal Liberation* (2nd edn). Jonathan Cape.

Smith, J (1992). Dissecting values in the classroom. *New Scientist* May 1992.

Smith, J.A. and Boyd, K.M. (1991). *Lives in the Balance: the Ethics of Using Animals in Biomedical Research.* Oxford University Press.

Smyth, D.H. (1977). *Alternatives to Animal Experiments.* Scolar Press.

The three Rs: developments in laboratory animal science. Replacement (M. Balls), Reduction (M.F.W. Festing), Refinement (P.A. Flecknell) (1994). *Laboratory Animals* 28, 193–231. Reprinted with additional references 2001.

UFAW (1994). *The Use of Animals in Scientific Procedures.*

Video: *The Right to Hope.* Seriously Ill for Medical Research.

Webster, J. (1994). *Animal Welfare: A Cool Eye Towards Eden.* Blackwell Science.

Zurlo, J, Rudacille, D and Goldberg, G (1994). *Animal and Alternatives in Testing: History, Science and Ethics.* Mary Ann Liebert.

# Chapter 3
# Health, safety and security

Researchers may find themselves exposed to numerous hazards in the course of their work. These hazards may be from the animals themselves, or equipment, chemicals, electricity, radiation or infectious agents found in the laboratory. The risk to which the researcher is exposed, however, depends on a combination of the nature of the hazard and how the hazard is contained to reduce or eliminate exposure. For example, a potentially hazardous compound may present only a minimal risk to personnel if handled in a safety cabinet, while wearing appropriate protective clothing. The competence and training of personnel and precautions taken to reduce exposure play an important part in controlling risks in the workplace.

## LEGAL FRAMEWORK

In the UK, the Health and Safety at Work Act 1974 imposes a responsibility on the employer to ensure safety at work for all their employees. Employers have to ensure so far as is reasonably practicable, the health, safety and welfare of their employees at work. This responsibility includes a duty to provide a safe working environment and premises, safe systems of work and appropriate training and supervision. Some groups of employees may require more care and supervision than others, for example disabled or pregnant workers. The employer's responsibility is usually only to his or her own employees and premises; however, it can be extended, for example, to visitors, students or contractors using the workplace, or to employees sent to work elsewhere.

Failure to ensure safe premises and working practices could result in a criminal prosecution or to an employee suing for personal injury. Details of any injuries sustained at work and the action taken by the employer should usually be recorded.

An employer should assess the level of risk as against the cost of eliminating that risk in deciding whether they have taken reasonable steps as far as they are able. Employers are obliged to consult employees either directly or through an elected representative on health and safety matters. Employers should have written rules and procedures covering basic health and safety requirements.

The Health and Safety at Work Act 1974 established the Health and Safety Commission and the Health and Safety Executive. The Commission is responsible for advising and authorising research and suggestions on putting into effect the provisions made in the Health and Safety at Work Act, as well as suggestions for passing regulations to support the provisions in the Health and Safety at Work Act and issuing codes of practice (CoPs). The Executive is responsible for providing information and advice to government ministers and to investigate breaches. The Health and Safety Executive and the Environmental Health Departments for the local authorities are responsible for enforcing the Health and Safety at Work Act 1974 and the various regulations. They can enter premises to investigate conditions or seize and destroy harmful substances. They can also prosecute employers or serve notices on them to improve working conditions, or in some cases serve notices that work should stop altogether. Table 3.1 shows a summary of relevant health and safety regulations.

**Table 3.1**    Summary of relevant health and safety regulations.

*Management of Health and Safety at Work Regulations 1999 (Management Regulations)*
These place an obligation on the employer to actively carry out a risk assessment of the work place and act accordingly. The assessment must be reviewed when necessary and recorded where there are five or more employees. It is intended to identify health and safety and fire risks.

*Workplace (Health, Safety and Welfare) Regulations 1992*
These deal with any modification, extension or conversion of an existing workplace. The requirements include control of temperature, lighting, ventilation, cleanliness, room dimensions, etc. The regulations also provide that non-smokers should be allocated separate rest areas from smokers.

*The Provision and Use of Work Equipment Regulations 1998*
These deal with minimum standards for the use of machines and equipment with regard to suitability, maintenance and inspection. The regulations also cover mobile work equipment since December 2002.

*The Manual Handling Operations Regulations 1992 (Manual Handling Regulations)*
These deal with the manual handling of equipment, stocks, materials, etc. Where reasonably practicable, an employer should avoid the need for his or her employees to undertake manual handling involving risk of injury.

*Personal Protective Equipment Work Regulations 1992 (PPE)*
These deal with protective clothing or equipment, which must be worn or held by an employee to protect against health and safety risks. It also covers maintenance and storage of such equipment. Employers cannot charge for such clothing or equipment, which must carry the 'CE' marking.

*The Health and Safety (Display Screen Equipment) Regulations 1992 (Display Screen Regulations)*
These introduced measures to prevent repetitive strain injury, fatigue, eye problems, etc. in the use of technological equipment. Every employer should make a suitable and sufficient analysis of each workstation and surrounding work environment to ensure it meets the detailed requirements set out in the Regulations. This includes eyesight tests on request, breaks from using the equipment and provision of health and safety information about the equipment to the employee.

*Working Time Directive and Working Time Regulations 1998*
These regulate the maximum working hours for workers, and require free health assessments to assess suitability to work particular hours. It also governs rest periods and breaks.

*The Reporting of Injuries, Diseases and Dangerous Occurrences Regulations 1995 (RIDDOR)*
Employers must notify the HSE or local authority about work accidents resulting in death, personal injury or sickness, where an employee is off work for more than 3 days. Records must be kept of all such accidents at the workplace for at least 3 years. Accident books must be kept, where an employer employs 10 or more people on the same premises.

*(Continued)*

**Table 3.1**   *(Continued).*

*Electricity at Work Regulations 1989*
These place a duty on an employer to assess risks involved in work activities involving electricity (this can even cover electrical appliances, such as kettles). All such equipment must be properly maintained.

*Fire Precautions (Workplace) (Amendment) Regulations 1999*
All workplaces should be inspected by the fire authority to check means of escape, firefighting equipment and warnings and a fire certificate issued.

*Health and Safety (First Aid) Regulations 1981*
Employers have to make adequate and appropriate provision for first aid.

*Noise at Work Regulations 1989 (Noise Regulations)*
These impose a duty on employers to reduce risk of damage to hearing of employees from exposure to noise.

*Ionising Radiation Regulations 1999*
These require employers to control exposure to sources of ionising radiation in the workplace and ensure areas where such work is carried out are properly supervised.

Under the provisions in the Employment Rights Act 1996, employees are protected from dismissal or victimisation by an employer for a health and safety-related reason.

Within the European Commission (EC), a number of Directives under the Treaty of Rome's Article 118A relate to health and safety and have been adopted by member states. At present, Community legislation relating to health and safety at work falls into three groups:

- Framework Directive 89/391/EEC, which contains general principles for health and safety organisation at the workplace. It outlines the responsibilities of employers and workers. Individual directives deal with specific groups of workers, workplaces or substances.
- Framework Directive 80/1107/EEC, which covers the health and safety of workers against the risks arising from exposure to chemical, physical and biological agents at the workplace. Individual directives deal with specific agents.
- Other directives containing exhaustive provisions unconnected to the framework directives, in respect of occupational activities or specific groups at risk. These include: The Chemical Agents Directive, Directives which protect workers from risks associated with exposure to BSE and TSE agents (97/59/EC and 97/65/EC) and Directive 97/42/EC, which deals with the protection of workers from exposure to carcinogens. The Workplace Directive contains minimum health, safety and welfare requirements for permanent workplaces. Directive 89/686/EC (The Use of Personal Protective Equipment (PPE) Directive) deals with the selection and maintenance of suitable protective clothing and other equipment. The Biological Agents Directive requires the notification to HSE of work involving certain dangerous pathogens, which includes genetically modified organisms (GMOs), cell cultures and human endoparasites. The Manual Handling of Loads Directive requires employers to eliminate the need for manual handling, where this may involve a risk of injury or to take steps to reduce the risk.

The EC updates directives, where it is necessary to take account of new risks or to allow for technical and scientific progress.

Occupational health and safety personnel need a detailed knowledge of legislation in order to be able to translate it into working practices. In many countries, some occupational diseases, such as occupational asthma and some zoonoses, must be reported to government agencies, and compensation may be awarded to personnel developing such occupational diseases. Employers are required to respond to employee risk factors, and may have to make difficult decisions about suitability for work both before and during employment. If appropriate action to protect employees is not taken, then the enforcement authorities can resort to legal action against the employer. Increasingly, insurance companies are requiring details of potential hazards and risks in the workplace, and evidence of suitable methods of control, before they will issue policies to employers.

## Control of Substances Hazardous to Health Regulations 1999

COSHH stands for the Control of Substances Hazardous to Health Regulations 1999. Hazardous substances are those that can harm health, if they are not properly controlled, for example, by using adequate ventilation. The definition of 'a substance hazardous to health' is broad and includes dust and animal allergens. Hazardous substances include substances used directly in research, for example cleaning agents, anaesthetic agents; substances generated during work activities, for example dust, fumes; and naturally occurring substances, for example blood, bacteria. Most commercial chemicals for which COSHH is relevant carry a warning label.

COSHH requires employers to perform the following:

- Identify hazardous substances in the workplace and assess the risks to health from using them. To evaluate the risk to health, the researcher needs to know what potential the substance has for causing harm, the chance of exposure occurring and how much personnel would be exposed to and for how long.
- Decide what precautions are needed before use.
- Prevent, or where this is not reasonably practicable, control exposure. Exposure can be prevented by changing the activity, so that the hazardous substance is not required or generated, or by substituting with a lesser hazard. If prevention is not reasonably practicable, exposure should be properly controlled using engineering controls or systems of work. PPE should be a last resort.
- Ensure control measures are used and maintained properly and that safety procedures are followed. Employees should use the control measures and report defects. Employers should ensure that controls are kept in good working order. Equipment should be examined and tested at suitable intervals.
- Monitor exposure to the hazardous substances. The concentrations of hazardous substances in the air should be measured in certain circumstances. Some substances including volatile anaesthetics have occupational exposure limits (OELs) (threshold limits for concentrations of hazardous substances in the air).
- Carry out health surveillance, where necessary. This may involve examinations by a doctor or nurse. Records must be kept of any health surveillance carried out.

- Ensure that employees are properly informed, trained and supervised. Employers should provide their employees with information and training about the nature of the substances they work with or are exposed to and the associated risks, and the precautions they should take, including details of control measures, their purpose and how to use them.

## Genetically modified organisms

These are the subject of particular concern, and are covered by specific sets of health and safety regulations. These are covered in more depth in Chapter 13. Work with GMOs is covered by the GMO (Contained Use) Regulations 2000. These regulations require that the GMOs are suitably contained, and that the risks to both human health and environmental safety are assessed and controlled. The human health risks are assessed under the GMO (Contained Use) Regulations 2000. For genetically modified micro-organisms (GMMs), the environmental risk assessment is undertaken under the COSHH Regulations; and for GMOs, the environmental risk assessment is undertaken under the GMO (Risk Assessment) (Records and Exemptions) Regulations 1996.

## Health and safety in animal facilities

Animal facilities may present specialised hazards that are unique. Such facilities are often isolated geographically from other areas of the institution, and the work may involve particular hazards not encountered in other parts of an establishment. It is particularly important that the safety policy for these units has been properly worked out and is familiar to all personnel involved. A set of local rules should be available in each unit, which covers both general and specific safety hazards in the area.

## THE HAZARDS

The major potential hazards to animal handlers can be divided into three groups:

1. allergy
2. infection
3. injury.

It is likely that all animal handlers will encounter at least one of these hazards during their careers. The problems involve both occupational health and occupational safety, and it is important that the institutional occupational health advisor (physician or nurse) and safety officer liaise closely in the investigation of occupational hazards and when deciding on appropriate control measures.

## Allergy to laboratory animals

Close contact with animals, their products and fur is generally unavoidable by animal technicians and research workers. However, between 10% and 44% of animal care workers suffer from allergic symptoms, and about 10% develop occupational asthma.

Allergies can have serious consequences for individuals in terms of health and future careers. Most allergies develop within 2 years of exposure, and up to half of those affected will develop signs so severe that they need regular treatment or are obliged to stop working with animals altogether. Anyone can develop an allergy, but it is more likely in atopics, who have an inherited tendency to develop IgE antibodies. Those with pre-existing allergies are more likely to develop animal allergies.

Allergy to laboratory animals (ALA) is commonly due to a Type 1 immediate allergic reaction, mediated through release of IgE antibody, occurring on exposure to allergen, either by direct contact or through inhalation. IgE sensitises tissue mast cells and basophils by binding to them, and these sensitised cells degranulate and release histamine and other inflammatory mediators on subsequent exposure to the allergen, leading to oedema, cell infiltration, mucus secretion and, in the lung, bronchoconstriction. Other mechanisms are involved less commonly, including IgG-mediated allergy, which may occur 1–12 h after exposure, and non-IgE-mediated allergy involving other immunoglobulins and giving rise to specific pathology, such as extrinsic allergic alveolitis.

A number of symptoms are commonly recorded in cases of ALA, including:

1.  Rhinitis (sneezing, running/blocked nose).
2.  Conjunctivitis (stinging and running eyes often with associated injection of the conjunctiva and local swelling of the eyelids).

These two symptom groups are the commonest associated with animal allergy.

3.  Skin effects.
    (a) Urticaria ('hives' or 'nettlerash').
    (b) Wheals (raised red areas around bites and scratches).
    (c) Eczema, particularly on the backs of the hands and occasionally the face.
4.  Asthma, characterised by a dry cough, wheezing and shortness of breath, which can persist after exposure ceases.
5.  Extrinsic allergic alveolitis.
6.  Anaphylactic reactions, which may be life threatening.

Rhinitis is the most common form of allergy, and many individuals will not make the connection with animals. Often, there is no progression to other symptom groups even on repeated exposure. People who are already asthmatic may just notice a slight increase in their need for bronchodilators.

Extrinsic allergic alveolitis may be acute or chronic. The acute form may resemble influenza, with sweating, cough, generalised muscle pains and malaise on exposure to the allergen, which resolves when exposure ceases. The chronic form is accompanied by an intermittent cough and increasing breathlessness. This is probably less common than asthma, but may be misdiagnosed.

Anaphylaxis is characterised by itching, hives, swelling of the face, lips and tongue, and occasionally laryngeal oedema and dyspnoea. There may be asthma and wheezing, and the subject may even go into shock, with bronchospasm, angio-oedema and hypotension, which may be life threatening. It may occur in animal handlers bitten by snakes or some insects, or in allergic individuals bitten by rodents. Death can occur through laryngeal oedema and hypoxia, if effective treatment is not instituted rapidly. Those likely to be affected must avoid exposure.

Since ALA is very common, regular health surveillance of animal handlers is required. Individuals identified as having major allergies prior to employment should perhaps be advised to seek alternative employment. Otherwise, regular symptom questionnaires and self-reporting of changes to occupational health advisers should identify those with developing allergies. Laboratory estimations of immunoglobulins and radio-allergo sorbent testing (RAST) may provide more specific information. In these circumstances, appropriate measures must be taken to control exposure, but if symptoms continue to progress despite the control measures, individuals may be wise to consider alternative careers.

## Causes of allergy

Several species are involved in ALA. The allergens in each case are different, and differences in the particle size and mode of spread lead to differences in the types of allergic symptoms noted and the appropriate control measures.

The rat is the species most commonly involved in ALA. The main allergens are a protein in urine and saliva. These are found in particles of varying size. Disturbance of rat litter leaves particles airborne for 15–35 min.

In mice, the main allergen is urinary protein.

In guinea pigs, the allergen is urinary protein, found on very small particles that can penetrate low into the respiratory tract.

In rabbits, the major allergen is a glycoprotein found in the fur. A protein found in urine and saliva is a minor allergen.

In cats, the main allergen is a protein from the sebaceous glands, which coats the hair shafts. It is also found in saliva. The particles are very small, and can go deeply into the lungs. The allergen is electrically charged and can stick to surfaces, such as walls and doors; these can, therefore, act as reservoirs for some time after the animals have left. Increasing air changes does little to reduce allergen concentrations.

In dogs, the main allergen is a protein found in saliva, hair and skin.

In pigs, signs of asthma and respiratory disease have been noted after exposure to pigs; however, this is more often due to ammonia than allergy.

In birds, rhinitis, asthma, hypersensitivity and pneumonitis have been reported after repeated exposure. Various proteins in droppings and serum have been implicated.

Horses are a potent source of allergens. Allergies have also been reported to fish and crustaceans. Allergy to non-human primates is uncommon. Sensitivity to cattle has been reported in farmers.

## Control

Although most allergens will produce symptoms in sensitised individuals at very low levels of exposure, there is some evidence that controlling levels may reduce the amount of animal allergy and its severity. The risk of developing allergy seems to be related to the duration of exposure, and exposure concentration, which is task related, cleaning out producing more allergens than simple handling. Pre-employment screening may identify those at risk, for example with a family history of allergies. Skin tests, RAST or enzyme-linked immunosorbent assay (ELISA) may be done to identify those with pre-existing allergies or IgE antibodies; these people may take appropriate precautions and low-risk assignments. Lung function testing to identify occupational asthma and to evaluate and monitor symptoms is advisable. Annual screening can detect those developing allergies so that intervention can be taken to prevent long-term difficulties. Workers with known risks should be assigned tasks that minimise exposure.

ALA remains a major problem despite control measures, but reducing exposure is still highly desirable.

The UK COSHH Regulations Approved CoP ideally requires elimination of the allergen, and where that is impossible, a series of measures designed to reduce exposure including:

(a) Totally enclosed processes and handling systems.
(b) Plant or processes or systems of work, which minimise the generation of, suppress or contain hazardous dust, fumes, micro-organisms, etc., and which limit the area of contamination in the event of spills and leaks.
(c) Partial enclosure with local exhaust ventilation.
(d) Local exhaust ventilation.
(e) Sufficient general ventilation. Effective ventilation can reduce the concentration of allergens, but only at reasonable stocking densities. More animals per area is equal to more allergens.
(f) Reduction of number of employees exposed and exclusion of non-essential access.
(g) Reduction in the period of exposure for employees.
(h) Regular cleaning of contamination from or disinfection of walls, surfaces, etc.
(i) Provision of means for safe storage and disposal of substances hazardous to health.
(j) Prohibition of eating, drinking, smoking, etc., in contaminated areas.
(k) Provision of adequate facilities for washing, changing and storage of clothing including arrangements for laundering contaminated clothing, to which may be added the requirement for PPE including respiratory protective equipment (RPE), which is only acceptable where other measures are already in place.

The Education Services Advisory Committee in the UK has produced two documents, which suggest specific ways of controlling animal allergens, and in particular concentrates on adequate general ventilation, specific ventilation for animal rooms, and especially designed cleaning systems to reduce the likelihood of aerosol production. PPE is essential for all people working with laboratory animals or entering the facilities and correct disposal or laundering of this is also required.

*Engineering controls*

A well-designed facility can reduce the level of exposure. Airborne allergen levels depend on the rate of production and the rate of removal. Production depends on the number of animals, removal depends on the ventilation. For rat allergens, increasing relative humidity can reduce the airborne allergen concentration. High-allergen exposure areas include:

• animal holding areas
• cleaning-out and cage-changing areas

- non-animal areas adjacent to animal areas, for example laboratories, offices, recreation areas, etc.

The allergen exposure levels in these areas can be reduced significantly by the use of purpose-designed equipment, and particular types of bedding can reduce exposure.

**Animal holding areas**   Open racking is the traditional type of animal accommodation, but offers little inherent protection from allergens. Particular types of caging can reduce exposure, for example filter-topped cages. These also offer some protection for the animals against disease. Placing transparent sliding curtains in front of open racks combined with directed room ventilation also reduces allergen exposure.

Animals can be held in various types of cabinets, such as allergen cabinets or ventilated filter cabinets (e.g. Scantainer, Scanbur), where the exhaust from the animals is drawn through the cabinet to the room extract, allowing efficient one-way air flow away from staff. These sometimes have HEPA filters and can significantly reduce exposure. These contain allergens and protect animals from disease.

With individually ventilated cage (IVC) racks, each cage has a filter top to prevent exposure of staff to allergens, and when in the racking each cage has its own filtered air supply, preventing cross contamination. Cages are changed and procedures carried out in a dedicated laminar flow cabinet designed to protect both animals and staff (see Chapter 6).

**Cleaning-out and cage-changing areas**   Mobile ventilated cleaning-out stations draw allergens away from staff and reduce exposure. Laminar air flow cabinets offer total containment of allergens.

### Systems of work

Workers need to know the risks and take proper measures to control and avoid exposure. Workers must keep to approved systems of work, which minimise their exposure to allergens. Frequent hand washing and showering on leaving the unit can help to control allergies. Air showers, which involve a blast of HEPA air, can prevent or reduce the spread of allergens to non-animal areas. These have the advantage that staff can enter in groups and no changing of clothes is required.

### Personal protective equipment

This is a last resort in control of allergy; however, advantage should be taken of gloves, coats, shoe covers, face masks and high-efficiency respirators. If engineering controls are unable to reduce allergen exposure to acceptably low levels, RPE will be required. Such equipment should be carefully chosen and comply with national standards, and individuals should receive training on fitting and using it. Those who are particularly allergic may require air-fed visors or helmets with high-efficiency filtration. However, for most individuals disposable dust masks, which must be discarded after usually 4–8 h use, will give sufficient protection to control symptoms. Simple surgical masks, however, are unlikely to be adequate.

The combination of appropriate control measures and adequate, specific and sensitive health surveillance should enable most workers affected by animal allergy to continue working. There will always be those who should be advised to avoid further exposure. Careful discussion will be required on a case-by-case basis with the occupational health adviser, and redeployment of those severely affected should be arranged.

# Infection

There are many well-known hazards from micro-organisms and parasites normally affecting animals, which can be transferred to humans. These range from the common gastrointestinal infections, such as *Campylobacter* and *Salmonella*, to rare but life-threatening diseases, such as haemorrhagic fevers (Marburg and Hantaan viruses) or Weil's disease (Leptospirosis). More than 150 of these zoonotic diseases have been recognised, with varying significance to humans. Modern research also produces new infection hazards, associated with emerging and re-emerging pathogens. Work with human viruses, viral vectors being used in gene therapies, or transgenic animals containing proviral DNA or receptors for human pathogens could all be potential hazards.

## *Zoonoses*

Hookworm infestation among the barefoot farmers of the developing countries is probably the commonest occupationally acquired disease in the world, and ringworm is a common zoonosis among farmers and those working with large animals, but there is little scientific data on the incidence of zoonoses in animal handlers in a research environment. Table 3.2 gives examples of zoonoses that may be encountered in animal facilities (after UK Education Services Advisory Committee, Health and Safety Commission 1992). Researchers working in the field may be exposed to unknown and potentially life-threatening hazards from wild animals, such as Lassa fever or Hantaan virus from rodents, or Filovirus infections (Ebola and Marburg) from wild primates in parts of Africa or the Far East. In such circumstances, it is vital for researchers to adhere strictly to safety precautions, such as the use of protective clothing and chemical restraint, and to ensure that all animals are examined by a veterinarian and screened for zoonotic diseases, wherever possible.

### *Prevention of zoonoses*

The risk of infection from research animals can be minimised by always obtaining animals with known health status from accredited sources and implementing regular health screening programmes to ensure their health is maintained, particularly where a COSHH assessment has identified a risk of zoonotic infection. Where health screening is impossible, for example with wild animals, they should be treated as though in quarantine. It is also essential to use suitable handling techniques to avoid bites and scratches.

**Table 3.2**    Examples of zoonoses in animal facilities.

| Organism | Animal source | Human disease | ACDP hazard group |
|---|---|---|---|
| *Campylobacter* | Various | Campylobacteriosis | 2 |
| *Chlamydophilia psittaci* | Sheep | Ovine chlamydiosis | 2 |
| | Birds | Avian chlamydiosis | 3 |
| *Coxiella burnetti* | Sheep and cattle | Q fever | 3 |
| *Cryptosporidium* | Sheep and cattle | Cryptosporidiosis | 2 |
| *Hantaan* virus | Rats | Korean Haemorrhagic fever | 3 |
| *Herpesvirus simiae* | Simians | Simian B disease | 4 |
| *LCM* virus | Mice | Lymphocytic choriomeningitis | 3 |
| *Leptospira* | Rats | Weil's disease (Leptospirosis) | 2 |
| *Microsporum* and *Trichophyton* | Various | Ringworm | 2 |
| *Salmonella* spp | Various | Gastroenteritis | 2 |
| (*S. typhi* and *paratyphi*) | (Fruit eating bats) | (Typhoid and paratyphoid) | (3) |
| *Shigella* spp | Primates | Bacillary dysentery | 2 |
| (*Shigella dysenteriae* type 1) | | | (3) |
| *Streptobacillus moniliformis* | Mainly rats and mice | Rat bite fever (Haverhill fever) | 2 |
| *Toxoplasma gondii* | Cats | Toxoplasmosis | 3 |
| *Bartonella henselae* | Cats | Catscratch disease (benign lymphoreticulosis) | – |

## *Particular hazards from simians*

The most dangerous zoonotic infections researchers are likely to contact are those that are carried by non-human primates. Simians carry a number of particularly pathogenic diseases, ranging from salmonellosis to tuberculosis, and the UK Medical Research Council has made particular recommendations with respect to simian herpesvirus (*Herpesvirus simiae*, B-virus) and simian retroviruses.

Simian herpesvirus occurs in Old World monkeys (but not Great Apes) and has caused at least 40 cases of disease in humans, most of which (70%) were fatal. Some human cases have occurred despite only minimal exposure to animals, when wearing appropriate protective clothing. Control methods include only using animals that have been screened for the disease and found to be negative for research projects. Different serological tests vary in their sensitivity and specificity, so care should be taken when interpreting single results. Avoidance of bites and spitting by careful handling and welfare techniques is also required.

Simian retroviruses are a complex group of related viruses. Both simian immunodeficiency virus (SIV) and simian T-lymphotrophic virus (STLV) are related to the equivalent human viruses, but at present it is unknown whether humans can be affected by SIV or STLV, although antibodies have been detected in exposed personnel. The rate of mutation of these viruses is high, leading to differences in *in vitro* and *in vivo* properties of different isolates. Appropriate containment levels are required for work with any immunodeficiency virus. The Advisory Committee on Dangerous Pathogens (ACDP) requires appropriate containment levels for work with immunodeficiency viruses: check with the ACDP before beginning such work. Antibodies to simian foamy virus have been detected in personnel working with non-human primates, but no associated disease has been reported.

## Working with pathogens

Many research projects involve the deliberate inoculation of animals with known pathogens, or working with tissues or body fluids. All such work should be considered potentially hazardous, and a COSHH assessment performed. Local rules can then be drawn up detailing methods for safe handling and disposal of the material. Material may be screened prior to inoculation to ensure no pathogens are present; but if this is impossible, assume the material is infected. Human blood and tissues should be screened for hepatitis B, hepatitis C and immunodeficiency viruses as a minimum. Animal tissues may have the potential for carrying pathogens, such as transmissible spongiform encephalopathies, and this needs to be considered.

Appropriate containment levels are mandatory for work involving introduced pathogens, and flexible film isolators, individually air-filtered ventilated cages or filter-topped cages may be used. Biohazard containment levels are determined by the severity of the disease caused to man, the mode of transmission, the availability of prophylaxis or therapy, and the risks of handling and caring for infected animals.

To help prevent biological hazards:

- avoid the use of sharps and take great care
- keep hands away from mouth, nose and eyes
- wear protective gloves and coat
- remove gloves and wash hands before leaving the animal areas
- use mechanical pipettes (not mouth pipettes)
- never eat, drink, smoke, handle contact lenses, take or apply medicines in animal areas
- take care to avoid creating splashes or aerosols in animal areas
- if creating aerosols, use a safety cabinet
- wear eye protection
- keep animal room doors closed
- decontaminate work surfaces promptly and wipe up spills
- decontaminate infected waste before disposal
- use secondary leakproof containers to transport samples.

In some cases, vaccination of the handler will be needed, for example those working with hepatitis B. Those working with *Vaccinia* or other poxviruses will need special advice. The ACDP recommends vaccination for those working with monkey pox, and a case-by-case assessment is required for people working with other poxviruses. Vaccination is contraindicated in pregnancy or for those with skin conditions, such as eczema.

People with immunodeficiencies pose a particular risk, and may not be able to be vaccinated as required. It is possible that the employer may have to take the decision to exclude these people from exposure to pathogens.

## *Health surveillance*

It can be difficult to identify individuals affected by micro-organisms encountered in the course of their work. It may be necessary to consider taking pre-employment serum samples for storage, particularly from people working with potentially life-threatening human viruses, such as human immunodeficiency virus (HIV) or hepatitis B, in order to rule out prior exposure. In any case, it is usual to take samples for storage from anyone who sustains a percutaneous injury involving contaminated blood or tissues.

# Injury

Most animal species, vertebrate and invertebrate, will react defensively if assaulted, and this can pose a hazard for the researcher. Animal handlers may sustain a variety of injuries from their charges, including the following.

**Traumatic injuries**    Farm animals by their sheer bulk can unintentionally cause considerable injuries including fractures, simply by treading on a foot, kicking or crushing. Smaller species may scratch. Injury may also be caused by lifting heavy animals and equipment, or twisting rapidly to catch a mouse escaping at high speed. Injuries may vary from very mild scratches or bruises to life-threatening physical injuries.

**Bites**    These may be as follows:

(a) Non-toxic, for example from pigs, dogs and small mammals. Even if the animal is a high-health laboratory bred mouse, bites can become infected with a variety of commensal pathogens including *Streptococci* and *Staphylococci*, which can be dangerous for humans.
(b) Toxic, for example snake, possibly lizard and spider bites. It is essential to have rapid access to appropriate medical advice in case of such injuries.

**Stings**    For example from fish, such as weavers, stone fish, scorpion fish, etc., coelenterates, echinoderms (starfish and sea-urchins), mollusca (cone shells) and arthropods (including bees, wasps, hornets and scorpions).

## *Prevention*

The prevention of injuries is difficult due to the unpredictable nature of many species. However, many injuries are preventable by good handling, and by taking into account factors that might trigger a traumatic event. For example, sudden noises or unfamiliar personnel may frighten an animal and cause it to react unpredictably. It is important to be aware of the animal's biology and behaviour in reducing the risk. The animal handler must understand the species they are working with, be aware of their habits and likely defensive tactics, and be trained to approach the species correctly. Strains of animals vary in temperament, and consideration should be given to selecting animals with placid temperaments. Specifically designed containment and caging facilities are required particularly with large animals when specimens are to be obtained. In the wild, anaesthetic dart techniques may be necessary to approach the animals safely.

Some species pose particular hazards. Non-human primates are strong, dextrous, intelligent and tenacious. They can pull on loose hair or neckties, and may throw things. The male of some species may be more aggressive than the female, but all species with young will react defensively to protect their offspring. Snakes and insects may bite, particularly when animals are surprised or disturbed by loud noises. Careless handling techniques without appropriate protective equipment can lead to injury.

Personnel are often unaware of the hazards associated with animal bites, such as infection, zoonotic diseases or contamination that could cause disease or spread to others. Medical attention should be sought, and the status of the animal checked for possible zoonoses. First aid facilities should be available in all animal handling premises, and individuals trained in first aid techniques to the appropriate national standard are required. They should have particular information about the nature of the animals and the likely injuries they could cause and, in the case of venomous species, particularly snakes, they will need training in specific first aid methods including standard procedures for containing the spread of venom. This may, for instance, include arterial tourniquet methods, which are inappropriate in other forms of first aid. Clear lines of communication to expertise via the local emergency facility are also required.

## MISCELLANEOUS HEALTH AND SAFETY HAZARDS AND RISKS

Animal handlers are exposed to a wide variety of other occupational hazards and risks similar to those that occur elsewhere. Wet floors in animal rooms can lead to slips and trips, and dim lighting or fixed light cycles may mean personnel are working in reduced lighting. The use of flammable solvents, and pressure vessels, such as autoclaves and gas cylinders in the laboratory poses additional hazards.

### Chemical hazards

Many chemicals are encountered in the laboratory, which may be flammable, corrosive, reactive, explosive or toxic, for example allergens, carcinogens, mutagens, teratogens or nephrotoxins. For most, there will be adequate information to perform a COSHH assessment. For unknown agents or new drugs, any information that is known about similar chemicals and data collected to date from preliminary toxicity studies can be used in risk assessment.

1. *Disinfection agents* may cause irritation of skin and mucous membranes, including the respiratory tract and/or sensitisation of the skin and lungs. Appropriate handling techniques are described by the manufacturers and should be available. Substances used for fumigation are covered by a separate Approved CoP under COSHH regulations.
2. *Chemotherapeutic agents*, particularly those used for large animals may require specific antidotes to be drawn up with a second person available in order to inject them rapidly. Other drugs may cause sensitisation if carelessly handled (e.g. prostaglandins), and some are carcinogenic (e.g. xylene), which require training in special handling and containment techniques. Some volatile anaesthetics have

been associated with abortion, cancer or liver disease (see Chapter 7 page 121 for Recommended exposure limits).
3. *General laboratory chemicals* may include mineral acids, alkalis, phenol derivatives, aromatic solvents, preservatives, fixatives and pesticides.

## Electrical hazards

Electrical hazards are ubiquitous in virtually all workplaces. Controls may be engineering controls, such as circuit breakers, or via standard operating procedures. Constant vigilance is needed to prevent accidents. Electrical apparatus should be inspected on a regular basis. Care should be taken when using sharp instruments close to a power cable, and plugs and sockets should not be contaminated with animal products, or allowed to get wet during cleaning.

Most jurisdictions have specific requirements to control the use of electricity at work. In the UK, the Electricity at Work Regulations 1989 apply.

## Radiation hazards

Animal workers may be exposed to radiation from equipment used to expose animals to alpha, beta, gamma, neutron or X-radiation. Alternatively, radioactive isotopes may be administered to animals and the animals themselves become a source. Such work is governed in the UK by the Ionising Radiations Regulations 1999. Organisations where ionising radiation is used have a Radiation Protection Adviser appointed, and this person needs to be consulted when work is to begin. Areas where work with ionising radiation is carried out may need to be designated 'controlled' or 'supervised' areas. In addition, the worker may be required to undergo regular health surveillance by an approved doctor.

Ultraviolet light, microwaves, lasers and other forms of non-ionising radiation all possess specific hazards, which require specific action to protect eyes and skin, and careful control by employers and employees. Class 4 lasers are particularly powerful and may pose a specific fire hazard as well as potentially causing damage to the eyes and skin even from reflection.

## Noise

Animal facilities are noisy places. Some animals, including pigs and dogs, and equipment, such as vacuum cleaners, can produce loud noises. Chronic exposure to loud sounds can impair hearing, typically reducing sensitivity to sounds above 2000 Hz. If conversation or talking on the phone is difficult, the noise is probably too loud. This can be controlled by engineering controls, where sound production is reduced through soundproofing or equipment design, or by administrative controls to reduce exposure, such as ear protection or reducing exposure times.

## Sharp instruments

Sharps injuries are common in animal handlers, partly due to the unpredictability of their charges. Percutaneous injury poses the risk of blood-borne transmissible disease or local infection. Care should be taken when handling sharps, and good animal handling and restraint techniques are needed. Disposal in appropriate containers is mandatory. Health and safety legislation may require containers constructed to a specific standard with subsequent disposal by special means including incineration in dedicated units.

Local laboratory practice in writing (local rules) should identify methods of handling and disposal of such instrumentation.

## Waste disposal

The cleaning of cages and the disposal of animal waste is a specialised technique, which needs to avoid the formation of aerosols of animal products in the environment. Such aerosols may settle only very slowly despite appropriate ventilation and will pose a hazard, particularly in terms of allergen content. Animal waste should be collected carefully, bagged in appropriate containers, labelled and disposed of according to national waste disposal regulations. It must not be treated like household waste. Carcasses and tissue specimens from animals may require double bagging in heavy gauge plastic bags of particular colour or labelling and should be collected for incineration by trained personnel.

Certain material associated with animal experimentation will require autoclaving prior to disposal by an appropriate route.

## LONE WORKING

Where there are identified hazards from occupations, there are particular risks in working alone. This is especially so for animal handlers, particularly in the field, with the possibility of severe injury or other potentially life-threatening hazards, such as snake bites or anaphylaxis. In all cases, workers must have a rapid means of communication to someone who can respond on their behalf. This is naturally much easier in a purpose-built facility in the middle of a centre of population, but may be impracticable in certain remote locations. Such workers accept the (theoretically) major risks associated with such work, but in order to make this judgement, they must be aware of the potential risks and make their own assessment in conjunction with their employer. Some lone workers carry alarms that are activated if they change position rapidly, and in certain areas carrying personal radios or portable telephones is a distinct possibility that should be considered. They should be sure that somebody knows where they are and not deviate from their plans, however tempting may be an alternative scenario. Checking into and out of animal facilities with security coded entrances is now common and an added reassurance for the lone worker.

## EMPLOYEE SECURITY

The very real problem associated with animal rights groups worldwide poses a considerable threat to the personal security of animal handlers. Animal facilities should be especially secure and will require high levels of entrance/exit control. The building should be designed so that breaking and entering is difficult or impossible and high levels of alarm systems connected to local police facilities are indicated.

Individual employees may wish their identity to remain confidential. In particular, the home addresses and telephone numbers of animal handlers should be kept completely confidential in secure storage. Such employees should not carry identification that indicates that they are animal handlers unless absolutely necessary. However, animal handlers (along with many other employees) may wish to carry a card indicating the nature of their work in general terms, and inform their doctor of their occupation. This should increase the 'index of suspicion' of a doctor or health facility to whom they are unknown, without identifying them as animal workers, if taken ill perhaps in a remote or strange location.

## SUMMARY

There are many potential hazards from research; however, the risks can be minimised by implementing simple control measures. Good housekeeping can help control many work-related hazards. Surfaces should be kept clean and clear from obstructions, waste and other materials. Food bags or waste should not be stored in corridors, where people may trip; floors should be left dry after cleaning. Using a vacuum when cleaning cages reduces the risk from airborne allergens. There are many potential hazards associated with research protocols, which may be related to the inherent dangerous qualities of the experimental agents, for example chemicals or virulent biological agents, or the complexity and type of the experimental operation, such as the need to create dust, dander or vapours. Having recognised and identified the hazards, it is possible to devise a protocol for minimising exposure. While the employer has overall responsibility under the Health and Safety at Work Act to ensure the health and safety of personnel, it is nonetheless also the responsibility of individuals to make sure that they conform to the local rules for their own safety and that of others.

## FURTHER INFORMATION

Advisory Committee on Dangerous Pathogens (1990). *Categorisation of Pathogens According to Hazard and Categories of Containment*. HMSO, London. ISBN 0-11-885564-6.

Advisory Committee on Dangerous Pathogens (1997). *Working Safely with Research Animals: Management of Infection Risks*. HMSO, London. ISBN 0-7176-1377-1.

Advisory Committee on Dangerous Pathogens and Advisory Committee on Genetic Modification (1990). *Vaccination of Laboratory Workers Handling Vaccinia and Related Poxvirus Infections for Humans*. HMSO, London. ISBN 0-11-885450-X.

Bland, S.M., Evans, R. and Rivera, J.C. (1987). Allergy to laboratory animals in health care personnel. *Health Problems of Health Care Workers*, 2(3). (ed. E.A. Emmett) State of the Art Reviews. Hanley & Belfus, Philadelphia.

Boulter, E.A., Kaler, S.S., Heberling, R.L., Guarjardo, J.E. and Lester, T.L. (1982). A comparison of neutralization tests for the detection of antibodies to *Herpesvirus simiae* (monkey B-virus). *Laboratory Animal Science* 32(2), 150–52.

Centers for Disease Control and Prevention Morbidity and Mortality Weekly Report (1997). *Non-human Primate Spumavirus Infections Among Persons with Occupational Exposure* 46(6).

Health and Safety Commission (1993). *Control of Substances Hazardous to Health. General Approved Code of Practice* (4th edn). HMSO, London. ISBN 0-11-882085-0.

Health and Safety Commission (1990). *What You should Know about Allergy to Laboratory Animals*. Education Services Advisory Committee. HMSO, London. ISBN 0-11-885527-1.

Health and Safety Commission (1992). *Health and Safety in Animal Facilities*. Education Services Advisory Committee. HMSO, London. ISBN 0-11-886353-3.

Health and Safety Executive (2002). *Control of Laboratory Animal Allergy*. Guidance note EH76. HSE Books, Suffolk. ISBN 07176-2450-1.

Holland, C. (ed.) (1997). *Modern Perspectives on Zoonoses*. Royal Irish Academy, Dublin.

ILAR (1997). *Occupational Health and Safety in the Care and Use of Research Animals*. National Academies Press, New York.

ILAR News (2003). Issue on Occupational Health and Safety in Biomedical Research, Vol. 44, No. 1.

Kibby, T., Power, G. and Croner, J. (1989). Allergy to laboratory animals: a prospective sectional study. *Journal of Occupational Medicine* 31, 842–46.

Medical Research Council (1990). *The Management of Simians in Relation to Infectious Hazards to Staff*. MRC Simian Virus Committee, London.

Royal Society of Chemistry (1992). *Hazards in the Chemical Laboratory* (5th edn). (ed. S.G. Luxon). RSC, London. ISBN 0-85186229-2.

Whitley, R.J. (1990). Cercopithecine herpes virus I (B virus). In *Virology* (2nd edn). (eds. B.N. Fields, D.M. Knipe *et al.*). Raven Press, New York.

Zangwill, K.M., Hamilton, D.H., Perkins, B.A., Regnery, R.L., Plikaytis, B.D., Hadler, J.L. *et al.* (1993). Cat scratch disease in Connecticut. Epidemiology, risk factors and evaluation of a new diagnostic test. *New England Journal of Medicine* 329(1), 8–13. ISSN 0028-4793.

# Chapter 4
# Pain, stress and humane end points

In order to satisfy the provisions of the Animals (Scientific Procedures) Act 1986 (ASPA), an assessment of the level of suffering that the animals under study may experience is required for consideration of the cost–benefit analysis. This judgement is also needed in order to assess the level of severity in the project licence application (see Chapter 2, The regulatory framework).

It is the responsibility of personal licence holders to look after the health and welfare of their animals. There are specific conditions attached to the project licence under which the work is done, which limit the amount of pain and discomfort any animal may experience. It is inevitable that some laboratory animals will experience discomfort as a result of some scientific procedures carried out on them, but pain is an unnecessary accompaniment to the majority of scientific procedures. Every effort must be made to identify the causes and to control the adverse effects of scientific procedures on animals. It is important to realise that pain or stress can produce a range of undesirable physiological changes, which may alter the rate of recovery from surgical procedures, and may affect the experiment itself. Section 5.5 of the ASPA requires that the most refined method possible shall be used causing the least pain, suffering, distress and lasting harm. This is reiterated in the project licence standard condition 6 and personal licence standard condition 12, which require that the personal licence holder takes precautions to minimise the pain, suffering, distress and lasting harm.

The evaluation of pain and distress is complex because thresholds and manifestations of pain and distress vary between species and between individuals within a species. The first stage in assessing an animal's well being is to become familiar with its normal appearance and behaviour. When doing 'hands on' training in the animal house, take time to observe the animals that you will be using in order to become familiar with their normal behavioural repertoire. Find out what the normal behaviour range is for the species you are working with, remembering that this may not be the same as the behaviour you observe in the laboratory due to the constraints of the captive environment (see www.ratlife.org). Animals have not evolved to live in cages.

## WHAT IS STRESS?

Certain levels of stress may not be detrimental to animals and indeed a low-physiological level of stress over which an animal has some control may be considered by some as enriching an otherwise boring life.

Physiological stress is that which occurs within normal physiological limits. The animal uses minimal effort to respond and is unconscious of this effort.

Overstress requires significantly more effort but the animal is still likely to be unconscious of it. It can be detrimental to biological processes, such as growth, in the longer term.

However, if the level increases to distress, considerable effort has to be put into the response, of which the animal is aware. The animal can be considered to be suffering.

Stress and distress in laboratory animals may be induced by painful or non-painful stimuli, including experimental methods, environmental factors or physiological disturbances. These factors contribute to the severity of the scientific procedure and impact adversely on animal welfare.

Pain is defined as an unpleasant sensory and emotional experience associated with actual or potential tissue damage. It can be divided into acute or chronic depending on the time scale over which it occurs. An animal will respond to a painful stimulus by modifying its conscious behaviour to avoid repetition of the painful situation that requires high-level central nervous system function. It will also exhibit automatic responses to protect the animal or a part of it; for example, withdrawal reflex, freeze or flight responses. It may also react to convey the experience to others in its group thus ensuring survival of some of the population. This may occur as vocalisation or by the release of pheromones, and this in itself may cause stress to other animals nearby, especially if they are unable to react as their normal behavioural repertoire would demand, for example by escaping to a safer place. The determination of what constitutes pain and distress is further complicated by the fact there are no universally agreed criteria for assessing what is, or is not, painful or distressing to an animal.

## ASSESSMENT OF PAIN AND DISTRESS

An animal's response to distress will be modified by a number of factors. Interpretation of the response will need to consider the following:

1. *The individual details of the animal, such as its species, age and origin.* These factors will, all, affect its response to painful stimuli. For example, a rabbit is far more stoical than a dog, since a prey species will be much better at hiding illness or injury than a predator species as this will be better for its survival, since predators will look for signs of weakness when hunting.
2. *The history of the animal and the establishment.* Take into account previous problems encountered, the course of the current problem, the environment in which the animal is kept, the procedures that have been carried out and any known current disease problems.
3. *Clinical examination of the animal to assess its current condition.* The extent of this may depend on the species you are working with. Take note of the following:
   – feeding behaviour (e.g. quantity, pattern of feeding)
   – physiological signs (such as heart rate, respiration rate, body temperature muscle tone and colour of mucous membranes)
   – biochemical signs (such as enzyme levels).
   If you suspect there may be intercurrent disease, contact the named veterinary surgeon for advice.
4. *Mental state.* Take notice if the animal appears dull, depressed, aggressive or hyperexcitable, especially if such traits are at variance with its usual behaviour.

The technician in charge of the animal will often be the best person to observe any changes in its temperament or its reluctance or otherwise to accept handling.

5. The *level of activity* of the animal may range from total inactivity to maniacal hyperactivity. Notice if there are any changes in gait, posture or facial expression.

6. *Vocalisation* will depend on the species and there are a wide variety of different noises produced by each species. The sound emitted may be outside the human auditory range and, therefore, go unnoticed but may be causing distress to others of the same species.

7. *Response to analgesics.* If a dose of an analgesic drug is administered and the animal's condition and demeanour improves, then this can be used as evidence that pain was indeed present.

All these are very general descriptions on how to assess distress qualitatively, and the interpretation of such parameters will vary quite widely between observers depending on their knowledge and experience of the species and the individual animal under observation. In making the judgement, it is necessary to consider the species, whether it is juvenile or adult, any normal physiological variation (e.g. pregnancy) and the animal's individual temperament.

Thus, the assessment of pain and distress in animals can be problematic, since it can be subjective and may be based on anthropomorphic assumptions that things which are distressing for humans will also be distressing for animals, which is not necessarily the case. This may lead to a tendency to overestimate the pain and suffering experienced by animals in some situations, and underestimate in others. Since this type of scoring is based on the subjective judgements of individuals, it is likely that two people with different backgrounds and experiences observing the same animal will give different scores. This can be avoided by having several observers score the animal at each point and average the scores, or by having all assessments performed by just one, or a few, experienced people. Vets, researchers or animal care staff can, with experience, become consistent in their markings and reduce this variation between assessors. However, it is better to consider how to quantify distress objectively in order to be able to judge whether it has been alleviated, to ascertain whether the degree of pain is within the severity banding of the project and to remove this inter-observer variability in making the assessment.

## QUANTIFICATION OF PAIN AND DISTRESS

Since it is impossible to distinguish between pain and other forms of distress, these are combined as a single assessment. A range of clinical signs are assessed, and given a score, and the overall score indicates the likelihood of whether the animal is suffering.

For a simple distress scoring (or welfare assessment) system (see General distress scoring sheet, Figure 4.1), monitor:

- appearance
- food and water intake
- clinical signs
- natural behaviour
- provoked behaviour.

| PARAMETER | ANIMAL ID | SCORE | DATE/ TIME | DATE/ TIME |
|---|---|---|---|---|
| **APPEARANCE** | NORMAL | 0 | | |
| | GENERAL LACK OF GROOMING | 1 | | |
| | COAT STARING, OCULAR AND NASAL DISCHARGES | 2 | | |
| | PILOERECTION, HUNCHED UP | 3 | | |
| **FOOD AND WATER INTAKE** | NORMAL | 0 | | |
| | UNCERTAIN: BODY WEIGHT ↓<5% | 1 | | |
| | INTAKE: BODY WEIGHT ↓10–15% | 2 | | |
| | NO FOOD OR WATER INTAKE | 3 | | |
| **CLINICAL SIGNS** | NORMAL T, CARDIAC AND RESPIRATORY RATES | 0 | | |
| | SLIGHT CHANGES | 1 | | |
| | T ± 1°C, C/R RATES ↕ 30% | 2 | | |
| | T ± 2°C, C/R RATES ↕ 50% OR VERY ↓ | 3 | | |
| **NATURAL BEHAVIOUR** | NORMAL | 0 | | |
| | MINOR CHANGES | 1 | | |
| | LESS MOBILE AND ALERT, ISOLATED | 2 | | |
| | VOCALISATION, SELF MUTILATION, RESTLESS OR STILL | 3 | | |
| **PROVOKED BEHAVIOUR** | NORMAL | 0 | | |
| | MINOR DEPRESSION OR EXAGGERATED RESPONSE | 1 | | |
| | MODERATE CHANGE IN EXPECTED BEHAVIOUR | 2 | | |
| | REACTS VIOLENTLY, OR VERY WEAK AND PRECOMATOSE | 3 | | |
| **SCORE** | IF YOU HAVE SCORED A 3 MORE THAN ONCE, SCORE AN EXTRA POINT FOR EACH 3 | 2–5 | | |
| | **TOTAL** | 0–20 | | |

**JUDGEMENT**
0–4    Normal.
5–9    Monitor carefully, consider analgesics or other treatments.
10–14  Suffering, provide relief, observe regularly. Seek second opinion from named animal care and welfare
       officer and/or named veterinary surgeon. Consider termination.
15–20  Severe distress, is this severity limit justified?

**Figure 4.1**   General distress scoring sheet.

At the start of the assessment, view the animal from a distance and note its natural appearance and undisturbed behaviour. Next, as you approach the animal, it should take notice of you and interact in some way. The nature of that interaction can be used to assess if the animal is responding normally. Finally, a detailed clinical examination can be carried out making appropriate clinical measurements (such as body weight).

If there is no deviation from the normal, for each parameter score 0. If there is mild deviation, score 1; moderate deviation, score 2 and substantial deviation, score 3. If three is scored more than once, give an extra one to each, making a maximum score of 20.

The use of such a system encourages regular close observation of the animal, leading to improved standards of animal care. If the animal is found to be deteriorating, then actively consider euthanasia before the experimental end point is reached. It is vital to remember to re-score the animal after giving analgesics or other treatments to ensure that the drugs have had the desired effect and the animal's condition has improved.

## Frequency of assessments

How often to use the scoring system to assess the animal depends on when signs are expected to occur and the length of time that they will persist. For example, in a toxicity study, the early signs are likely to be due to the primary effects of a substance on a particular tissue or cell, which depends on the physical and chemical characteristics of the test substance. Secondary effects occur after the compound has been taken into the body and undergone metabolism in the cells. The effects of this may occur at cellular level, organ level or affect the whole animal and may be manifested in a variety of physiological and behavioural effects. Tertiary effects may not be related directly to the interaction of the compound itself within the body, for example if a compound induces diarrhoea, the animal may become dehydrated, if it does not drink; and it is the dehydration that will cause the death of the animal. Signs that occur shortly before death may be due to the secondary effects of the substance but are more likely to be due the tertiary effects. Carcinogenicity studies may involve a necessary assessment of tertiary effects and provide needed experimental data, but the majority of toxicity studies are to determine the primary and secondary effects; the tertiary effects provide little additional information. The combination of the type of clinical signs and their duration can be used to assess the severity of the procedure and the intensity of suffering of the animal. The observations should, therefore, be frequent enough to identify any animals that are showing the defined set of signs of distress to enable euthanasia to be carried out in a timely manner. It is also scientifically useful to collect as much data as possible on clinical signs, and any unobserved animal deaths will represent lost information on the compound under test and a reduction in the quality of the scientific information yielded.

## DEFINING THE HUMANE END POINT

By definition, procedures carried out under the ASPA will have the potential to cause pain, suffering, distress or lasting harm; so it is necessary to address how these adverse effects might be controlled or prevented. There are three possible end points to every experiment.

**Experimental end point**   The experiment has simply run its course, and adequate experimental data have been collected.

**Error end point**   Sometimes mistakes happen that invalidate the experiment and, therefore, it has to be ended prematurely; there is no point in continuing, since any data generated will be erroneous.

**Humane end point**   The animal is killed at a defined point to limit its suffering. Waiting until the animal dies should be avoided as the end point for animal experiments. Use should be made of defined alterations to the animal's usual state, such as behavioural changes, changes in body temperature, body condition or weight loss. Continual refinement of the point of intervention should always be sought and implemented.

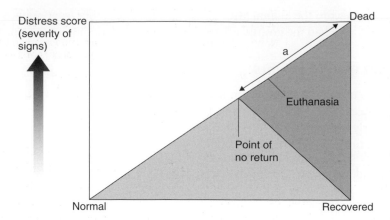

**Figure 4.2**    Application of the humane end point.

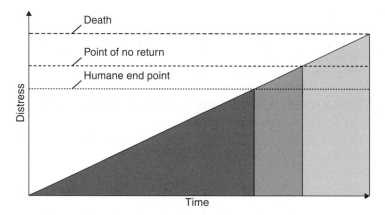

**Figure 4.3**    Humane end point: area under the curve equates to the suffering endured by the animal.

In Figure 4.2, the procedure involved would ultimately result in either the recovery or the death of the animal. For simplicity, a linear relationship has been shown between the suffering of the animal (severity of signs), to which a numerical figure is given in the distress score, and the time course of the procedure. After the development of a certain set of signs assessed to give the distress score, the animal passes the point of no return and at that point it is unnecessary to continue to death. Since it will not recover now, it may be possible to collect all the required data at this point. The experiment should, therefore, be designed to make the time line 'a' as long as possible to allow more time for intervention, so the animals can be euthanased before they suffer and reach the high-distress scores at the terminal stages of the procedure. The area under the curve equates to the total amount of suffering the animal endures (see Figure 4.3). By defining a humane end point, this suffering can be considerably reduced by euthanasia of the animal at an early point. Well-designed experiments detect very early signs of distress, allowing the definition of a point at which adequate data can be collected, but the suffering of the animals is kept to a minimum. The application of a

| Parameter | Subjective assessment | Objective assessment |
|---|---|---|
| Subjective, e.g. behaviour | Normal/abnormal | Assign numerical score based on degree of abnormality |
| Objective, e.g. body weight | Light/heavy | Measure parameter and note actual changes |

**Figure 4.4**   Differentiating between subjective and objective assessments.

defined humane end point will thus utilise a lower severity limit than would be needed if the procedure were allowed to run its full course. The precise time at which to kill the animal must be based on the appropriate clinical judgement, assessing the degree of suffering and the potential loss of data. Ideally, the maximum achievable information should be obtained from each animal, while suffering and distress are kept to the minimum. Utilising this concept of the humane end point will refine the procedure and reduce the costs to the animals, improving the justification and the cost–benefit equation for the experiment.

For both ethical and experimental reasons, it is important to keep adverse effects to a minimum, but in order to minimise them they must first be recognised and quantified, that is, it is necessary to assess the distress objectively. Objective methods of assessing pain and distress in animals are valuable for several reasons:

- they allow potential refinements and new research techniques to be evaluated critically
- they allow real judgements to be made about the need for and efficacy of analgesics
- they allow the implementation of humane end points.

Objective assessment involves looking at the chosen parameters and quantifying what is observed, whereas subjective assessment relies on the observer's opinion, which will necessarily vary from person to person. In addition to the assessment method, the parameters themselves can also be either subjective or objective (see Figure 4.4). Many assessment systems have been described for use in animals that involve studying a range of parameters and assigning a numerical score depending on the divergence from normal. However, this depends on the observer's opinion of normality, which may simply be what they 'normally see'. Sometimes, quite abnormal states may be classified by some observers as normal, for example stereotypic behaviours in captive animals are frequently misjudged as normal since they occur commonly.

## DEVELOPMENT OF DISTRESS SCORING SYSTEMS

In practice, scoring systems can be valuable tools in keeping the costs to animals in biomedical research to a minimum. However, the system outlined in Figure 4.1 is very general. Many research projects produce changes in just one organ system, and a general scoring system, such as the one described here, may not be sensitive enough to pick up specific indicators of distress in these cases. To overcome this, the parameters are modified to include only those specific changes that are anticipated in the particular project. Pilot studies are important to develop these more specific assessment sheets, and it may be necessary to modify the chosen system as the experiment progresses. The list of clinical signs to be assessed for a particular scientific procedure should be developed through experience and to a large extent will be unique to the specific husbandry system, the species or strain and to the specific experiment.

A scheme of scoring clinical signs for recognition and assessment of adverse effects on animals during scientific procedures has been shown to have a number of benefits including:

- Closer observation of animals by all staff at critical times in the experiment. This increases awareness of the potential adverse effects and allows for the appropriate use of methods of alleviation.
- Subjective assessments are avoided and opinion is both more structured and more evidence based, thus promoting more fruitful dialogue between scientists and animal care staff.
- Providing assistance with making a valid cost–benefit analysis in the justification of a procedure.
- Consistency in scoring is increased.
- Combinations of signs can be used to indicate the overall severity of the procedure and the continued assessment will determine the effectiveness of any therapies given to alleviate the adverse effects.
- The assessment will allow retrospective review of procedures to assess which experimental models cause the least pain and distress and will, therefore, help to further refine procedures in the future, to develop better systems of animal care, yielding better science and better animal welfare.
- The use of scoring systems assists with the training of new personnel in how to assess adverse effects on animals.

## Examples of specific distress scoring systems

### *Rat model of emphysema*

In this experiment, there may be some peracute (sudden) deaths that are impossible to predict using the general scoring sheet in Figure 4.1. Animals reaching score of 14 do not recover, but the critical period is the first 24 h. The problems seen are principally respiratory signs and the score sheet is not sensitive enough to identify the animals that are succumbing. The modified score sheet in Figure 4.5 gives more value to the respiratory parameters and the degree of dehydration, and is sensitive enough to allow these animals to be identified before they are in extremis. A humane end point can then be applied, so the animals are euthanased before suffering any more.

### *Experimental allergic encephalomyelitis in the mouse*

In this model, there are a number of scoring systems to assess the neurological effects of experimental allergic encephalomyelitis (EAE) to define an experimental end point (e.g. Figure 4.6), but these do not take into account the effect of the disease on the general health and well being of the animal. Neurological deficits appear from day 10–15 and follow a predictable course, which may be chronic and relapsing, allowing the

| PARAMETER | ANIMAL ID | SCORE | DATE/ TIME | DATE/ TIME |
|---|---|---|---|---|
| **APPEARANCE** | NORMAL | 0 | | |
| | GENERAL LACK OF GROOMING | 1 | | |
| | PILOERECTION, FRESH OCULAR AND NASAL DISCHARGES | 2 | | |
| | PILOERECTION, HUNCHED UP | 3 | | |
| | ABOVE AND EYES HALF CLOSED | 4 | | |
| **NATURAL BEHAVIOUR** | NORMAL | 0 | | |
| | MINOR CHANGES | 1 | | |
| | LESS MOBILE AND ISOLATED, BUT ALERT | 2 | | |
| | RESTLESS OR VERY STILL, NOT ALERT | 3 | | |
| **HYDRATION STATUS** | NORMAL | 0 | | |
| | ABNORMAL PINCH TEST | 5 | | |
| **CLINICAL SIGNS** | NORMAL RESPIRATORY RATE AND PATTERN | 0 | | |
| | SLIGHT CHANGES, INCREASED RATE ONLY | 1 | | |
| | INCREASED RATE WITH ABDOMINAL BREATHING | 2 | | |
| | DECREASED RATE WITH ABDOMINAL BREATHING | 3 | | |
| | MARKED ABDOMINAL BREATHING AND CYANOSIS | 4 | | |
| **PROVOKED BEHAVIOUR** | NORMAL | 0 | | |
| | MINOR DEPRESSION OR EXAGGERATED RESPONSE | 1 | | |
| | MODERATE CHANGE IN EXPECTED BEHAVIOUR | 2 | | |
| | VERY WEAK AND PRECOMATOSE | 3 | | |
| | **TOTAL** | 0–19 | | |

**Figure 4.5**   Modified distress scoring sheet with respiratory parameters.

| GRADE 0 | NORMAL |
|---|---|
| GRADE 1 | LOSS OF RIGHTING REFLEX/TAIL PARALYSIS |
| GRADE 2 | INCOMPLETE HIND LIMB PARALYSIS |
| GRADE 3 | COMPLETE HIND OR FRONT LIMB PARALYSIS |
| GRADE 4 | MORIBUND |

**Figure 4.6**   Neurological effects of EAE to define experimental end point.

long-term benefits of treatments to be studied. Affected animals that do not die usually recover, which makes defining a humane end point difficult, since animals may develop quite severe disease but then recover fully. The neurological scoring system alone is too specific and needs to be combined with an assessment of general distress to determine the humane end point, since some animals with severe neurological deficits maintain body condition and general well being, whereas some with relatively minor neurologcial disorders are sometimes generally much more affected and show

ANIMAL NUMBER

| DATE AND TIME | SCORE | | | | | | | | | | | | | | | |
|---|---|---|---|---|---|---|---|---|---|---|---|---|---|---|---|---|
| **SURFACE AREA OF ULCERATION** | | | | | | | | | | | | | | | | |
| <50% OF TUMOUR | 1 | | | | | | | | | | | | | | | |
| 50–80% OF TUMOUR | 2 | | | | | | | | | | | | | | | |
| >80% OF TUMOUR | 3 | | | | | | | | | | | | | | | |
| **DEPTH OF ULCERATION** | | | | | | | | | | | | | | | | |
| SURFACE LAYER OF SKIN ONLY | 1 | | | | | | | | | | | | | | | |
| EXTENDING BELOW DERMIS | 2 | | | | | | | | | | | | | | | |
| ~50% TUMOUR DEPTH | 3 | | | | | | | | | | | | | | | |
| ~FULL DEPTH OF TUMOUR | 4 | | | | | | | | | | | | | | | |
| **VISUAL APPEARANCE** | | | | | | | | | | | | | | | | |
| DRY WITH SCAB | 1 | | | | | | | | | | | | | | | |
| WET, SEROUS EFFUSION | 2 | | | | | | | | | | | | | | | |
| WET, BLEEDING | 3 | | | | | | | | | | | | | | | |
| WET, PURULENT | 4 | | | | | | | | | | | | | | | |
| **CLINICAL CONDITION** | | | | | | | | | | | | | | | | |
| POOR GROOMING | 1 | | | | | | | | | | | | | | | |
| SCRATCHING AFFECTED SKIN | 2 | | | | | | | | | | | | | | | |
| SOLITARY, HUDDLED BEHAVIOUR | 5 | | | | | | | | | | | | | | | |
| **TOTAL (MAX = 16)** | | | | | | | | | | | | | | | | |

**JUDGEMENT**
3–6   Continue careful monitoring.
7–10  Consider killing by Schedule 1 method. If necessary, seek second opinion of NACWO or NVS.
        If not sacrificed observe on at least a daily basis.
11–16  Kill by Schedule 1 method.

**Figure 4.7**   Scoring sheet for evaluation of tumour ulceration.

signs of poor well being. Thus, the end point is defined, when an animal shows one or more of the following:

- weight loss > 30%
- failure to eat or drink for >24 h
- EAE score > grade 3 for 24 h.

## Evaluation of tumour ulceration

For more details of evaluation of tumour ulceration see Figure 4.7. This system takes into account the area and depth of the ulceration and the pathology of the ulcer in addition to the overall condition of the animal.

## Distress and condition scoring for neonatal mice and rats

The need for objective methods for assessment of welfare in the neonatal rodent arises because of the huge number of new mutant and transgenic strains that are being created. Many misconceptions exist regarding the sentience and welfare of neonatal rodents. Studies have shown that sensory nerves are present in the skin and skeleton of rats from

| PARAMETER (NEONATES) | ANIMAL ID | SCORE | DATE/TIME | AGE |
|---|---|---|---|---|
| APPEARANCE/COLOUR (SEE COLOUR CHART) | NORMAL (PINK) | 0 | | |
| | PINK/BLUE ABDOMEN | 1 | | |
| | PINK/PALE EXTREMITIES | 2 | | |
| | BLUE/PALE | 3 | | |
| SURFACE TEMPERATURE | WARM | 0 | | |
| | ? | 1 | | |
| | COLD | 2 | | |
| NATURAL ACTIVITY | WRIGGLING ++ | 0 | | |
| | WRIGGLING + | 1 | | |
| | ± | 2 | | |
| | STILL | 3 | | |
| REFLEXES/RESPONSE TO TOUCH | +++, RIGHTING REFLEX + | 0 | | |
| | ++, RIGHTING REFLEX ± | 1 | | |
| | + | 2 | | |
| | − | 3 | | |
| MILK IN STOMACH | ++ | 0 | | |
| | + | 1 | | |
| | − | 2 | | |
| TOTAL SCORE (NEONATES) | 0–13 | | | |
| PARAMETER (MOTHER*) | ANIMAL ID | SCORE | DATE/TIME | AGE |
| NEST BUILDING | GOOD NEST MAKING | 0 | | |
| | SOME NEST MAKING | 1 | | |
| | NO NEST | 2 | | |
| RETRIEVAL OF YOUNG | ALWAYS | 0 | | |
| | SOMETIMES | 1 | | |
| | NEVER | 2 | | |
| TOTAL SCORE (MOTHER) | 0–6 | | | |

*NB: Include milk score.

<u>JUDGEMENT</u>: Neonate
0–4  Good.
5–8  Fair.
9–12  Poor.
Always assess maternal factors as well. Maternal score 5–6 = Will these animals need fostering?

**Figure 4.8**  Distress and condition scoring for neonatal mice and rats.

late gestation onwards, and the newborn nervous system mounts a clear response to pain, although its responses may not be predictable or organised. Neonates can perceive painful stimuli even if they do not possess the cognitive ability to interpret them. Failure to provide adequate analgesia in the neonate may result in unnecessary distress or have knock-on effects later in life by producing central sensitisation to pain. The small size and lack of development of neonates in many species makes the problem rather complex, since examination is at best difficult and at worst may lead to cannibalism by the mother. Using the same principles as those used for adult animals, a system for assessing the welfare of neonatal rodents from day 0–5 is shown in Figure 4.8.

The selected criteria are:

- colour
- surface temperature
- natural activity
- reflexes/response to touch
- the presence or absence of milk in the stomach.

Since some strains are poor mothers and others are good mothers, the score is related to the natural ability of the mother to look after her young. This is assessed by looking at milk in the stomach as above, nest making and young retrieval. Awarding scores of 0–2 or 0–3 in each category, scores of 0–13 for the neonates and 0–6 for mothering ability are arrived at.

It is essential to take care to wash hands between litters, rubbing them in soiled bedding prior to handling the animals and to handle the neonates as little as possible.

The best way to assess colour is to roll the animal onto its side and look at the lateral chest area. This area stays pink up to day 5 even in pigmented animals. To ensure the colour judgement is unbiased, match the colour to paint colour charts. Normal animals will fall into particular colour ranges depending on their age, and it is possible to compile a chart of normal and abnormal colours for comparison. Animals are then awarded a colour score based on the best match.

For natural activity, observe the litter in the nest. This allows a comparison of activity between animals within a litter, and between litters. Marked differences will be found between strains. For example, factor XIII transgenics were noticeably less active at day 4 than BALB/c nudes.

To assess the righting reflex, turn the animals over. At day 0–1, 'normal' animals will stretch their limbs out and attempt to turn over. By day 3–4, they can turn over immediately. Some transgenic strains may have more difficulty doing this.

In some cases, individuals who score overall between five and nine are found to fall into the colour range for animals 1 or 2 days younger. These animals may improve over the following few days, but the assessment indicates a lack of maturity and a need for careful monitoring.

A method for assessing the welfare of neonatal rodents allows the identification of strains and individuals which are weak or disadvantaged, and thus a reasoned judgement about the effects of any genetic modification. Steps can then be taken to improve their welfare and increase their chances of survival, for example by altered husbandry practices, or they can be humanely killed if their welfare is compromised.

### Welfare assessment of rats post-thyroidectomy

For an example of a post-operative monitoring scheme, see Figure 4.9. For further information on post-operative management, see Chapter 9.

## Other distress assessment records

Some assessment systems do not use a numerical score but set out key clinical signs against time in the score sheet. The sign is then recorded as being present or absent as

| PARAMETER | | SCORE | POST-OPERATIVE TIME (MINUTES) | | | | | | |
|---|---|---|---|---|---|---|---|---|---|
| | | | 0 | 10 | 20 | 30 | 60 | 120 | |
| GENERAL (MOBILITY, REACTIVITY, COAT CONDITION, EYES, EATING AND DRINKING) | ABNORMAL | 3 | | | | | | | |
| | NORMAL | 2 | | | | | | | |
| | | 1 | | | | | | | |
| RECURRENT LARYNGEAL NERVE DAMAGE | RESPIRATORY FAILURE* | 3 | | | | | | | |
| | RESPIRATORY DYSFUNCTION | 2 | | | | | | | |
| | NORMAL RESPIRATION | 1 | | | | | | | |
| HYPOCALCAEMIA | COMPLETE STIFFNESS | 3 | | | | | | | |
| | WEAKNESS AND MILD STIFFNESS | 2 | | | | | | | |
| | NORMAL | 1 | | | | | | | |
| HAEMORRHAGE | HAEMATOMA, WHITE MMS | 3 | | | | | | | |
| | SLIGHT HAEMATOMA | 2 | | | | | | | |
| | NORMAL | 1 | | | | | | | |
| PAIN | SEVERE UNCONTROLLED LOCAL PAIN | 3 | | | | | | | |
| | SOME LOCAL PAIN | 2 | | | | | | | |
| | NO PAIN | 1 | | | | | | | |

INTERVENTIONS:
Any score of 3  Immediate Schedule 1 killing
Any score of 2  Closer monitoring, specific treatment required (e.g. extra oral calcium, give analgesics)
Any score of 1  Normal
*Only likely to occur immediately post-operatively

**Figure 4.9**   Score sheet to evaluate the welfare assessment of rats post-thyroidectomy.

a '+' or '−' sign (or '+/−' if the observer is in doubt). Convention dictates that a negative sign indicates normality, whereas a positive sign indicates a compromised welfare state. By utilising this method, a score sheet can be visually scanned and an appreciation of more plusses or minuses quickly made, which is more time efficient when dealing with large numbers of animals, such as in toxicity testing. However, for some procedures a more detailed quantitative assessment of each clinical sign is more appropriate.

When the level of pain and distress has been scored, records must be kept to ensure the procedure is kept within the severity limit allocated to the procedure and to the severity banding on the project licence. If this severity is exceeded, the Home Office Inspector must be informed. For experiments where the animal's condition is expected to deteriorate, the use of the distress scoring chart is invaluable in fixing the humane end point to a certain limit when the animal must then be humanely destroyed.

European Commission (EC) Directive 86/609 requires in Article 5 that the well-being and state of health of protected animals shall be observed by a competent person to prevent pain or avoidable suffering, distress or lasting harm, and in Article 12 requires particular justification for experiments that may cause severe pain. The UK ASPA requires that procedures are classified as being of mild, moderate or substantial severity and that these limits are not exceeded. However, these are subjective terms open to interpretation. Without a supporting structure and scales of reference, these requirements are of limited operational value, since when left to their own devices some researchers will use purely subjective assessments, which are open to debate, or no method of assessment at all. Pain and distress caused by scientific procedures are predictable and should be easily avoided or relieved, but even if there is unexpected distress, objectively measuring pain and distress in animals is not impossible. The challenge is for us to decipher the state of the animal from the information available. If any doubt exists, then the welfare of the animal must come first, and the responsibility for this lies with the personal licensee.

## FURTHER INFORMATION

Association of Veterinary Teachers and Research Workers (1986). Guidelines for the recognition and assessment of pain in animals. *Veterinary Record* 118, 334–38, and published by UFAW.

Berdoy, M. (2002). *The Laboratory Rat: A Natural History*. www.ratlife.org.

Beynen, A.C., Baumans, V., Bertens, A.P.M.G., Havenaar, R., Hesp, A.P.M. and Van Zutphen, L.F.M. (1987). Assessment of discomfort in gallstone bearing mice: a practical example of the problems encountered in an attempt to recognise discomfort in laboratory animals. *Laboratory Animals* 21, 35–42.

Committee on Regulatory Issues in Animal Care and Use, Institute for Laboratory Animal Research, National Research Council. *Definition of pain and distress and reporting requirements for laboratory animals, Proceedings of the workshop.* 22 June, 2000.

Costa, P. (1996). Neurobehavioural tests in welfare assessment of transgenic animals. Harmonization of Laboratory Animal Husbandry. In *Proceedings of the Sixth FELASA Symposium*, Basel, Switzerland.

Council of the European Communities. (1986). *Directive on the Approximation of Laws, Regulations and Administrative Provisions of the Member States Regarding the Protection of Animals Used for Experimental and Other Scientific Purposes (86/609/EEC).*

Derrell Clark, J., Roger, D.R. and Calpin, J.P. (1997). Animal well being: I General considerations, II Stress and distress, III An overview of assessment, IV Specific assessment criteria. *Laboratory Animal Science* 47, 564–97.

FELASA Working Group on Pain and Distress (1994). Pain and distress in laboratory animals. *Laboratory Animals* 28, 97–112.

Fitzgerald, M. (1994). Neurobiology of fetal and neonatal pain. In *Textbook of Pain* (3rd edn). (eds. P.D. Wall and R. Melzack). Churchill Livingstone, Edinburgh.

Flecknell, P.A. (1994). Refinement of animal use – assessment and alleviation of pain and distress. *Laboratory Animals* 28, 222–31.

Hawkins, P. (2002). Recognizing and assessing pain, suffering and distress in laboratory animals: a survey of current practice in the UK with recommendations. *Laboratory Animals* 36, 378–95.

Lloyd, M.H., Wolfensohn, S.E. and Thornton, P.D. (2000). Quantitative assessment of welfare in experimental animals: the development and use of scoring systems. In *Progress in the Reduction, Refinement and Replacement of Animal Experimentation*. (eds. M. Balls, A.-M. van Zeller and M.E. Halder). Elsevier Science.

Moberg, G.P. (1999). When does stress become distress? *Lab Animal* 28, 22–26.

Morton, D.B. and Griffiths, P.H.M. (1985). Guidelines on the recognition of pain, distress and discomfort in experimental animals and an hypothesis for assessment. *Veterinary Record* 116, 431–36.

National Research Council (1992). *Recognition and Alleviation of Pain and Distress in Laboratory Animals*. A report from the Institute of Laboratory Animal Resources. National Academy Press, Washington.

Orlans, F.B. (1996). Invasiveness scales for animal pain and distress. *Lab Animal* 25(6), 23–25.

Report of the Laboratory Animal Science Association Working Party. (1990). The assessment and control of the severity of scientific procedures on laboratory animals. *Laboratory Animals* 24, 97–130.

Sisask, G., Bjurholm, A., Ahmed, M. and Kreicbergs, A. (1995). Ontogeny of sensory nerves in the developing skeleton. *Anatomical Record* 243(2), 234–40.

UKCCCR (1997). *Guidelines on the Welfare of Animals Used in Experimental Neoplasia*. From PO Box 123, Lincoln Inn Fields, London WC2A 3PX

Van der Meer, M., Baumans, V. and van Zutphen, L.F.M. (1996). Use and welfare aspects of transgenic animals. Harmonization of Laboratory Animal Husbandry. In *Proceedings of the Sixth FELASA Symposium*, Basel, Switzerland.

Wallace, J., Sanford, J., Smith, M.W. and Spencer, K.V. (1990). The assessment and control of the severity of scientific procedures on laboratory animals. *Laboratory Animals* 24, 97–130.

# Chapter 5
# Humane methods of killing

## INTRODUCTION

Experimental animals may need to be killed for a variety of reasons. The Animals (Scientific Procedures) Act 1986 (ASPA) requires that at the end of a series of regulated procedures, the animals used be killed immediately by the person who carried out the procedures, except in particular circumstances. In addition, any animal that is suffering severe pain, which cannot be alleviated, must be humanely killed immediately. Animals may also be killed if their health gives cause for concern, if they have reached the end of their breeding life, if they are unwanted stock or if tissues and blood are required. Killing an animal is always an unpleasant task for the operator, but it does not have to be unpleasant for the animal, provided it is carried out competently, swiftly and humanely.

The 1986 Act states that 'an animal shall be regarded as continuing to live until the permanent cessation of the circulation or the destruction of the brain'; therefore, any method of killing used must ensure that one or both of these criteria is met. The Act imposes restrictions on the methods of killing, which may be employed for experimental animals, or any stock animals of a species listed in Schedule 2, which are surplus to requirements. Schedule 1 to the Act lists standard methods of humane killing (see Table 5.1). Killing an experimental or a stock animal using a method listed in Schedule 1 for that particular type of animal is not a regulated procedure; so neither a project nor personal licence is required to carry this out. However, the person carrying out the killing must be competent to do so without causing distress to the animals involved. If a method of killing is used which is not in Schedule 1 or if one of the listed methods is used for an animal for which it is not deemed appropriate, then it becomes a regulated procedure, and must be authorised on both project and personal licences. For stock animals, where no such licences exist, an additional condition is needed on the certificate of designation in order to authorise a non-schedule 1 method of killing.

The certificate holder is required to make sure that someone is available at all times to perform humane killing, and that they are trained and competent in the methods used. Records must be kept of animals killed by a Schedule 1 method at designated scientific procedure establishments.

The current version of Schedule 1 came into effect in 1997, and a supplementary Code of Practice (CoP), The Humane Killing of Animals under Schedule 1 to the ASPA, replaces the information contained in Chapter 4 of the *Home Office Code of Practice for the Housing and Care of Animals Used in Scientific Procedures* (published in 1989). Schedule 1 lists methods, which are straightforward and can be applied consistently, the aim of which is either to produce instantaneous death or a rapid loss of

**Table 5.1**   Schedule 1 – appropriate methods of humane killing.

1. Subject to Paragraph 2 below, the methods of humane killing listed in Tables A and B below are appropriate for the animals listed in the corresponding entries in those tables only if the process of killing is completed by one of the methods listed in sub-paragraphs (a) to (f) below:

   (a)  Confirmation of permanent cessation of the circulation.
   (b)  Destruction of the brain.
   (c)  Dislocation of the neck.
   (d)  Exsanguination.
   (e)  Confirming the onset of rigor mortis.
   (f)  Instantaneous destruction of the body in a macerator.

2. Paragraph 1 above does not apply in those cases where Table A specifies one of the methods listed in that paragraph as an appropriate method of humane killing.

| A  Methods for animals other than fetal, larval or embryonic forms | Animals for which appropriate |
|---|---|
| 1.  Overdose of anaesthetic using a route and an anaesthetic agent suitable for the size and species of animal | All animals |
| 2.  Exposure to carbon dioxide in a rising concentration | Rodents, rabbits and birds up to 1.5 kg |
| 3.  Dislocation of the neck | Rodents up to 500 g<br>Rabbits up to 1 kg<br>Birds up to 3 kg |
| 4.  Concussion of the brain by striking the cranium | Rodents and rabbits up to 1 kg<br>Birds up to 250 g<br>Amphibians and reptiles up to 1 kg (with destruction of the brain before the return of consciousness)<br>Fishes (with destruction of the brain before the return of consciousness) |
| 5.  One of the recognised methods of slaughter set out below, which is appropriate to the animals and performed by a registered veterinary surgeon, or, in the case of Paragraph (ii) below, performed by the holder of a current licence under the Welfare of Animals (Slaughter or Killing) Regulations 1995<br><br>   (i)  Destruction of the brain by free bullet, or<br>   (ii) Captive bolt, percussion or electrical stunning followed by destruction of the brain or exsanguination before return of consciousness | Ungulates |

*(Continued)*

**Table 5.1**   (*Continued*).

| B Methods for fetal, larval and embryonic forms | Animals for which appropriate |
| --- | --- |
| 1.  Overdose of anaesthetic using a route and anaesthetic agent appropriate for the size, stage of development and species of animal | All animals |
| 2.  Refrigeration, disruption of membranes, maceration in apparatus approved under appropriate slaughter legislation or exposure to carbon dioxide in near 100% concentration until they are dead | Birds Reptiles |
| 3.  Cooling of fetuses followed by immersion in cold tissue fixative | Mice, rats, rabbits |
| 4.  Decapitation | Mammals and birds up to 50 g |

consciousness that persists until death. The CoP is due for revision and Schedule 1 is currently under review.

## PREPARATION FOR HUMANE KILLING

As with any regulated procedure, humane killing requires a certain amount of preparation. Points to be considered are given below.

### *Practice*

Any method of killing can cause distress if badly performed, so staff must be suitably trained and competent in the methods they will be using. Humane killing is included in Module 2 of accredited training courses (see Chapter 1).

### *Handling*

Animals must be handled carefully and competently without causing them distress (see Chapter 6), until unconsciousness has occurred. Staff must be trained and competent to hold animals properly and securely. Some methods of killing may require two or more people to hold the animal, so make sure that there are sufficient people available to do the job properly. Animals will often be calmer, if held by a person with whom they are familiar.

### *Location*

If an animal is frightened but conscious it may exhibit total immobility or it may show behavioural responses, such as vocalisation, struggling, urination, defaecation, anal sac emptying and muscle tremor. Any fear or distress experienced can be communicated by sound or smell to other animals, causing distress. Some of these responses may even be exhibited by unconscious animals before death occurs. It is most important that animals are removed to another room away from the group before they are killed.

*Equipment*

Some methods of killing require equipment, such as anaesthetic induction chambers, carbon dioxide cylinders, bottles of anaesthetic agents, needles and syringes or firearms. It is essential to make sure that any equipment is clean, prepared and ready for use at the start, and that the operator is fully trained and competent to use it.

## SCHEDULE 1 METHODS (TABLE 5.1)

Schedule 1 is in two parts, Part A and Part B as described below. Part A describes methods suitable for animals other than fetal, larval and embryonic forms, and Part B methods for fetal, larval and embryonic forms. Note that killing pregnant animals is usually considered to kill the fetuses, so killing a dam by a Schedule 1 method would not require licence authority. However, the subsequent use of any live fetuses more than halfway through gestation for scientific study would require authority. Newborn animals fall under Part A.

## A  Animals other than fetal, larval and embryonic forms

### *Overdose of anaesthetic*

An overdose of anaesthetic, using a route and agent suitable for the species and size of animal, is considered to be suitable for all animals. With modern anaesthetic agents and combinations used (see Chapter 7) there is generally a fairly wide safety margin, and indeed with some anaesthetics it is actually quite difficult to kill an animal using a reasonable volume or concentration. When carrying out euthanasia it is, therefore, important to select the agent carefully.

For *injection*, the drug of choice for euthanasia is pentobarbitone, which indicates its unsuitability as an agent for safe, reversible anaesthesia. It is usually presented as a 20% solution (200 mg/ml) and is administered at a dose of at least 140 mg/kg. It is preferable to give it intravenously for the most rapid action. If it is not possible to locate a vein in a conscious animal, it may be necessary to sedate it first with an agent administered by an easier route (note that this may constitute a non-schedule 1 method and require licence authority). When the sedative has taken effect and the animal can be handled more easily, the pentobarbitone can be administered intravenously to kill it quickly and humanely. In the smaller species it may be administered intraperitoneally, using a suitably sized needle (see Chapter 9). Pentobarbitone must not be given intramuscularly as it is very irritant to the tissue and this will cause pain, and it is also not recommended for intracardiac administration unless the animal has first been rendered unconscious by some other agent.

For *inhalation*, the animal is exposed to a high concentration of an anaesthetic agent, for example halothane or isoflurane. Ideally, this is used in an induction chamber, with the agent piped in from an anaesthetic machine to ensure the even distribution of vapour. The animal must be physically separated from the liquid agent, since volatile anaesthetics can be highly irritant to mucous membranes. Depending on the agent chosen and the concentration used, unconsciousness usually occurs quite rapidly but death may take rather longer. It is important to ensure that the animal is left in the chamber for long enough, and to confirm that it is dead, since if it is removed too soon and allowed to breathe room air, it may recover. The chamber should be designed so that the animal can be easily observed, and so that it can be easily cleaned between batches of animals to remove all traces of urine and faeces, which contain pheromones by which the animals communicate stress. Placing the animals on disposable paper, which can be replaced each time, is a simple way of controlling this potential stress factor. Chambers of this type should always be used in an extraction cabinet or with a suitable ducting system to keep the volatile agent away from the operator. Inhalation is suitable for small animals, but it can be difficult to restrain larger animals, and diving animals can hold their breath for long periods making induction unacceptably slow. Newborn animals are resistant to hypoxia and can take an unacceptably long time to die.

For immersion, animals (such as fishes, small amphibia and *Octopus vulgaris*) are immersed in an agent, such as tricaine methanesulphonate (MS 222), which is then absorbed percutaneously. As for inhalation, the animal must be left in the solution for an adequate length of time to ensure that death has occurred when it is removed.

## *Exposure to carbon dioxide*

Exposure to a rising concentration of carbon dioxide causes animals to become unconscious due to a direct narcotic effect of the carbon dioxide then, as the concentration increases, they die from hypoxia. Unconsciousness occurs more rapidly in smaller animals, so Schedule 1 restricts the use of carbon dioxide to the killing of rodents, rabbits and birds up to 1.5 kg in weight. The concentration of carbon dioxide used for euthanasia must be *rising*, otherwise the inhalation of high concentrations of carbon dioxide produces an unpleasant fizzing sensation in the nasal passages, and may even cause pain. The animals should be placed in a chamber, which is easy to clean and gives a clear view of the animals inside, containing room air. It is important that the chamber is not overcrowded. The flow of carbon dioxide should then be turned on and gradually increased, displacing the air. After use, the chamber must be inverted to tip out all the residual carbon dioxide since it is heavier than air and will sink to the bottom of the chamber. If this is not done and animals are put into the chamber when the concentration is already high or if the concentration is increased too rapidly, they will exhibit respiratory distress as they fight for breath. Solid dry ice should not be used, and carbon dioxide coming from a gas cylinder may be uncomfortably cold for the animal, so a delivery system that also warms the gas is to be preferred.

There is considerable debate about the suitability of carbon dioxide for humane killing. Numerous studies in pig and poultry have indicated that it is aversive to breathe (see, e.g. Gregory *et al.*, 1987; Leach *et al.*, 2002), and animals killed by this method frequently exhibit epistaxis and damage to the nasal mucosa. If animals huddle together, some animals may be held in pockets of air and avoid the gas, therefore remaining alive or suddenly being exposed to high concentrations. Unintended recovery after apparent death from carbon dioxide has also been reported, so death must be confirmed by exsanguination or dislocation of the neck. If carbon dioxide is to be used effectively and humanely, it must be used properly, and there should be standard operating procedures in place, which must be followed. Neonatal animals and cold-blooded vertebrates are resistant to hypoxia, and diving birds and mammals can hold their breath for long periods, so the use of carbon dioxide is not recommended in these animals. While carbon dioxide can be a quick and simple method for the euthanasia of large numbers of animals, practical considerations should not take precedence over animal welfare, and alternative methods may be more humane. For example, although not currently included under Schedule 1, mixtures of gases containing high proportions of argon and nitrogen have been found to be less aversive than carbon dioxide and very effective at humane killing.

## Physical methods

These methods should cause immediate loss of consciousness through physical trauma to the brain. If carried out properly, they are often more humane than some chemical methods, since death is very quickly achieved. However, they may be distasteful to the person carrying them out, and this leads to a tendency to be rather hesitant. However, human feelings should not be allowed to influence the choice of the most humane techniques, and manual dexterity and an ability to handle the animal confidently are essential to minimise any apprehension. It is essential to make careful observations of the method being carried out by a competent and experienced person, then practise on dead animals, before carrying out these methods on live animals.

### Dislocation of the neck

This method is appropriate for rodents up to 500 g, rabbits up to 1 kg and birds up to 3 kg. If carried out correctly, this causes extensive damage to the brainstem and instantaneous unconsciousness. Dislocation must be carried out quickly and with confidence, otherwise there might not be complete separation of the cervical vertebrae and the animal may experience distress or pain. For small rodents, put the animal on a surface which it can grip, place a pencil or similar object firmly across the back of the neck, take a firm grasp around the hindquarters or the tail and pull sharply. The neck will be dislocated and the animal will die instantly. For larger rodents and lagomorphs, hold the body firmly in one hand, the head in the other and pull sharply with a rotating action. It may be preferable to sedate these animals prior to cervical dislocation. For larger birds, hold the legs or body in one hand, and pull the neck sharply down and backwards with the other. It may be necessary to wrap the bird to prevent involuntary flapping, and to confirm death by severing the major vessels in the neck.

### Concussion

Striking the back of the head renders the animal unconscious, following which death must be ensured by dislocation of the neck or by exsanguination. As with dislocation of the neck, confidence in handling the animal and manual dexterity are required to carry out this method without causing distress to the animal. Support the animal by the hindquarters and swing the body downwards such that the back of the head comes sharply into contact with a hard surface, such as a workbench. Considerable training and practise on dead animals is required to ensure competence with this method, and it is difficult to ensure that animals are stunned consistently. Concussion may be used for rodents and rabbits up to 1 kg, birds up to 250 g, amphibians and reptiles up to 1 kg and fishes. For amphibia, reptiles and fishes, the brain must be destroyed immediately following concussion, as in these species the brain is very tolerant to hypoxia, and it cannot otherwise be guaranteed that concussion is irreversible or that unconsciousness will last until death.

### Recognised methods of slaughter

Ungulates may be killed under Schedule 1 by one of the standard methods of slaughter, such as use of a free bullet, a captive bolt or electrical stunning followed by destruction of the brain or exsanguination. However, these methods are controlled by other pieces of legislation and are, therefore, only available to veterinary surgeons or licensed slaughtermen, who have been appropriately trained and issued with the relevant licences.

## B Fetal, larval and embryonic forms

The ASPA covers immature forms from particular stages of development. For mammals, birds and reptiles, this is the halfway point of gestation or incubation, and for amphibia, fish and *Octopus vulgaris*, the point at which they become capable of independent feeding. Schedule 1 describes methods of humane killing that can be used for these forms, which take into account the degree of development of the nervous system in the various animals. Some species are highly developed at birth and, therefore, require special consideration during the last few days of gestation or incubation, whereas others are less well developed and are less able to perceive pain at this stage.

### Overdose of anaesthetic

This may be used for all animals. An anaesthetic agent appropriate for the size and stage of development of the animal should be chosen. In large fetuses or embryos, anaesthetics may be given by the intravenous or intraperitoneal routes; smaller animals and larvae may be immersed in anaesthetics.

### Refrigeration, disruption of membranes, maceration or exposure to 100% carbon dioxide

These methods can be used for birds and reptiles. In birds, cooling to below 4°C is effective, but reptile embryos are resistant to hypothermia and hypoxia, so death must be ensured by overdose of anaesthetic, maceration or immersion in tissue fixative.

## *Cooling followed by immersion in fixative*

Mouse, rat and rabbit fetuses may be chilled until movement has stopped, then immersed in cold (4°C) tissue fixative.

## *Decapitation*

This is a humane and quick method, which can be used for mammals and birds up to 50 g weight which are not well developed, using a strong pair of sharp scissors.

# OTHER METHODS

Other methods of killing may be employed, if there is a scientific need. These will require authority on both personal and project licences.

## Microwaves

These can be used to fix brain metabolites without losing anatomical integrity. Specialist apparatus is required, and careful technique. The microwaves are focused on particular areas of the brain, producing death very rapidly.

## Electrical stunning

This is used in ungulates under Schedule 1, but may also be used for other species, such as poultry or rabbits. It requires specialist equipment, and death must be confirmed using another method.

## Pithing

This may be carried out in unconscious fish, amphibia or reptiles. A sharp needle is inserted through the foramen magnum and agitated to destroy the brain. This requires technical skill in order to ensure rapid death, and must *not* be carried out in conscious animals.

## Rapid freezing

Liquid nitrogen is used in situ or following decapitation to freeze the brain. The animal must be rendered insensible first, as it can take up to 90 s to freeze deep structures.

## Decapitation

This may not be humane in conscious animals, because of the length of time it takes for the decapitated head to lose consciousness, particularly in cold-blooded vertebrates. If this method is required for scientific reasons, there must be particular justification, and consideration given to sedating or anaesthetising the animal first. Decapitation for animals other than fetal, larval and embryonic forms is not included in Schedule 1.

## CONFIRMATION OF DEATH AND DISPOSAL OF CARCASES

After carrying out any method of killing it is vital to check that the animal is dead before disposing of the body. Thus, the process of killing must be completed by one of the following six methods:

1. Confirmation of permanent cessation of the circulation, for example, by severing the major vessels.
2. Destruction of the brain with a permanent loss of brain function.
3. Dislocation of the neck.
4. Exsanguination.
5. Onset of rigor mortis.
6. Mechanical disruption by instantaneous destruction of the body in a macerator.

Carcases from research institutes are generally classed as clinical waste and as such must be disposed of correctly either by maceration or in yellow clinical waste bags that go for incineration. There will be local rules in the work area relating to the method of disposal and these must be followed.

## CHOICE OF METHODS

When choosing a method of humane killing, consider the following points:

1. Death must occur without producing pain.
2. The time required to produce loss of consciousness must be as short as possible.
3. The time required to produce death must be as short as possible.
4. The method must be reliable and non-reversible.
5. There must be minimal psychological stress on the animal.
6. There must be minimal psychological stress to the operators and any observers.
7. It must be safe for personnel carrying out the procedure.
8. It must be compatible with the requirements of the experiment.
9. It must be compatible with any requirement to carry out histology on the tissues.
10. Any drugs used should be readily available and have minimum abuse potential.
11. The method should be economically acceptable.
12. The method should be simple to carry out with little room for error.

Table 5.2 lists recommended methods of euthanasia for different species.

Euthanasia is not necessarily the most difficult part of the procedure for the animal, indeed if carried out competently it can be easier for the animal than any parts of the procedure that may have caused pain, suffering or distress. However, euthanasia is frequently the most difficult part for the researcher, particularly if the animal has been used on a long-term project and is one of the higher species. By becoming a personal licence holder, you must accept that you are responsible for taking that animal's life, and feeling compassion is a necessary part of that responsibility. Whichever method of humane killing is chosen, it is very important to be confident and competent to carry it out swiftly and humanely. However, if there is any hesitancy, animals may experience unnecessary distress. No one should be expected to carry out a method of humane killing with which they are uncomfortable. So, if in doubt, do not do it.

**Table 5.2**  Recommended methods of euthanasia for experimental animals.

| | Overdose of anaesthetic | | | Carbon dioxide | Cervical dislocation | Concussion | Slaughter (free bullet, captive bolt, electrical stunning) | Decapitation | Pithing | Cooling and immersion in fixative | Refrigeration, disruption of membranes, maceration |
|---|---|---|---|---|---|---|---|---|---|---|---|
| | By injection | By inhalation | By immersion | | | | | | | | |
| Rodents | **** | **** | | *** | *** | *** | | * ! | | | |
| Rabbits | **** | * | | ** | *** | ** | ** ! Electrical stunning | * ! | | | |
| Carnivores | **** | *** | | | * ![a] | * ! | ** ! Captive bolt | | | | |
| Primates | **** | | | | | | | | | | |
| Large animals | **** | * Young animals | | | | * ! | **** | | | | |
| Birds | **** | *** | | *** | *** | ** | * !Electrical stunning | * ![a] | * ![a] | | |
| Reptiles | **** | | | | *** | *** | **** ! Captive bolt | * ![a] | * ![a] | | |
| Amphibia | *** | | **** | | *** | *** | | * ![a] | * ![a] | | |
| Fish | ** | * | **** | | ** ! | *** | | * ![a] | * ![a] | | |
| Fetal larval and embryonic forms | **** | | | **Birds and reptiles | | | | *** Mammals and birds up to 50 g | | *** Mice, rats, and rabbits | ***Birds and reptiles |

**** Recommended; *** generally acceptable; ** sometimes acceptable; * use if other methods not possible; ! Non-schedule 1 methods (these require personal and project licence authority); [a] only use on unconscious animals.

# FURTHER INFORMATION

Gregory, N.G., Moss, B.W. and Leeson, R.H. (1987). An assessment of carbon dioxide stunning in pigs. *Veterinary Record* 121, 517–18.

Home Office Code of Practice (1997). *The Humane Killing of Animals under Schedule 1 to the Animals (Scientific Procedures) Act 1986*. HMSO. ISBN 0-10-265397-6.

Ikarashi, Y., Maruyama, Y. and Stavinoha, W.B. (1984). Study of the use of the microwave magnetic field inactivation for the rapid inactivation of brain enzymes. *Japanese Journal of Pharmacology* 35, 371–87.

Leach, M.C., Bowell, V.A., Allan, T.F. and Morton, D.B. (2002). Aversion to gaseous euthanasia agents in rats and mice. *Comparative Medicine* 52(3), 249–57.

Recommendations for euthanasia of experimental animals. *Report of a Working Party in Laboratory Animals* (1996) 30, 293–316 and (1997) 31, 1–32.

Shalev, M. (2002). OLAW clarifies PHS policy regarding use of carbon dioxide for euthanasia of small laboratory animals. *Lab Animal Europe* 2(8), 13–14.

Stavinoha, W.B., Frazer, J.W. and Modak, A.T. (1978). Microwave fixation for the study of acetylcholine metabolism. In *Cholinergic Mechanisms and Psychopharmacology*. (ed. Jenden, D.J.). Plenum Publishing Corp, New York; pp. 169–79.

# Chapter 6
# Introduction to laboratory animal husbandry

## SELECTION OF ANIMALS

Research animals may come from a wide variety of sources. They may come from within the same facility that the experiments are being carried out, from another animal facility within the same Certificate of Designation (e.g. another animal unit of the same university), from colleagues or collaborators at another research institute working in the same field, from a commercial supplier or from the wild. Species listed in Schedule 2 to the Animals (Scientific Procedures) Act 1986 (ASPA) (which covers most of the commonly used species) must come from an establishment designated under the Act, unless an exemption has been granted.

First one needs to decide which species of animal to use. A number of procedures can be done effectively *in vitro* on cells in culture, on insects (such as *Drosophila*) or on species such as zebra fish. About 85% of procedures are carried out on rodents, but even after deciding on the species, and this is the only detail required on the project licence, there are other decisions to be made, such as which stock or strain.

Rodents can be supplied as an *outbred stock*, which are colonies of genetically undefined animals usually maintained as closed colonies. The term 'genetically undefined' means that the genotype of an animal at any given locus is usually unknown. Such animals usually have good fertility, with a good growth curve, a large litter size and so are easy to produce. They are, therefore, cheaper and more readily available than inbred strains. (Outbred animals are known as 'stocks', whereas inbred ones are known as 'strains'.)

An *inbred strain* is produced by 20 or more consecutive generations of brother × sister mating, producing animals that are 99% homozygous. Examples of inbred strains of mice and rats are shown in Table 6.1. Due to inbreeding depression there is a reduction in reproductive performance, survival and general fitness characteristics. These include lower weight (Table 6.2), lower litter size (Table 6.3), a higher pre-weaning mortality and a tendency to be more aggressive. Production, therefore, requires much more by way of planned colony management than for outbred stocks. The effects of inbreeding depression are most noticeable in the first few generations of brother × sister mating. Once an inbred strain is established, no further inbreeding depression occurs. An *F1 hybrid* is produced by mating two inbred strains.

A *mutant* is an outbred stock carrying a mutant gene, such as nude or obese. The maintenance of mutant stocks depends on whether the mutant is 'dominant' or 'recessive' and whether homozygous mutant animals of one or both sexes are viable and fertile. Breeding systems are more complex to produce mutants because of harmful

**Table 6.1**  Examples of inbred strains of rodents.

| Inbred mice | Inbred rats |
| --- | --- |
| BALB/c | BN/Ss |
| CBA/Ca | DA |
| C3H/He | F344 |
| C57BL/6J | LEW |
| DBA/2 | PVG |

**Table 6.2**  Table showing variation between strains for weight of female mice at different ages.

| Age (days) | DBA/2 | BALB/c | MF1 |
| --- | --- | --- | --- |
| 21 | 8.3 g | 10.0 g | 14.0 g |
| 28 | 12.0 g | 13.3 g | 18.8 g |
| 35 | 13.8 g | 16.0 g | 22.0 g |

**Table 6.3**  Mean litter size born of inbred strains* of mice compared to outbred stocks†.

| Strain | Litter size born |
| --- | --- |
| A/J* | 5.37 |
| BALB/c* | 6.09 |
| CBA/Ca* | 5.73 |
| C3H/He* | 6.01 |
| C57BL/6* | 7.60 |
| C57BL/10* | 6.39 |
| DBA/1* | 4.11 |
| DBA/2* | 4.53 |
| NZB* | 6.15 |
| NZW* | 4.82 |
| SJL* | 6.33 |
| 129* | 5.22 |
| MF1† | 11.33 |
| TO† | 9.64 |

recessive genes, which may increase perinatal death and thus reduce productivity; therefore, mutants are considerably more expensive to buy. Additionally, special housing requirements may be necessary to protect susceptible mutants from infection.

A *transgenic strain* results from foreign DNA being introduced into early-stage embryos in such a way that it becomes incorporated permanently into the host DNA. The first transgenic animals were developed in the early 1980s. *Knockout animals* are transgenic animals that have been produced by inactivating an existing gene. (See Chapter 13 for more details on Genetically modified animals.)

The nomenclature system of names and terminology is extremely important. Nomenclature for mice was introduced in 1952. Before that a single strain could be known under several different names and as strains were passed between investigators, confusion occurred. Definition of the genetic background of the animals is important to ensure the reproducibility of data and should be included in the methodology for the experiment.

## HEALTH MONITORING

As in any field of science, the merit of animal experiments depends on the rigid adherence to principles of scientific method. By following these principles, data produced will be both reliable and reproducible. However, living organisms are complex and can be subject to wide variations in biological response to apparently insignificant influences.

Disease prevention should be a prerequisite of any animal experiment for three reasons:

1. *For animal welfare:* Infectious agents have the ability to cause ill health and possibly death thus compromising the welfare of the animals. Even sub-clinical infection can introduce greater variation between individuals thereby increasing the numbers of animals required to produce statistically significant results.
2. *For scientific quality:* Overt or sub-clinical infection is likely to affect experimental results, so reducing reliability and reproducibility of the research.
3. *For safety:* To safeguard health of laboratory and research staff as some animal pathogens are transmissible to humans.

It is, therefore, customary to monitor the health of animals used in laboratories. The researcher should be aware of the pathogen status of the animals used, not just initially, but throughout the course of study. The animals may not show clinical signs when they arrive, but may harbour pathogens that are capable of severely compromising the health of the animal when it is subjected to experimental stress. Alternatively, the infection may never cause clinical disease but may induce microscopic or biochemical changes that have profound effects on research data and increase biological variability. If it is recognised that an animal is unwell but that the changes are unrelated to the procedure, it will be necessary to consult the named veterinary surgeon (NVS) in order to investigate the causes of the disease and obtain advice on treatment.

## Effect of disease on research

While some infectious agents are pathogenic and will induce clinical signs of disease in laboratory animals with morbidity and/or mortality, many micro-organisms induce only mild disease or no illness at all, particularly in cases of endemic disease. However, these cases are still important since the experimental procedures, which cause stress and immunosuppression, or environmental factors, such as transportation or changes in diet, may convert sub-clinical infection into clinical problems. Also different strains of mice may show varying sensitivity to an infectious agent with some strains having asymptomatic infection while others may show moderate to severe clinical signs. In general, the symptoms will be more serious in immunodeficient animals. The infectious agents do not only impact on the whole animal. Many will also affect experiments conducted on isolated organs or cells. They can persist in cells, tumour lines and other biological materials for prolonged periods of time and, thus, affect *in vitro* experiments or can be reintroduced back into whole animals with the passage of such contaminated material in animals. Thus, the detection and elimination of such agents affect each one of the three Rs, namely, replacement, reduction and refinement; eradication of infection will improve the quality of *in vitro* work, reduce the number of animals that have to be used and improve the welfare, if animals used are in good health.

As most infections are sub-clinical and modifications of research results due to natural infections often occur in the absence of clinical disease, the lack of a clinical indication of the infection has only limited diagnostic value. It is prevention of infection, not just clinical disease, which is important. The presence of unwanted micro-organisms and the suitability of a group of animals for a specific experiment can only be demonstrated by a comprehensive health monitoring programme. The data generated by this programme constitutes part of the experimental data and should be available for consideration in the interpretation of the test results. Thus, the health monitoring information should be included in the publication of experimental results. There should be microbiological standardisation of laboratory animals in order to produce better and more reliable results of experiments with fewer animals. For details of the effects of rodent infections on experimental data, see the report of the working party on hygiene of the GV-SOLAS (German Laboratory Animal Science Association) on implications of infectious agents on results of animal experiments, also available via www.lal.org.uk.

## Sources of disease

The most important source of infection is other laboratory animals, often due to population density and the turnover of animals within a unit. Animals entering a unit should be of known health status and come from accredited breeders. Accompanying such animals should be a report on their microbiological status and housing. There are various terms used to describe the microbiological status of laboratory animals, which in turn indicates the type of housing in which they are maintained. *Germ-free* (axenic) animals are free of any associated life and are maintained in isolators with no contact with the outside world. *Gnotobiotic* animals have one or more associated non-pathogenic micro-organisms, the identity of which is known. These animals are also maintained in isolators with no contact with the outside world. *Specific pathogen-free* (SPF) animals are free from *specified* pathogens. The SPF designation requires that the absence of the listed pathogens is supported by regular monitoring for those pathogens. These animals are maintained in barrier units that use a combination of construction, equipment (e.g. individually ventilated cages), operating procedures (including showering facilities, the provision of sterilised food, water and bedding) and restricted access to the unit to minimise any potential contact with those specified pathogens. *Conventional* animals carry normal microbial flora that is undefined. Their housing has less strict access and operating conditions. However, they are still monitored for the main animal pathogens. *Wild-caught* animals have an unknown microbial flora and are likely to carry pathogens that may cause disease to both staff and other animals.

To ensure research animals remain free from disease it is necessary to consider the potential sources of infection, of which there are many. Other animals brought into the unit should be considered first, particularly in large facilities with multiple users. A well-run facility will have a standard operating procedure (SOP) that should be followed for all incoming animals in order to protect the health of those already in the unit. Examine the health profile from the supplier and ask what tests were carried out, who did them and how the interpretation was arrived at. It is surprising how often two batches of serum from the same animals, sent to two different laboratories will come back with two different answers on the disease profile. Environmental sources of contamination include water, food and bedding; all of which may, therefore, require sterilisation before being given to the animals. Find out if the water supply for the animals is purified, and if so, how this is carried out, and what methods are used for checking it has been done effectively. Find out how the food that is going to be given to your animals is being stored, and check that there is adequate protection from contamination by wild rodents or birds, which may introduce disease (e.g. *Salmonella*). Ensure that the method of storage prevents depletion of vitamin levels or the development of moulds or toxins. Look at the quality of the bedding and ask how the microbiological quality is assured. Ensure that the ventilation rates comply with the Home Office Code of Practice (CoP) and are adequate to remove any build-up of ammonia from within the room, which will predispose to respiratory disease. Find out how often the air filters are changed and ensure this is done frequently enough. Check that all your equipment is clean and will not spread disease to your animal. Examples of potential sources of contamination include such items as anaesthetic face masks, clippers, gloves/dirty hands, white coats and gavage cannulae. Cell lines and serum may be contaminated and should be screened before bringing them into units for use in animals. During transportation, animals should be protected from infection where possible by transporting them in filter-protected cages. Good hygiene procedures should be followed at all times in the animal unit.

Rodents, and many other species, are generally supplied with a health profile from the breeder. If the animals are to be kept only short term it may not be necessary to do any more, but if they are kept long term, continual regular screening will be necessary to ensure they have not picked up extra infections. If the animal is kept under conditions to prevent entry of disease it is important to maintain these barriers and not to bring micro-organisms into the unit.

Some animals may have predisposing factors, such as a genetic variant, which contribute to the development of disease. For example BALB/c mice are more susceptible to lethal ectromelia infection than the C57BL/6 strain. Genetic monitoring of inbred colonies is vital to ensure that this predisposition remains a constant factor within the experimental model. The susceptibility of transgenic strains may be difficult to predict due to changes in the immune system (see Chapter 13, page 277 for further information). Nutritional status of the animal will also be a factor in sus-ceptibility to disease and must be considered carefully. However, the single most important predisposing factor in the laboratory animal is *stress*, which leads to immunosuppression and the subsequent development of disease. It is, therefore, very important to do everything possible to reduce the stress caused to your animals.

## Health monitoring methods

Health monitoring of laboratory animals is a fundamental part of disease prevention used to determine their pathogen status and general health. Animals received from a commercial breeder will normally be accompanied by a health monitoring report that should be examined. Such reports state whether pathogenic bacteria or fungi have been isolated and to which viruses, if any, antibodies have been detected. Always note the date of such reports, as they will only reflect the health status of a population at the time of testing.

The health of your animals can be monitored passively or actively. Passive moni-toring is studying information that is readily available from the population, without actually killing animals simply for the purpose of health screening. All animals that die unexpectedly, all animals that produce unusual experimental results and a pro-portion of all animals used terminally should be examined routinely. The scope of this examination will depend on the facilities readily available at the institute, but the minimum will be a gross post-mortem. It may be possible, and is certainly desirable, to add to this routine bacteriology, parasitology, serology, and histology. A routine faecal screen from the live animal can also be useful in detecting various sub-clinical infections.

In active health monitoring, animals are taken from the population at regular inter-vals. Blood is taken for serological testing for a number of viral infections and some bacterial infections and they undergo full post-mortem examination to detect any other infections. *Sentinel* animals can also be used to monitor the population. These are animals of the same species whose bacterial, parasitic and virological burden is already defined. This is extremely important, for example, you may need to specif-ically request *Helicobacter*-free animals for health screening when ordering them from the suppliers. They are housed in cages on the lower shelves of the racks of the experi-mental population, and exposed to their dirty bedding. They will then be exposed to the same pathogens and they can be sampled to determine their pathogen status, which will reflect the status of the original experimental population. Immunodeficient animals (e.g. nude mice) do not produce sufficient amounts of antibodies to give reli-able test results and are, therefore, not suitable for serological testing, although they may be used for bacteriological and parasitological investigations. Sentinel animals should be at least 10 weeks old and should have been housed in the unit for at least 4 weeks.

### *Sampling strategies*

The determination of the number of animals to be screened for infection is very important and depends on the assumed rate of infection and the randomness in the sampling. There is a natural inclination to keep the sample size small on grounds of economy and availability, but it must be sufficiently large to give the required level of confidence in the results. Table 6.4 (from ILAR 1976) shows that if 10 animals are randomly selected and the infection rate of the agent in question is 40%, then there is a 99% probability that at least one infected animal will be found in that sample size. For single agents it is, therefore, possible to determine the necessary sample size reasonably accurately, but for health screening for multiple agents, which may have very different infection rates, it is impossible to maintain the same degree of precision. Routine sampling is usually based on assumed infection rates of around 40–50% in order to keep sample sizes reasonable but the limitations of this need to be recognised.

Since the population must be sampled randomly, this involves taking animals from different cages, racks and shelves, of different sexes and different ages. It is advisable to use two age groups since younger animals will have a higher parasite load. Young adults will be best for detecting recent viral infections and retired breeders give an indication of the history of the colony. The Federation of European Laboratory Animal Science Associations (FELASA) guidelines give advice on the frequency of testing, which can vary between monthly and annually depending on circumstances.

**Table 6.4**   Probability of detecting infection in a sample of animals.

| Sample size ($N$) | Assumed infection rate (%) | | | | | | | | | | | |
|---|---|---|---|---|---|---|---|---|---|---|---|---|
| | 1 | 2 | 3 | 4 | 5 | 10 | 15 | 20 | 25 | 30 | 40 | 50 |
| 5 | 0.05 | 0.10 | 0.14 | 0.18 | 0.23 | 0.41 | 0.56 | 0.67 | 0.76 | 0.83 | 0.92 | 0.97 |
| 10 | 0.10 | 0.18 | 0.26 | 0.34 | 0.40 | 0.65 | 0.80 | 0.89 | 0.94 | 0.97 | 0.99 | |
| 15 | 0.14 | 0.26 | 0.37 | 0.46 | 0.54 | 0.79 | 0.91 | 0.95 | 0.99 | | | |
| 20 | 0.18 | 0.33 | 0.46 | 0.56 | 0.64 | 0.88 | 0.95 | 0.99 | | | | |
| 25 | 0.22 | 0.40 | 0.53 | 0.64 | 0.72 | 0.93 | 0.98 | | | | | |
| 30 | 0.25 | 0.45 | 0.60 | 0.71 | 0.79 | 0.96 | 0.99 | | | | | |
| 35 | 0.30 | 0.51 | 0.66 | 0.76 | 0.83 | 0.97 | | | | | | |
| 40 | 0.33 | 0.55 | 0.70 | 0.80 | 0.87 | 0.99 | | | | | | |
| 45 | 0.36 | 0.69 | 0.75 | 0.84 | 0.90 | 0.99 | | | | | | |
| 50 | 0.39 | 0.64 | 0.78 | 0.87 | 0.92 | 0.99 | | | | | | |
| 60 | 0.45 | 0.70 | 0.84 | 0.91 | 0.95 | | | | | | | |
| 70 | 0.51 | 0.76 | 0.88 | 0.94 | 0.97 | | | | | | | |
| 80 | 0.55 | 0.80 | 0.91 | 0.96 | 0.98 | | | | | | | |
| 90 | 0.60 | 0.84 | 0.94 | 0.97 | 0.99 | | | | | | | |
| 100 | 0.63 | 0.87 | 0.95 | 0.98 | 0.99 | | | | | | | |
| 120 | 0.70 | 0.91 | 0.97 | 0.99 | | | | | | | | |
| 140 | 0.76 | 0.94 | 0.99 | | | | | | | | | |
| 160 | 0.80 | 0.96 | 0.99 | | | | | | | | | |
| 180 | 0.84 | 0.97 | | | | | | | | | | |
| 200 | 0.87 | 0.98 | | | | | | | | | | |

$$N = \frac{\log(1 - \text{probability of detection of infection})}{\log(1 - \text{assumed infection rate \%})}.$$

## *Technique for routine post-mortem examination*

If a post-mortem examination is to be of any value then it must be conducted thoroughly. While it may not be feasible to dissect the carcase minutely, it is desirable to examine the whole cadaver and remove and inspect each organ. It may then be necessary to submit portions of diseased tissues to a laboratory for further investigation. The basic procedure is the same for all species with minor variations depending on the size of the animal involved.

### *Procedure*

1. Weigh the animal and examine the external appearance of the carcase. Make a note of the body condition, and examine all external orifices for any abnormalities or discharges. Examine the feet, tail and skin for any lesions and note any evidence of vomiting, diarrhoea or dehydration. If samples of skin are required for parasitological investigation, take them at this stage.
2. Lay the animal out on its back, pin the feet if necessary, or incise the axillae and over the femoral heads so the limbs can be forced downwards to support the carcase. Swab the ventral surface liberally with disinfectant to reduce bacterial contamination and prevent pollution of the area with dander and fur.
3. Make a midline skin incision from mandible to pubis and reflect the skin away from the midline. Remove the muscles over the thorax and open the chest cavity by holding the xiphisternum and cutting through the costochondral junctions on each side. Reflect the sternum and ribs anteriorly to expose the underlying viscera. Observe any abnormalities such as fluid in the pleural cavity or pericardium. Open the trachea and note any inflammation or fluid inside.
4. Open the abdominal wall with a straight midline incision and reflect the wall sideways. Again, note any obvious changes such as liver abscessation or fluid in the peritoneal cavity.
5. Grasp the trachea and oesophagus, cut across and lift upwards to remove the heart and lungs, easing away any dorsal connections. Cut across the oesophagus as it passes through the diaphragm and remove the thoracic viscera for a more thorough examination on a separate tray. Look for areas of discolouration, altered texture, adhesions or other abnormalities. Open the length of the trachea, oesophagus, and bronchi. Cut through the lung lobes and squeeze gently to see if there is any fluid present in the lung parenchyma. Open the heart by incising from the apex of the left ventricle up into the left atrium and into the aorta, and from the apex of the right ventricle up into the right atrium and into the pulmonary artery. This method ensures that the heart valves and endocardium can be examined undamaged by the dissection.
6. Examine the intestinal tract carefully noting such facts as whether the stomach is full or empty, whether the gut is full of gas, fluid or solid matter or any areas of inflammation. Remove the intestinal tract and place on a separate tray for more detailed examination later. Examine the mesenteric lymph nodes and the inside surface of the stomach and the length of the intestinal tract.
7. Cut around the dorsal surface of the liver to remove it and cut through the lobes. Examine the cut surface for variations in the normal architecture.

8. Examine the uro-genital tract. Incise the kidneys longitudinally and inspect the internal structure. Peel off the capsule.
9. The eviscerated carcase should then be examined for any other abnormalities such as enlarged joints or lymph nodes. If the history indicates it, the head can be removed to take out the brain for detailed inspection.
10. Ensure the carcase and viscera are correctly disposed of and the area thoroughly cleaned and disinfected.

## Which diseases to monitor

It is not practical or cost effective to test for all known infectious agents so testing, of necessity, has to be selective. The threat of disease either clinical or sub-clinical should be perceived as serious by all those involved in order for screening to be carried out effectively and for barriers to be maintained. The choice of agents to test for is based on pathogen significance and likelihood of interference with research and includes:

- Any zoonotic diseases should be the first priority in screening. This will enable any necessary precautions to be taken to prevent spread of disease to humans.
- The second group of diseases to look for will be those that might be present as sub-clinical infections but which will cause overt clinical disease when the animal is subjected to an experimental stress.
- The third group to consider are those diseases whose presence, whether clinically evident or only sub-clinical, will interfere with, and may invalidate the experiment. For example, this may be the presence of a viral infection that has no effect on the animal but elevates certain enzyme levels, the measurement of which may form part of the experimental study.

A discussion with your NVS will aid in designing a sensible screening programme which will be cost effective. The cost of health monitoring in experimental units may seem high, but as a proportion of the total cost of the experiments it is a justifiable and indeed an essential means of enhancing the reliability of the experiments. Before embarking on a screening programme it is important to be prepared for the possibility of positive results, and to consider what action will need to be taken if the result shows the presence of certain infections. Health screening of the animals should not be a theoretical exercise and action should be taken if positive results are found; otherwise it is a waste of time, money and animals not just in terms of health screening, but possibly for the whole experiment. The epidemiology of the disease must be understood in order to know how frequently to test, what samples to take and how to deal with a positive result if it should be found. The programme will need to be re-evaluated once the status of the colony is known, as subsequent tests may need to be done less frequently, or only certain groups of the population tested, after the initial screen. Screening can be a very costly and laborious task but this should not be used as an excuse to ignore the possibility that infections exist which may be of concern to personnel, detrimental to the animals' welfare and to the validity of the science being carried out. Monitoring laboratories should follow the principles of Good Laboratory Practice (GLP) and the FELASA guidance for the accreditation of laboratory animal diagnostic laboratories. The recommendations of FELASA for health monitoring in each species should be followed. The purpose of health monitoring is to supply the researcher with data on variables that might influence the outcome of an experiment. Therefore, these data are part of the experimental work and must be considered during the interpretation of the experimental results. The results of health monitoring should, therefore, be included in scientific publications.

## SUPPLY OF LABORATORY ANIMALS

### General considerations

One aim of the ASPA is to guarantee the quality of laboratory animals and to provide safeguards, ensuring that, whenever possible, the animals used have been specifically bred for the purpose. Schedule 2 lists those animal species that may only be obtained from an establishment that has been designated under the Act for breeding or supplying. A Certificate of Designation will only be issued for such premises if they meet the required standards of husbandry and animal care as laid down in the Home Office CoP for the Housing and Care of Animals in Designated Breeding and Supplying Establishments. This CoP also requires that regular health-monitoring programmes be implemented in breeding establishments, to ensure that laboratory animals remain disease free. Many commercial breeders now exist, which can deliver high-quality, high-health laboratory animals. Details of these suppliers in the UK and the rest of Europe may be found in the *Laboratory Animals Buyers Guide*, published by Laboratory Animals.

### Importation of Schedule 2 animals

The introduction of Schedule 2 animals from non-designated premises requires prior permission from the Secretary of State at the Home Office, so this applies to all such animals imported from abroad. The importation of animals from overseas is also controlled by the Rabies (Importation of Dogs, Cats and Other Mammals) Order 1974 of the Animal Health Act 1981, and an import licence must be obtained in advance from the Department of the Environment, Food and Rural Affairs (DEFRA). Rabies susceptible animals are required to enter 6 months of quarantine on arrival, unless imported under the Balai Directive (see below). Quarantine premises are inspected and authorised by a DEFRA official, and the overall responsibility for the maintenance of animals in quarantine falls to the appointed veterinary supervisor. Accurate records must be kept of introductions, births and deaths during the quarantine period, and the veterinary supervisor should be informed of any morbidity or mortality in the animals while in quarantine.

The importation of animals from certain registered establishments in other member states of the European Union (EU) may fall under European Commission (EC) Directive 92/65/EEC (the Balai Directive). Animals that can be shown to have been born in the holding of origin and which are free from rabies may be imported under this Directive without the need to enter quarantine. Details may be obtained from DEFRA. Importation of embryos, ova and semen may be carried out under the

Importation of Embryos, Ova and Semen Order 1980 in accordance with the current DEFRA guidelines.

## TRANSPORT OF LABORATORY ANIMALS

### Legislation and transport regulations

The transport of animals within the UK and the European Union is regulated by the Welfare of Animals (Transport) Order 1997 (WATO 97), and EC Council Directive 91/628/EEC on the Protection of Animals During Transport. You are advised to read the WATO 97 and the *Guidelines for the Care of Laboratory Animals in Transit, Laboratory Animals* (1993), 27, 93–107. New guidelines from LASA are in preparation.

The importation or export of laboratory animals must comply with the relevant international legislation and transport regulations. For animals travelling by air, the IATA Live Animals Regulations define the responsibilities of shippers and carriers and container requirements, and are updated annually. The needs for individual species are listed, including those covered by the Convention on International Trade in Endangered Species (CITES). These regulations have been adopted as standard by many countries including the UK. For importation of rabies susceptible animals, the rabies control legislation applies (see above).

Exportation of animals will require authority to discharge them from the controls of ASPA if they are under project licence (see Chapter 11, page 226) This especially applies to transgenic animals (see Chapter 13).

### General considerations

WATO 97 requires that all animals shall be accompanied by an Animal Transport Certificate stating:

- the name and address of the transporter
- the name and address of the owner of the animals
- the place that the animals were loaded, and their final destination
- the date and time the first animal was loaded
- the date and time of departure.

Arrangements for the transport of animals should ensure that their well-being is not jeopardised, and that they arrive at their destination in good health. Attention should be paid to the following points:

1. *Health and welfare prior to shipment.* Sub-clinical infections could become clinical during transport, so they should be examined by a competent person before despatch.
2. *Design of containers.* These should provide comfort and minimise stress to the animals. They must be leak-proof and escape-proof, and be such that the animals cannot damage themselves during transport. They should prevent contamination with microbes, and be able to be disinfected.
3. *Environmental conditions.* There must be adequate ventilation within the container. Vents should be placed on opposite sides of the containers and in such a

position that they cannot be occluded. The temperature should be within the thermo-neutral zone for the animal.

4. *Bedding.* Bedding should provide comfort and absorb moisture, insulating the animal against temperature changes and vibrations.

5. *Food and water.* Animals should generally have free access to food and water until immediately prior to despatch, except dogs and cats, which may be starved for 4 h. Rodents and rabbits need free access to food and water throughout the period of transport. Water should be available, and provided in leak-proof containers, or as mash, gel, fruit or vegetables. Juveniles and lactating animals may have particular needs. For journeys longer than 24 h or over 50 km, special feeding, watering and inspection arrangements need to be made, and written feeding, watering and resting instructions should accompany the animals.

6. *Duration and type of transport.* It is best if dedicated vehicles and staff are used for transportation. Personnel should be responsible, experienced and competent. Vehicles should be insulated and air conditioned, with a ventilation system which is independent of the main engine. Alarms should warn of failures of the heating and ventilation system. The vehicle needs to be able to be cleaned and disinfected thoroughly, and back-up systems should be available in case the vehicle breaks down. Animals should be examined by a competent person as soon as they arrive, and the transport should be arranged in advance so that animals can be unboxed and placed in fresh ready-prepared cages immediately on arrival.

7. *Experience and training of personnel.* Staff need to be familiar with the needs of the particular species. WATO 97 states that any carrier, who transports vertebrate animals for a journey of over 50 km, shall ensure that the personnel entrusted with the animals includes at least one person who has either specific training or equivalent practical experience with that species.

8. *Number of animals per container.* Sufficient space should be provided such that animals will not feel any discomfort, taking into consideration the conditions that will prevail during transport. Animals to be transported together should be the same age and sex, and from the same source. Species should not be mixed in containers, and animals should not be transported in the same vehicle as their natural predators. Care must be taken when transporting horned animals to prevent injury.

9. *Long journeys.* Journeys over 50 km for large animals require a written route plan authorised by the DEFRA specifying food and rest stops as appropriate. In addition, the transporter requires separate authorisation.

Diseased or injured animals should only travel for treatment, diagnosis or emergency slaughter. Pregnant animals will not normally be transported during the last fifth of pregnancy. Surgically prepared animals, neonates, nursing animals and animals with genetic defects may need extra care.

Some animals, such as non-human primates and wild animals, may need to be acclimatised beforehand to the conditions which will prevail during transport.

## HANDLING LABORATORY ANIMALS

Good animal handling techniques will reduce the risk of injury from bites and scratches, and will increase the confidence of both the handler and the animal, thus reducing stress to all those involved. All animals will respond in some way to the presence of a human and most species can recognise individuals and will be nervous of strangers. It is, therefore, important for the licensee to establish a friendly relationship with the animal to reduce nervousness on both sides. An animal that is confident and relaxed with its handler will be more co-operative enabling procedures to be carried out more easily. Some aspects of handling will vary according to the species. A brief description of techniques for each species can be found in the remainder of this chapter, but with each it is essential to get advice and assistance from people with previous experience.

## INTRODUCTION TO LABORATORY ANIMAL HUSBANDRY

The laboratory is far from being the natural environment for the animals that are kept there. Laboratory animals do not have the freedom to move away from adverse conditions, to search for food and water, or to find a better nesting site. All their physiological and behavioural needs must be supplied by the laboratory environment. These needs are not optional; they must be catered for or poor health will result. Caging or housing needs to keep terrestrial mammals dry, clean and warm. There must be adequate room to allow a normal range of movement, without overcrowding, and there must be free access to food and water. Cages must be made from harmless material, which is easily cleaned and sterilised, and must be able to withstand attempts to escape. Some animals are particularly adept at chewing through plastic cages or removing food hoppers to escape.

*Guidelines on the Care of Laboratory Animals* are published by the Home Office, and can be found in the *Code of Practice for the Housing and Care of Animals Used in Scientific Procedures*, and the *Code of Practice for the Housing and Care of Animals in Designated Breeding and Supplying Establishments*. However, note that these documents are due for revision following on from alterations proposed to Appendix A to the *Convention on the protection of vertebrate animals in experimental and other scientific procedures* (see Chapter 2). For those in the US or in institutes working to the Association for the Assessment and Accreditation of Laboratory Animal Care International (AAALAC) standards, the *National Research Council Guide for the Care and Use of Laboratory Animals* is the accepted text. These documents give details of recommended environmental conditions, and include minimum cage sizes and stocking densities.

### The five freedoms

Regard should be had to best practice as enunciated by the Farm Animal Welfare Council and the desirability of ensuring the five freedoms:

- freedom from thirst, hunger or malnutrition
- freedom from discomfort
- freedom from pain, injury and disease
- freedom to express normal behaviour
- freedom from fear and distress.

# An overview of caging types

Rather than conventional shoebox cages on open shelving or racks, housing for laboratory rodents is now frequently designed in such a way as to offer microbiological containment. This may be done because it is required as a strategy for the containment of animals that may pose a risk to human safety, because they are carrying biological agents that fall into hazard groups categorised by the Advisory Committee on Dangerous Pathogens. Sometimes the principal requirement is to protect staff from animal allergens, or it may be to prevent the spread of organisms between animals in order to maintain their SPF status, perhaps to allow animals of different microbiological backgrounds to be housed in close proximity. Sometimes the caging equipment does not achieve the desired result, because the exact requirements have not been properly assessed.

## Flexible film isolators

An isolator is like a large plastic bubble, which is sealed from the outside world. Filtered air is supplied, and equipment and food are passed in through a port that allows disinfection of the packaging prior to entry into the isolator. Isolators operate under negative or positive pressure, offering complete environmental protection against the spread of pathogens in or out of the isolator, so animals of different health status can be housed within the same room, in different isolators. They are mobile but do not make good use of available floor space. They must be alarmed in case of failure of the air supply and they can be difficult to work with.

## Filter top cages

Cages are held on an open rack, but covered with individual filters. Some containment of micro-organisms is achieved with well fitting lids, but the microenvironment in the cage is compromised as there is restricted airflow. The filter top should only be removed in a safety cabinet, which can make them difficult to work with.

## Ventilated cabinets

These are similar to sealed cupboards with their own filtered air supply. The cabinet operates under negative pressure. Inside, filter top cages are generally used. They are easy to install, relatively cheap and mobile but can present a risk when the cabinet doors are open or at cage changes.

## Individually ventilated caging systems

These are cages with filter tops held in a specialised rack that allows each cage to receive its air supply individually. Air is forced into or drawn out of the cage through nozzles adjacent to the lid. Cages can be held at positive or negative pressure, depending on the nature of the barrier. The pressure is variable and is determined by whether or not the cage is sealed. Air movement through the nozzles produces sound, but in general the lower the air speed, the lower the noise level is likely to be. The fans and filters used may be connected directly to the cage rack within the animal room, or may be sited remotely within a service plant room. If fans are situated on the cage rack, vibration may be transmitted to the cage. Whatever the design, it is crucial to install an alarm system, and consideration of procedures in the event of a breakdown or power failure will be necessary.

The containment provided by the cage system must be maintained while the cage is cleaned or the animals examined. These procedures are, therefore, carried out in ventilated workstations or safety cabinets. There are three classes:

- *Class I*, protects the operator
- *Class II*, protects the animal and the operator and has an easy access open front
- *Class III*, in effect is a totally sealed box.

Individually ventilated caging (IVC) systems are complex cage systems that rely on engineering to support the animals' environment. If this equipment is to fulfil its objectives thorough staff training is required, ranging from simple husbandry procedures to prevent damage to cages, to knowing how to ventilate a rack of cages when a fan unit breaks down. SOPs are required for IVC and safety cabinets to ensure that the required level of containment is maintained.

The IVC provides the animal with an environment that is controlled for ventilation, temperature and relative humidity. The containment provided by an IVC may be beneficial: the quality of the science may be improved by using healthier animals, enabling fewer animals to be used more effectively. However, there are drawbacks since this type of caging makes the animal more remote from the staff. The animal technician cannot see the animal as easily and cannot hear or smell the animal, all valuable sources of information when assessing its overall condition. The welfare of the animals will depend on the qualities and skills of the staff employed.

## Use of bedding materials

Bedding materials may be used to provide warmth and comfort, and to improve sanitation. The bedding must be harmless, that is, non-toxic and non-irritant, hygienic, absorbent, easily disposable, cheap and readily available, and easy to use. Bedding should be changed as often as is required to maintain a clean environment.

There is currently much debate on whether it is acceptable to keep rodents on wire-bottomed cages rather than solid-bottomed cages. The *Home Office Guidelines for the Housing and Care of Animals* does not specify, but does state, 'Bedding and nesting material should be provided, unless it is clearly inappropriate'. Maintenance costs for animals in solid-bottomed cages with bedding are higher than for mesh cages since there are the costs of the bedding, labour costs and disposal costs to be considered. The life of polycarbonate plastic cages depends on factors such as chemical exposure, washing temperature and autoclaving, which will vary depending on cleaning frequency; but it is undoubtedly less than for stainless steel cages. The exposure of staff to health risks from bedding need not be an issue with modern waste-handling systems. The welfare and comfort of the animals should also be part of the caging choice decision, since if the caging leads to stress in the animals, the research results will be invalid and the cost–benefit analysis of the ethical review decision to carry out the work will be altered. However, there are few data in this area. Rodents prefer to sleep in bedding on a solid floor but awake animals spend more time exploring the wire-bottomed area. No significant differences in physiological data between the two have been found. The preference of rodents for one type or another depends on species, strain, sex, age and group composition. It will also be affected by the gauge of the wire in the bottom of the cage, the mesh size, the wire shape and, in solid-bottomed cages, the type and quantity of bedding. Further objective work is needed in the area to clarify what would be in the welfare interest of the animals (Stark, 2001).

Laboratory animal bedding material is often overlooked, compared to other elements in the animal's immediate environment, with respect to its relative importance. Extreme precaution is taken in controlling research variables, such as using microbiologically clean animals, feeding them sterilised diets, filtering and purifying the water and filtering the air. Despite this, animals are quite often put onto the 'cheapest' bedding material available in an effort to cut costs. Research animals live in confined environments, and may be in direct contact with the bedding and their waste material 24 h a day. Bedding production plants are not under the same degree of scrutiny as diet production mills. Therefore, the appropriate choice of material is very important.

No single type of bedding material is the best for all applications. Owing to the many variables involved due to differing environmental situations in housing (type of caging, humidity levels, air changes per hour in the room, air changes per hour within each cage, species in a given cage, number of animals per cage, size or age of animals, and the type of research being performed), it is nearly impossible to compare one bedding type with another. It is impossible for a manufacturer to recommend a specific amount of material that should be put into each cage that is appropriate for all possible combinations of species, cage populations, and user-specific environmental situations. That decision has to be left to the individual facility.

The following is a brief comparative summary of the major types of bedding materials.

## Wood products

Wood materials and by-products, due to their relatively low price, are the most common bedding material. Due to the high temperatures used in the drying process, they are relatively low in microbiological contaminants, assuming correct storage and handling conditions. Softwoods (such as pine and cedar) should be avoided, due to the presence of resins and aromatic hydrocarbons, which can cause elevated liver enzymes. Hardwoods include maple, beech, birch and aspen (e.g. Harlan 7090 Sani Chips). Due to the density and small particle size of wood chips, rodents cannot make nests in them. *Shredded* aspen is also made from hardwood, but has the added advantage that rodents can make nests in it due to the shredded texture and longer strands of wood.

Although wood products are cheaper, they are poorer performers in absorption, dust levels and in ammonia control. Wood products absorb slowly, dry slowly, and even with ideal airflow, ammonia levels can rise. Small chips have been known to clog automatic water valves. If air circulation is poor, or static cages are used, cages generally must be changed two to three times per week with this type of bedding.

## Corn cob products

Corn cobs are both middle-priced and mid-range performers. They absorb a little better than wood, but still tend to dry slowly. Moisture absorption is from the bottom up, which keeps animals drier but can soil cage bottoms quicker, leading to the need to clean, scrape or de-scale cages more frequently. Dust levels are generally low, but this depends on the quality of the cleaning equipment at the point of manufacture. Cobs tend to contain a higher levels of moulds and biological activity, because of the nature of the raw material. Due to the lower dust and higher absorbency relative to wood, cobs are preferred for use in micro-isolator units. There are fewer reports of clogged water valves with cobs. However, animals cannot make nests in cobs, because of density and particle size, making cobs gravel like. They may be obtained in different particle sizes (e.g. Harlan 7092 is 1/8 in and Harlan 7097 is 1/4 in).

## Paper products

Paper bedding materials are the most absorbent materials available, and are available as either pelleted or non-pelleted.

### Non-contact paper pellets

Pelleted paper bedding (e.g. Teklad 7094), is for use as a non-contact bedding material, such as for use in trays under suspended wire cages or as a litter material for cats or ferrets. Pelleted paper tends to be dusty, which can create problems if used as contact bedding.

### Paper bedding products

Paper bedding materials that are not pelleted tend to be the best overall performers for use in a wide variety of applications. Since paper products are the most absorbent, this allows for the longest interval between cage changes. In ventilated rack systems with mice some products will allow a cage change interval of up to 2 weeks. Dust levels of non-pelleted paper bedding are the lowest. The softer, fluffier texture of these materials makes them the environmentally 'friendliest' materials, maximising the ability for rodents to make nests. This feature makes paper bedding materials the preferred choice for breeding mice. Unit pricing of paper bedding materials tends to be higher than the other options. However, since fewer cage changes are needed, the labour saving and reduced costs of waste disposal will usually more than offset extra expense.

## Enrichment bedding materials

A relatively new category of bedding materials has been created in order to provide additional environmental enrichment. These are made from paper, cotton or a combination of the two so that they are shreddable. These products may be added to the cage to supplement existing bedding if wood chips or corn cobs are used. Some

| MATERIAL | PRICE | DUST | ABSORBENCY | AMMONIA CONTROL | OVERALL PERFORMANCE |
|---|---|---|---|---|---|
| HARDWOODS | LOW | MODERATE | LOWEST | LOW | MODERATE |
| CORN COBS | MODERATE | LOW | MODERATE | MODERATE | MODERATE |
| PELLETED PAPER | HIGH | HIGH | HIGH | HIGH | HIGH |
| PAPER PULP | HIGH | LOW | HIGH | HIGHEST | BEST |
| ENRICHMENT PADS | HIGH | LOW | HIGHEST | HIGH | HIGH |

**Figure 6.1**   Bedding performance summary chart.

products such as compressed cotton pads will provide all of the necessary bedding material in an accurate, pre-measured amount. Dust levels are low, and cleanliness and convenience are high. Rodents experience enrichment in shredding the pads, and have large amounts of clean, dry absorbent material with which to make nests. Products such as Harlan 6900 iso-PADS come pre-irradiated for additional convenience (see also Figure 6.1).

## Environment

Several factors contribute to the quality of the environment. The temperature, humidity, ventilation and lighting intensity must be maintained at a level appropriate for the species. The lighting level should be monitored both in the room and in the cages. The light level in cages on the top row of a rack may be significantly brighter than in other cages, which can be a problem for albino animals that have little pigment in the retina. For these animals, light levels above 60 lux can cause retinal damage. It is advisable to cover the top row of the rack to reduce the light level, and to keep the whole population in a uniform environment since variation in light level may affect the experimental results. Noise levels should be monitored. Animals' ears do not necessarily respond to the same range of frequencies as human ears. The room may seem quiet to people, but there may be sound uncomfortably loud in the ultrasound range which can be detected by rodents. Therefore, the intensity and frequency of the noise in the room should be assessed.

It is essential to cater for both the physiological and the psychological needs of the animals. The animal must have freedom to express as much natural behaviour as possible, including play and social contact if appropriate. The inability to exhibit a full range of natural behaviours is deleterious to health and welfare causing poor psychological well-being. This leads to chronic distress, and a reduced repertoire of natural behaviour and high levels of stereotyped or disorganised behaviour, and an inability to respond appropriately to changes in the environment. Environmental enrichment caters for the behavioural needs of the animals, and improves their health and welfare as much as any other environmental factor. The provision of play articles or bedding may be a simple way to achieve environmental enrichment, allowing the expression of normal behaviour, and improving the welfare of the animals (see Figures 6.2–6.5 and 15.3). Reports from the Animal Procedures Committee stress that environmental enrichment is crucial to the quality of life. A laboratory animal only spends a small

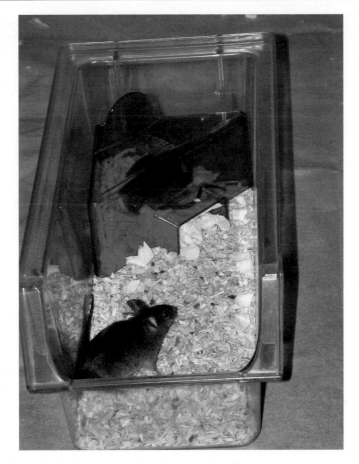

**Figure 6.2**    Example of environmental enrichment for mice.

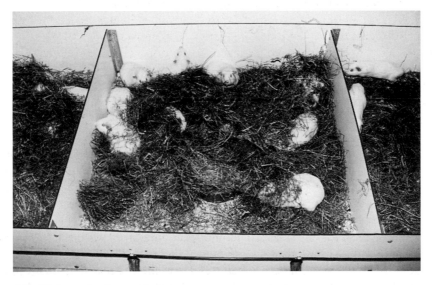

**Figure 6.3**    Guinea pigs housed in floor pens.

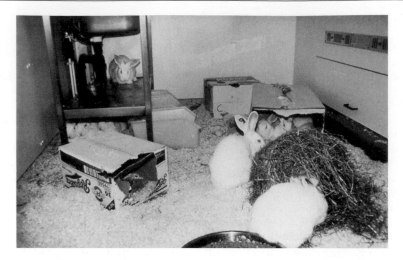

**Figure 6.4**    Floor housed rabbits with examples of environmental enrichment.

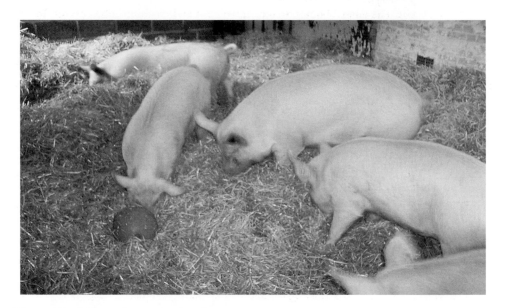

**Figure 6.5**    Indoor pigs rooting in substrate.

proportion of its life as an active research subject. Animal welfare considerations require that proper regard be paid to the quality of the animal's whole life, which involves more than just ensuring the conditions are hygienic and the animal is in good physical health. Some thought should be given to what environment the animal would choose to satisfy all its needs, and as close a match as possible should be provided by the laboratory (see www.ratlife.org). There are a multitude of papers describing provision of environmental enrichment techniques for the various species of laboratory animals. For a good review see Dean, 1999 which stresses the importance of challenging historical practices and including environmental enrichment as part of study design.

# FURTHER INFORMATION

Anderson, R.S. and Edney, A.T.B. (eds.) (1991). *Practical Animal Handling*. Pergamon Press, Oxford.

Biological Council Animal Research and Welfare Panel (1992). *Guidelines on the Handling and Training of Laboratory Animals*. Universities Federation for Animal Welfare.

Bhatt, P.N., Jacoby, R.O., Morse H.C. and New, A.E. (eds.) (1986). *Viral and Mycoplasmal Infections of Laboratory Rodents: Effects on Biomedical Research*. Academic Press, Orlando.

Coates, M.E. and Gustafssen, B.E. (eds.) (1984). *The Germfree Animal in Biomedical Research*. Laboratory Animals Ltd., London.

Clark, H.E., Coates, M.E., Eva, J.K., Ford, D.J., Milner, C.K., O'Donoghue, P.N., Scot, P.P. and Ward, R.J. (1977). Dietary standards for laboratory animals: Report of the LAC Diets Advisory Committee. *Laboratory Animals* 11, 1–28.

Clough, G. (1982). Environmental effects on animals used in biomedical research. *Biological Review* 57, 487–523.

Clough, G. (1984). Environmental factors in relation to the comfort and well-being of laboratory rats and mice. In *Standards in Laboratory Animal Management*, pp. 7–24. *Proceedings of a LASA/UFAW Symposium*. UFAW, Herts.

Clough, G. (1999). The animal house; design, equipment and environmental control. In *The UFAW Handbook on the Care and Management of Laboratory Animals* (7th edn). Blackwell Science; pp. 97–135.

Dean, S. (1999). Environmental enrichment of laboratory animals used in regulatory toxicology studies. *Laboratory Animals* 33, 309–27.

FELASA Working Group on Animal Health (1998). FELASA recommendations for the health monitoring of breeding colonies and experimental units of cats, dogs and pigs. *Laboratory Animals* 32, 1–17.

FELASA Working Group on Health Monitoring of Rodent and Rabbit Colonies (2002). Recommendations for the health monitoring of rodent and rabbit colonies in breeding and experimental units. *Laboratory Animals* 36, 20–42.

FELASA Guidance Paper for the Accreditation of Laboratory Animal Diagnostic Laboratories (1999). *Laboratory Animals* 33, S1:19–38.

FELASA Working Party Report (1999). Health monitoring of non-human primate colonies. Recommendations of the FELASA Working Group on Non-Human Primate Health. *Laboratory Animals* 33, S1:3–18.

Fletcher, J.L. (1976). Influence of noise on animals. In *Control of the Animal House Environment*. Laboratory Animal Handbooks Vol. 7. (ed. T. McSheehy). Laboratory Animals Ltd., London; pp. 61–62.

Gamble, M.R. (1982). Sound and its significance for laboratory animals. *Biological Review* 57, 395–421.

Institute of Laboratory Animal Resources (1976). Long term holding of laboratory rodents. *ILAR News* 19, L1–25.

King, J.O.L. (1978). *An Introduction to Animal Husbandry*. Blackwell Scientific Publications.

Krinke, G.J. (2000). *The Laboratory Rat*. Academic Press.

Laboratory Animal Breeders Association of Great Britain Limited (LABA) and Laboratory Animal Science Association (LASA) (1993). Guidelines for the care of laboratory animals in transit. *Laboratory Animals* 27, 93–107.

Lindsey, J.R. (1998). Pathogen status in the 1990's: abused terminology and compromised principles. *Laboratory Animal Science* 48, 557–58.

Manser, C.E., Broom, D.M., Overend, P., Morris, T.H. (1998). Operant studies to determine the strength of preference in laboratory rats for nest boxes and nesting materials. *Laboratory Animals* 32, 36–41.

National Research Council (1995). *Nutrient Requirements of Laboratory Animals*. National Academy Press.

*National Research Council Guide for the Care and Use of Laboratory Animals* (1996). National Academy Press, Washington DC.

Report of the Working Party on Hygiene of the GV-SOLAS on implications of infectious agents on results of animal experiments (1999). *Laboratory Animals* 33, S1:39–87.

Roe, F.J.C. (ed.) (1983). *Microbiological Standardisation of Laboratory Animals*. Ellis Horwood, Chichester.

Stark, D.M. (2001). Wire-bottomed versus solid bottomed rodent caging issues important to scientists and laboratory animals specialists. *Contemporary Topics* 40, 11–14.

Svendsen, P. and Hau, J. (eds.) (1994). *Handbook of Laboratory Animal Science: Vol. 1. Selection and Handling of Animals in Biomedical Research*. CRC Press.

## WEBSITES

http://jaxmice.jax.org/index.shtml
http://www.informatics.jax.org/mgihome/nomen/
http://www.defra.gov.uk/
http://www.eulep.org/Necropsy_of_the_Mouse/index.php

# Chapter 7
# Anaesthesia of laboratory animals

When carrying out procedures on animals it will frequently be necessary to perform them under anaesthesia because the procedure itself would otherwise be painful, or simply to provide some restraint of the animals. Schedule 2A to the Animals (Scientific Procedures) Act 1986 (ASPA) states that 'All experiments shall be carried out under general or local anaesthesia, unless the giving of the anaesthetic would cause more trauma than the experiment itself or the giving of an anaesthetic is incompatible with the experiment' (e.g. a behavioural experiment). Thus, the default position is that anaesthesia will be used. In Section 19b of the project licence the anaesthetic code will dictate what level of anaesthesia should be used. The options available are as follows:

- AA: No anaesthesia.
- AB: (Local or general) anaesthesia with recovery.
- AC: Anaesthesia without recovery.
- AD: Use of neuromuscular-blocking agents.

Successful anaesthesia does not depend simply on the types of drugs, doses and routes of administration used. A good standard of animal care must also be maintained, both pre- and post-operatively, including reduction in stress and provision of pain control. All these factors must be taken into account when designing an anaesthetic regime. If proper care is not taken during an anaesthetic, then recovery may be prolonged. Semi-conscious animals may lie in their urine or faeces and develop skin lesions, or get bedding material in their eyes and noses. Their cage mates may attack them, and they may remain inappetant for long periods if recovery is slow. These and other problems, such as post-operative pain, are distressing for the animal, and can be avoided by good intra-operative and post-operative care.

## CHOOSING AN ANAESTHETIC

Numerous issues currently confront us regarding the selection and appropriate use of anaesthetic drugs in laboratory animals. Traditional issues have centred on how to produce safe, effective anaesthesia in a cost-effective manner, but to these we must now add new considerations that have evolved due to a continuous effort to provide better anaesthetic care. The primary reasons for giving an anaesthetic are to provide humane restraint, which may require some modification of the animal's behaviour and level of conciousness by *narcosis*; a reasonable degree of *muscle relaxation* to facilitate procedures; and most importantly, sufficient *analgesia* to prevent the animal experiencing pain. These three elements make up the classical triad of anaesthesia (see Figure 7.1). The production of analgesia in many instances is the single most

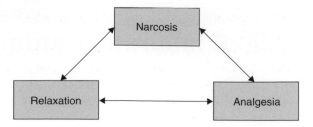

**Figure 7.1**    The classical triad of anaesthesia.

important drug effect. An additional requirement is the desire for anaesthetic drugs to produce antistress effects by influencing and inhibiting the release of cytokines from tissues damaged by surgery, and to modify the typical stress hormones, such as cortisol, ACTH and catecholamines. There is evidence that production and release of stress-related substances will produce pain and hypersensitise the nervous system to otherwise non-painful stimuli, promote the inflammatory response and inflammation, which will delay wound healing, and depress the immune response to infection.

In summary, the combination of drugs selected to produce ideal anaesthesia should include a behavioural modifier, a muscle relaxant, an analgesic and a stress reducer. This will be achieved by *'balanced anaesthesia'*, which means the administration of drugs in combinations, including premedicants, inhalation and injectable anaesthetics and analgesics, in order to produce stable anaesthesia and to reduce the potential side effects of any individual drug.

The effects of the anaesthetic must be consistent and repeatable. The drugs must have a wide safety margin, both for the animal and the user. Health and safety of the user must be safeguarded by controlling operating room pollution by volatile agents. Good anaesthetic practice is essential to ensure the scientific validity of any study using animals. Animal models are carefully defined to have the smallest degree of unwanted variation. If the animal is to recover from experimental surgery, it must return to physiological normality, or a pre-defined state of abnormality, as rapidly as possible. Pain, fear, distress, inappetance, hypothermia, hypoxia or respiratory acidosis, which may occur with poor anaesthesia, does not make for a good animal model. So physiological stability and minimal deleterious effects are required during the anaesthetic. An anaesthetic regime should be selected which interferes as little as possible with the experiment, and either does not alter the measurements being recorded or alters them in a consistent manner, which can be accounted for. There is evidence that many anaesthetic drugs can be given simultaneously to produce a synergistic (supra-additive) effect while at the same time decreasing the probability and seriousness of the side effects. It is also known that the choice of anaesthetic drug will affect the rate of recovery from anaesthetic and the rate of wound healing. Injectable drugs have been developed whose pharmacological and physiological effects may be relatively easily controlled due to their very short half-lives or their reversibility, but it must be realised that it is most unlikely that the pharmaceutical industry will ever develop the ideal anaesthetic drug.

These factors are forcing us to re-evaluate anaesthetic practices. No single answer will be universally applicable but the problem must be approached in a practical manner and techniques must be constantly refined in the light of new advances to achieve the required aims of the anaesthesia.

Anaesthetic regimes of different durations and depths will be required for different procedures, and some anaesthetic drugs will be contraindicated in certain protocols. Therefore, advantage should be taken of the wide variety of anaesthetic drugs and combinations available, rather than sticking to one or two methods, which will not be best suited to all experimental protocols.

When choosing an anaesthetic regime, it must be remembered that surgical techniques and anaesthesia have effects on the physiology of the animal. Surgical procedures have potentially major disruptive effects, which can be prolonged. The stress of surgery results in corticosteroid release, and levels can remain high for several days. The more invasive the surgery, the greater the stress response, which is designed to assist the animal in overcoming injury, but may be undesirable in the experimental subject, and unnecessary if peri-operative care is good.

The physiological effects of different anaesthetic regimes may be quite minor compared with those produced by the experimental surgery, so the possibilities of short-term minor alterations in experimental results should not be used as an excuse for adhering to an unsuitable anaesthetic technique. The anaesthetic should be chosen when all factors potentially influencing the protocol have been considered.

## PRE-OPERATIVE CARE

Animals which are healthy and disease free are clearly less likely to have problems during anaesthesia than those with overt or sub-clinical disease. Those with respiratory infections in particular should be avoided. It is best to use animals of known health status (see Chapter 6), but this may not be possible, and sometimes a previous experimental procedure may have altered the health of the animal. Either way, animals should be given a *clinical examination* prior to anaesthesia to rule out infectious and non-infectious diseases. The thoroughness of the examination depends on the species, the procedure and the likely duration of anaesthesia. As a minimum, the respiratory and cardiovascular systems should be examined. In small species, this can be achieved simply by careful observation of the animal noting the rate and character of the breathing and the colour of the extremities. Animals should be eating normal quantities of food and water (for normal values, see Section 2: Species), and show no obvious signs of disease.

Animals need to become acclimatised to their surroundings, possibly for 1–2 weeks before starting procedures, or normal physiological stress responses will result in abnormal experimental measurements. Adequate pre-operative *training* of animals to accept the procedure calmly, and sensible *individual animal selection* will reduce the stress placed on the animals. The temperaments of individual animals vary and some will be more suited to certain types of procedure than others.

*Fasting* prior to anaesthesia is not required in some species, such as rodents, since they cannot vomit and would become rapidly hypoglycaemic if deprived of food. If there is an experimental reason for fasting, such as for upper gastrointestinal tract surgery, the stomach will only be empty if coprophagy is prevented. Careful and *expert handling* of the animals is important. The fear and stress associated with movement from the animal-holding room to the operating theatre should be considered. Anaesthesia aims to provide humane restraint and an absence of pain, but unnecessary distress should not be caused while trying to achieve these aims.

The objectives of premedication include:

- to decrease *fear* and *apprehension*, to aid in stress-free induction
- to *reduce the amounts* of other anaesthetic agents required to induce general anaesthesia, so reducing their undesirable side effects
- to assist a *smooth recovery* from anaesthesia
- to *reduce salivary and bronchial secretions*, and to block the vaso-vagal reflex, in which bradycardia occurs due to endotracheal intubation and handling of the viscera
- to *reduce post-operative pain*.

## PRE-ANAESTHETIC DRUGS

### Narcotic analgesics (opioids)

Opioid analgesics interact at opioid-receptor sites in the central nervous system (CNS) and other tissues. There are three main receptor sites: $\mu$ (mu), $\kappa$ (kappa) and $\sigma$ (sigma). Most of the clinically used opioids interact with the $\mu$ receptors providing analgesia as well as respiratory depression, miosis (pupillary constriction), reduced gastrointestinal motility and euphoria. These drugs are potentially addictive, so most of them are controlled drugs under the Misuse of Drugs Regulations 1985 (amended 2002). Lower doses cause depression of the CNS, but high doses cause excitement, hence the potential for abuse of these drugs. Overdoses cause coma and death. There is a population of $\mu$ receptors ($\mu_1$, $\mu_2$, etc.), which explains the differences in action of the various analgesics. Stimulation of the receptors results in modulation of ionic conductance through cell membrane channels preventing the release of the neurotransmitters, which are responsible for the pain signal. Morphine, fentanyl and alfentanil are examples of potent agonists; codeine and pethidine are less potent agonists. Increasing the dose of a pure agonist increases the analgesia produced, but will also increase the respiratory depression. Pentazocine, buprenorphine and butorphanol are regarded as mixed agonist–antagonists (partial agonists), showing a wider range of activity. However, the respiratory depression produced by the partial agonists is also limited and these drugs are less liable to abuse. Partial agonists will also antagonise pure agonists to a certain extent. This can be useful in that a partial agonist like buprenorphine will antagonise the side effects of morphine, such as respiratory depression, but will maintain analgesia. This is sometimes known as sequential analgesia and is used to control residual respiratory depression caused by the initial injection of the pure agonist. Buprenorphine produces good sedation and analgesia, although it has a slow onset of action, but it lasts for 8 h. It is useful for producing sedation, alone or with phenothiazines, as part of premedication, but is used primarily for analgesia. It is the opioid analgesic of choice for most laboratory species. Diprenorphine and nalorphine are also partial agonists but closer to pure antagonists, reversing all of the effects of the agonist but retaining a degree of intrinsic activity that is expressed at higher doses. Naloxone is a pure antagonist having no sedative or analgesic action at recommended doses but capable of reversing the effects of an agonist. An overdose of buprenorphine may cause respiratory depression, which can be reversed with naloxone, but this will reverse all the analgesic effects as well as the respiratory depression. It is, therefore, better in many circumstances to counter the respiratory depression with doxapram, which is a respiratory stimulant, thus limiting the undesirable effect physiologically rather than by opposing pharmacological actions. There are major species differences in the responses elicited by opioid analgesics.

## Tranquillisers, sedatives or hypnotics

There is considerable confusion surrounding the definitions of these and there is no single classification of such terms. A hypnotic may be defined as a depressant of the CNS, which enables the animal to sleep more easily or more deeply, whereas a sedative relieves anxiety and is associated with drowsiness, thus making it easier for the animal to get to sleep. A tranquilliser removes anxiety without causing this sedative effect of drowsiness. However, many drugs fall into more than one classification, the difference usually being dependent on dose and on the species in which it is used. Classification is now usually in three categories: anxiolytic, antipsychotic and sedative/hypnotic, although the benzodiazepines fall into both the anxiolytic and sedative/hypnotic groups. The antipsychotic drugs were previously called neuroleptics (e.g. butyrophenones, phenothiazines). This multiplicity of definitions is confusing and it is much more important to understand the major actions of the drugs and appreciate how this will affect their use rather than to be able to categorise them. All of these drugs potentiate the action of anaesthetics, hypnotics and narcotic analgesics, so are useful in calming the animal before induction of anaesthesia and in reducing the dose of other drugs required to produce surgical anaesthesia.

### Phenothiazines

Examples for phenothiazines include acepromazine, chlorpromazine. All of these drugs cause hypotension and a fall in body temperature. Care should be taken with aged animals, those with impaired cardiovascular function or those with a history of epileptiform-type seizures.

### Butyrophenones

Examples for butyrophenones are fluanisone, azaperone. These are more potent than phenothiazines but less hypotensive. They are primarily used as a component of neuroleptanalgesia.

### Benzodiazepines

Examples for benzodiazepines include diazepam, midazolam. In some species (rabbits, rodents) these cause marked sedation, together with good skeletal muscle relaxation, and are potent anticonvulsants. There are minimal effects on the cardiovascular system. They potentiate the action of many anaesthetics and narcotic analgesics and are a valuable adjunct to many anaesthetic regimes.

### $\alpha_2$-Agonists

These drugs act on $\alpha_2$-adrenoceptors and produce dose-dependent sedation. There is marked bradycardia resulting from sino-atrial and atrio-ventricular heart block in response to initial drug-induced hypertension, which is then followed by moderate hypotension. Hyperglycaemia and polyuria also occur with the all drugs in this group.

Examples of $\alpha_2$-agonists are given below.

### Xylazine

This produces potent depression of the CNS leading to sedation, narcosis, unconsciousness and eventually to general anaesthesia with increasing doses. It is used to produce sedation or for premedication, as it can markedly reduce the quantity of anaesthetic required. It is not recommended for use before induction with Saffan or barbiturates as the combination produces severe respiratory depression. Its main use is in combination with ketamine to produce general anaesthesia.

### Medetomidine

This is a very potent and specific $\alpha_2$-agonist that produces sedation, analgesia and bradycardia. It also causes vasoconstriction in the periphery so blood pressure is maintained despite the fall in heart rate although it may decrease slightly after a few hours. Respiratory rate may also fall slightly. Medetomidine can cause heavy urination, so care must be taken to prevent the animal becoming wet, hypothermic or even dehydrated. Cyanosis may be apparent, with venous blood being very dark. Despite this, blood oxygen saturation remains high. The duration and degree of sedation and analgesia are dose dependent. Medetomidine is synergistic with ketamine and opioids, such as fentanyl. It also markedly reduces the dose of inhaled agents required. The most important feature of medetomidine is the existence of a reversal agent, atipamezole. This is a specific $\alpha_2$-antagonist and can also be used to reverse xylazine. Therefore, the animal will wake up in a few minutes and potential problems with depressed respiration and hypothermia are avoided.

### Romifidine

Romifidine can be administered in combination with butorphanol or ketamine to produce anaesthesia, or used alone for sedation. It is particularly used in the larger species.

## Anticholinergics

These block parasympathetic stimulation and decrease salivary and bronchial secretions, which is especially important in smaller animals. They can protect the heart from vagal inhibition, which causes bradycardia, and may occur when viscera are handled. There is recent evidence to suggest that they may also cause some bradydysrhythmias and their use is falling out of favour somewhat at present. The agent of choice is atropine sulphate or glycopyrronium, which is useful in neurological research since it does not cross the blood–brain barrier. In ruminants the anticholinergics make the saliva more viscid and are, therefore, contraindicated.

## GENERAL ANAESTHESIA: INHALATION OR INJECTION?

This is often the first choice made by an anaesthetist. Rather than immediately discarding one group of techniques, the possibility of using both methods should be considered.

Frequently, injectable agents are used for induction, and inhaled agents for maintenance of anaesthesia. The advantage of maintaining the animal on gas is that control of anaesthesia is excellent with this system. The use of constant infusion techniques with the ultra-short-acting injectables can provide a similar degree of control. Inhaled agents are mainly eliminated by the lungs, whereas injectable agents may need to be metabolised by the liver, and excreted by the kidneys. This process can be prolonged for some drugs. Recovery is, therefore, usually more rapid from inhaled agents, which is important in regaining normal physiology, to control post-operative hypothermia and fluid or electrolyte imbalance. Many of the newer injectable anaesthetics have specific reversal agents, which speeds recovery and overcomes many of these potential problems. It is better to have a rapid recovery and provide adequate post-operative analgesia, than to have prolonged anaesthesia.

If injectable agents are used, it is sometimes wrongly presumed that an anaesthetic machine is not needed. Oxygen supplementation is, therefore, not given, and hypoxia may well develop, particularly in long-term anaesthesia lasting for more than 1 h. The respiratory depression induced can lead to hypercapnia and acidosis. Similarly, endotracheal intubation may only be considered if the animal is to be connected to an anaesthetic machine and ventilated. However, the ability to administer oxygen and control ventilation, if required, helps control many potential difficulties encountered in anaesthesia.

Reversal of overdose of anaesthetic is quicker and usually more successful with inhalation agents than injectable ones, so reducing mortality.

Other factors influencing the choice of anaesthetic include the species involved, the length of the procedure, the depth of anaesthesia required and the nature of the procedure.

# GENERAL ANAESTHETIC DRUGS

## Inhaled agents

### *Administration of a volatile agent*

#### *Anaesthetic machines*

It is essential to have an anaesthetic machine with an appropriate vaporiser for long-term inhalation anaesthesia. These allow precise control of the amount of volatile anaesthetic agent delivered to the patient, and therefore allow precise control of the depth of anaesthesia. They are available with varying degrees of sophistication, from an oxygen cylinder on a trolley with a vaporiser to a workstation with multiple gas cylinders and facilities for forced ventilation.

Every research laboratory should have a purpose made vaporiser that will deliver a known concentration of the anaesthetic vapour over a given range of flow rates and temperatures. Each vaporiser is calibrated for a particular agent (e.g. halothane or isoflurane) and should not be used with the wrong agent. Gas from a compressed gas cylinder is then passed continuously over the volatile agent in the vaporiser. Either pure oxygen or oxygen combined with nitrous oxide is used. The anaesthetic properties of the nitrous oxide will reduce the amount of volatile agent that is required.

The animal, if it is a small rodent, is placed in the induction chamber and the anaesthetic machine will deliver known concentrations of anaesthetic to the animal within the chamber. This should have transparent sides, for easy observation, and be easy to clean. Disposable tissue should be placed on the floor of the chamber, and it should be cleaned thoroughly between animals, or the smell of the previous occupant could cause distress. Chambers are simple and convenient for small rodents, but should not be used for larger animals such as rabbits or cats.

The components of the anaesthetic machine include:

- *Gas cylinders:* These are available in several sizes. Oxygen is delivered in black cylinders with white collars, nitrous oxide in blue cylinders and carbon dioxide in grey cylinders.
- *Reducing valve:* A reducing valve attaches to the gas cylinders to ensure that a constant low pressure of gas is delivered to the flowmeter.
- *Flowmeter:* The flowmeter monitors the amount of gas flowing to the patient. It consists of a graduated glass tube with a bobbin, which floats at a level determined by the amount of gas passing through the tube. The tube is calibrated such that the top of the bobbin is in line with the marking indicating the flow rate of the gas. The bobbin should rotate in the tube. This rotation can be detected by observing a small spot, which is painted in the centre of the bobbin. Each flowmeter is calibrated specifically for a particular gas.
- *Vaporiser:* From the flowmeter, gas passes into a vaporiser, which contains the volatile anaesthetic. The carrier gas is diverted into the vaporiser to collect the vapour. The amount of gas passing into the vaporiser can be controlled, thus changing the concentration of anaesthetic delivered to the patient. The calibrations on each vaporiser are specific for a particular volatile agent, due to the differing physical properties of the agents.

Inhaled anaesthetics are volatile compounds that are allowed to vaporise, and the vapour is then inspired and has specific effects on the CNS. The concentration in the CNS starts low and gradually builds up as more anaesthetic is administered until the CNS concentration is the same as the concentration in the lungs, and anaesthesia is achieved. This can be a slow process, that is, induction can be slow. There is a time lag between inhaling the vapour and the onset of anaesthesia. The speed of onset will depend on the concentration of vapour in the inspired gas and on the properties of the particular agent used, such as boiling point or lipid solubility. To increase the speed of induction, particularly with the slower agents, the concentration of vapour in the inspired gas may be increased to a level which, if it were maintained, would cause excessive depression of the CNS and death. This is known as the 'induction concentration'. As soon as anaesthesia is achieved, the inspired concentration must be reduced to a 'maintenance concentration'.

Once the animal is anaesthetised, as judged by lack of movement and reflexes and monitoring the rate and depth of breathing, it can be removed from the chamber. For most procedures, the volatile agent is then administered via an endotracheal tube or face mask at a suitable maintenance concentration for as long as required (see Table 7.1 for suitable concentrations). For procedures lasting less than 1 min, maintenance may not be required.

**Table 7.1**   Use of volatile agents in rodents and rabbits.

| Anaesthetic | Concentration (%) | |
|---|---|---|
| | Induction | Maintenance |
| Halothane | 2.0–4.0 | 0.8–2.0 |
| Isoflurane | | |
|    Small animals | 2.0–3.0 | 0.25–2.0 |
|    Large animals | 3.0–4.0 | 1.5–3.0 |

Use of a face mask for induction of anaesthesia, as may be employed for larger species, can be resented by the animal. Stress can be reduced by administering a sedative or tranquilliser as a premedicant in the home pen, before induction, allowing sufficient time for it to reach maximum effect, and/or by using an injectable agent for induction before using the volatile agent for maintenance.

### Anaesthetic circuits

In order to maintain an animal with volatile anaesthetic, a system is required to deliver gases from the anaesthetic machine to the animal. Use should be made of a suitable circuit. Examples are shown in Figures 7.2–7.7. The particular one chosen will depend on the size of the patient, the site of the operative field, whether intermittent positive pressure ventilation (IPPV) is to be used, and personal preference.

Traditionally breathing systems have been described as open, closed, semi-open and semi-closed. These terms are now outdated and too ill defined to be of practical value as small alterations in the geometry of the system or the fresh gas flow can lead to confusion. The classification is, therefore, divided into two broad groups – those that contain the means to absorb carbon dioxide and those that do not.

### Partial rebreathing systems

These do not absorb carbon dioxide, so there is the potential for rebreathing expired carbon dioxide-containing gas. This is of physiological consequence, if the carbon dioxide-containing part of the gas enters the animal's alveolar space. A lightly anaesthetised animal will respond to rebreathing of alveolar gas by increasing ventilation to maintain a near normal alveolar carbon dioxide concentration. The fresh gas flow needed to prevent rebreathing in these systems is defined as the flow, which prevents both ventilation rate and arterial carbon dioxide changes.

### (i) Ayres T-piece

This circuit has minimal resistance and little dead space and is the circuit of choice for rodents up to 3 kg bodyweight. The open tube acts as the reservoir and there are no valves. The exhaled gases are pushed out of the open end of the reservoir tube by fresh gases flowing in from the anaesthetic machine during the expiratory phase.

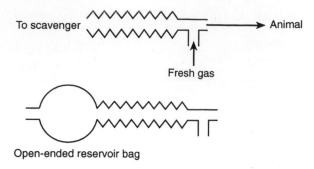

**Figure 7.2**   Ayres T-piece.

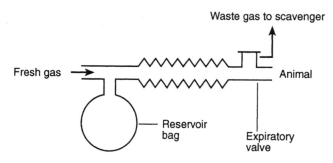

**Figure 7.3**   Magill circuit.

The capacity of the reservoir tube should be at least equal to the tidal volume of the animal. Ventilation may be carried out by occluding the end of the tube or by modification to include an open-ended bag.

### (ii) Magill circuit

Initially during expiration the dead-space gases pass down the corrugated tubing while fresh gases entering the system flow into the reservoir bag. As the system fills, the pressure increases to a level at which the expiratory valve opens and then expired alveolar gas escapes through the valve. A fresh gas flow of 80–90% of minute volume (respiratory rate × tidal volume) should be used. This circuit is only suitable for animals of 10 kg and over because the valve causes high resistance and it has a relatively high dead space. It is a widely used circuit for animals between 10 and 40 kg.

### (iii) Co-axial circuits

- *Bain's co-axial circuit:* This is a modification of the T-piece where the fresh gas inflow pipe runs inside the reservoir limb. It is suitable for animals of 3–10 kg and a minimum flow rate of 100–300 ml/kg/min is needed to prevent rebreathing.
- *Lack co-axial circuit:* This uses the alternative arrangement in which fresh gas flows up the outer tube and expiration takes place down the inner tube. This was designed to aid scavenging of the expired gas but restricts its use to spontaneously breathing animals as it cannot be used with controlled ventilation.

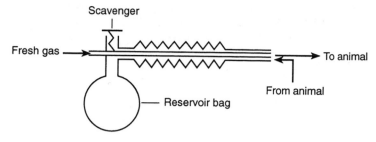

**Figure 7.4**    Bain co-axial circuit.

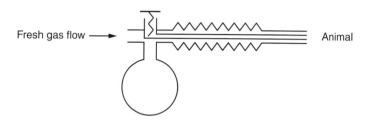

**Figure 7.5**    Lack co-axial circuit.

Care must be taken with co-axial circuits not to use tubing of too small a bore so that excessive demands are made on the animal's respiratory efforts. It is also possible for the inner tube to become detached from either the machine or the animal, resulting in a very large dead space. These circuits must always be examined carefully and tested immediately before use.

*Rebreathing systems*

These are systems in which the carbon dioxide in the exhaled gases is absorbed by soda lime so that the anaesthetic vapour can be re-circulated with the addition of fresh oxygen. The gas flow in closed systems is, therefore, significantly reduced and the re-use of the expired anaesthetic vapour makes them very economical to use. Nitrous oxide should not be used with closed systems, since it is impossible to monitor the concentration in the recycled gas. The disadvantage of the closed method of administration is the resistance to respiration caused by the packed soda lime. This makes the use of these systems unsuitable for animals under 15 kg in weight, and the conservation of heat in the system may give rise to heat stroke in sheep.

(i) *To and fro system:* The Water's canister containing soda lime is placed between the animal and the reservoir bag to absorb the carbon dioxide. This increases the dead space and so it is only suitable for animals over 15 kg. The dust from the soda lime may be inhaled and cause inflammation in the respiratory tract.

(ii) *Circle systems:* In these, there is a circular flow of gas controlled by two unidirectional valves. They were designed for large animals as there is high resistance in the system but there are some lightweight systems that may be used on animals

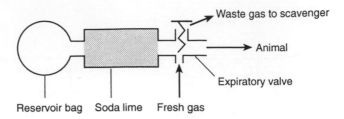

**Figure 7.6**   To and fro system.

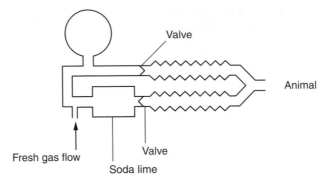

**Figure 7.7**   Circle system.

5–10 kg, although the preference is generally to use non-rebreathing systems in such animals.

The quantity of oxygen piped into the circuit depends on the needs of the animal (which depends on its body weight), and the type of circuit. For all except closed circuits, the expired air is not re-inhaled, that is, rebreathing should not occur. If the oxygen flow rate is too low, rebreathing may occur, and carbon dioxide can build up to dangerous levels as there is no method of removing it. It is essential, therefore, to have a high enough flow rate to remove the alveolar gas when it is expired. As shown in Figure 7.8, for the Ayre's T-piece, the exhaled gases are swept out of the open end of the reservoir tube by the fresh gases flowing in during the expiratory phase. The part of the circuit immediately adjacent to the animal is known as the 'dead space' and should be minimised in order to reduce the amount of gas that has to be removed to ensure there is no rebreathing of alveolar gas.

## Anaesthetic delivery systems

The anaesthetic vapour and carrier gas is delivered to the animal in one of several ways.

### (i) The face mask

The vaporiser is connected at the end of the tubing, to a face mask to deliver the anaesthetic. This must be snugly fitting over the nose and mouth but not rub the eyes. The disadvantages of this are that gas invariably leaks from around the mask, contributing to pollution of the atmosphere, so it should be used in a flow hood or use made of

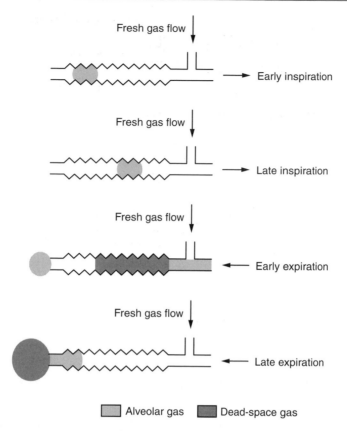

Fresh gas flow

→ Early inspiration

Fresh gas flow

→ Late inspiration

Fresh gas flow

← Early expiration

Fresh gas flow

← Late expiration

☐ Alveolar gas    ■ Dead-space gas

**Figure 7.8**  Prevention of rebreathing with the T-piece, fresh gas flow must exceed at least twice the animal's minute volume.

purpose-made face masks for small rodents, which incorporate a gas-scavenging system and are, therefore, safer to use. Face masks require a flow rate of three times the animal's minute volume.

### (ii) Induction chamber

The induction chamber is a simple and very convenient way to induce anaesthesia in small rodents. It is a simple box with transparent sides, so that the animal can be observed during the induction, and the box should be easy to clean between animals. The inlet pipe is at low level and the extract at high level, since the volatile agents are heavier than air. Anaesthesia is induced by piping in the induction concentration of the agent (see Table 7.1). Once the animal has lost its righting reflex, is immobile in the chamber and breathing regularly, the concentration can be reduced to the maintenance concentration and the animal can be removed from the chamber. Anaesthesia will persist for a brief period of about 1 min so that short procedures (such as tail biopsy or ear punch) can be carried out immediately. If longer periods of anaesthesia are required, then the animals can be transferred to a face mask or an endotracheal tube placed so that a maintenance concentration of anaesthesia can be administered for as long as is necessary.

## (iii) Endotracheal tubes

When using circuits, animals are normally intubated using a rubber or plastic tube inserted into the trachea. These are available in many different sizes for different species, with or without an inflatable cuff, which is used to make an airtight seal in the trachea ensuring that the gases stay in the circuit and reducing leakage. The tube will provide a patent airway so that artificial respiration may be given if required. Endotracheal intubation requires skill, which may be easily learned, and in some species the use of an appropriate laryngoscope. The lubricated tube should be passed over the tongue and epiglottis, and through the larynx. Once the tube is in situ, the cuff is inflated to seal the trachea and prevent the animal from being able to breathe around the tube. For tubes smaller than 5 mm diameter, inflatable cuffs should not be used, as these reduce the size of the airway, and in small animals this is undesirable.

The size of tube used depends on the size of the animal, but as a rough guide, adult beagles will need a 9- or 10-mm tube, with a cuff, cats need a 3–5-mm tube without a cuff, and rats need a modified urinary catheter. Dogs, cats and primates may be intubated while lying in left lateral recumbency (right-handed operator). An assistant holds the head and neck extended and lifts the upper jaw. The operator pulls the tongue forward and down, and usually the larynx can then be visualised. The tube is then passed gently through the glottis into the trachea. In cats, the larynx should be sprayed with local anaesthetic prior to passage of the tube to prevent laryngeal spasm.

Pigs have a particularly long larynx, and a laryngoscope is required for intubation. This illuminates the larynx and also holds down the tongue and epiglottis.

Rabbits can be intubated via surgical implantation of an endotracheal tube in the trachea in non-recovery situations, or by passing a tube carefully into the mouth. The tube is inserted in the mouth to one side of the incisors, as far as the glottis. The tube is then advanced into the larynx during the inspiratory phase of respiration. Another method requires an assistant to stand in front of the prone rabbit holding its head up and pulling the tongue forward. The operator stands behind the rabbit, and advances the tube gently as far as the glottis, then passing the tube into the trachea during inspiration.

## Health and safety

Volatile anaesthetic agents pose some risk to human health. Prolonged exposure is thought to cause hepatotoxicity and abortion, among other side effects. Each volatile agent has a defined occupational exposure limit (OEL) the level of which should not be exceeded, and so it is necessary to use either an active or passive scavenger system. A length of tubing attached to the expiratory port of the circuit can be used to duct waste gases to the outside, either actively or passively. Alternatively, the apparatus may be used in an extraction cabinet, although this may cause problems with adequate access to the animal. Another option is to use a fluosorber, which actively scavenges the volatile agent using charcoal. Portable scavenging units are available from IMS (International Market Supply). Remember the canister must be weighed regularly and changed when it is exhausted and that the fluosorber will not remove nitrous oxide.

All anaesthetic equipment must be regularly serviced to ensure the correct quantities of vapour are delivered. Also the machine must be checked before each anaesthetic is given to ensure the following:

- *Oxygen* cylinders are full, spare cylinders are available, and a key to turn them on is available.
- *Flowmeters* are working.
- The *vaporiser* is working and contains enough volatile agent.
- The *emergency oxygen* flush is working.
- A *suitable circuit* is correctly attached and has been tested.
- *Endotracheal tubes* are in good condition.
- The *scavenging system* is attached and functional.
- Any *monitoring equipment* is set up properly.

Only once all these have been checked should the animal be anaesthetised.

## Volatile agents

Volatile agents are delivered to the patient from an anaesthetic machine using oxygen, or a mixture of oxygen and nitrous oxide, as the carrier. There are several volatile agents available.

**Halothane**    Halothane is a non-flammable liquid, which is very potent, but has a high therapeutic index. It is non-irritant to the mucous membranes, so causes little increase in salivary and bronchial secretions. It has a cardiodepressant effect, reducing heart rate and blood pressure, and it sensitises the heart to the dysrhythmic effects of catecholamines. There tends to be some shivering on recovery. It is the cheapest of the modern volatile agents. The OEL is 10 ppm.

**Isoflurane**    Isoflurane has similar physical properties to halothane, but is slightly less soluble in blood and so induction and recovery are more rapid. Isoflurane is metabolised far less in the liver (0.2%) than halothane (20%), the majority being excreted unchanged via the lungs.

Halothane induces liver microsomal enzyme systems whereas isoflurane does not, so the latter is more suitable for studies requiring normal liver metabolism. Although changes in peripheral arterial blood pressure are similar with both anaesthetic agents, the fall in blood pressure observed with isoflurane is primarily due to vasodilation rather than the myocardial depression that is found with halothane. This property in association with less sensitisation of the myocardium to adrenaline makes isoflurane the agent of choice in small laboratory animals. The maximum exposure limit for personnel is higher than for halothane at 50 ppm making it safer to use.

**Enflurane, Desflurane (I653) and Sevoflurane**    Enflurane, desflurane (I653) and sevoflurane are all used in human anaesthesia, but they offer no significant advantages over isoflurane for the majority of procedures while being considerably more expensive.

**Nitrous oxide**   All of the above mentioned agents produce smooth induction and whichever is chosen may be used in conjunction with nitrous oxide gas. Nitrous oxide is not potent enough for induction of anaesthesia in most species, and is, therefore, unsuitable for use alone or with neuromuscular-blocking agents. However, it has minimal cardiovascular and respiratory effects, so if used with a volatile agent it reduces the required concentration of that agent, reducing its side effects. It is used $60:40$ or $50:50$ with oxygen to deliver the volatile agent. After prolonged anaesthesia, 100% oxygen should be given for 5–10 min, or oxygen can be displaced from the lungs by the nitrous oxide as it is breathed off, causing diffusion hypoxia, which can lead to suffocation.

The required concentration of volatile agent does not depend on the weight of the animal, but on the agent itself and the species in which it is used. Therefore, heavier animals do not necessarily need a higher concentration of anaesthetic, although the larger farm species generally require higher concentrations than small rodents (see Table 7.1).

Provided that anaesthesia has not been prolonged, recovery from gaseous anaesthesia is usually rapid, but if animals have been maintained on volatile agents for 1 h or more, full recovery can take more than 15–20 min. The speed of recovery varies depending on the attention, which has been given to controlling the depth of anaesthesia during surgery, by varying the concentration of agent delivered to the patient. Generally, as anaesthesia progresses, the concentration of anaesthetic can be reduced slightly. After major surgery, a further reduction in depth can be made during suturing of subcutaneous (s.c.) tissues and skin, so reducing recovery time following completion of surgery. This ability to vary the depth of anaesthesia is one of the major advantages of using inhalation agents.

## Injectable agents

### General considerations

Injectable agents are given either intravenously (i.v.), that is, go directly into the bloodstream, or via another parenteral route from which they are absorbed into the blood. They are particularly useful for the induction of anaesthesia, which can then be maintained by inhalation, or for short-duration anaesthesia. The i.v. injections usually act very rapidly, producing loss of consciousness almost immediately. The calculated dose is administered slowly, allowing time for the drug to circulate before deciding whether more is required. The drug can, therefore, be administered to effect and titrated to the exact requirements of the animal. However, most injectable anaesthetics are administered to small rodents by the intraperitoneal (i.p.) route as a single dose. When this route is used, absorption can be slow and unpredictable, residual drug effects persist for long periods and full recovery can be prolonged. There is also the possibility of accidental injection into a blood vessel or major abdominal organ, which could have serious consequences.

There are difficulties associated with the use of injectable agents for the induction of anaesthesia. Skill is required to perform i.v. injections, particularly in small rodents, and it takes time and practice to acquire these skills. For injectable agents more than inhaled agents, the level of anaesthesia achieved depends on the level of stimulation of the animal at the time. An animal that is given an injection and left undisturbed may be apparently deeply anaesthetised, but once surgery starts it may respond by reflex movements of the limbs and an increase in the depth and rate of breathing. This does not necessarily mean that a further injection of anaesthetic is required; if more is given, and surgery then stops and the animal is no longer stimulated, there is a risk that the level of anaesthesia will become dangerously deep. This phenomenon also occurs with inhaled agents, but to a lesser degree. *It is, therefore, important to be familiar with the techniques required for the administration of injectable agents, and the type of anaesthesia obtained, and to develop the necessary skills for monitoring accurately the depth of anaesthesia.*

## Recovery

With inhaled agents, if an overdose is given, the vaporiser can simply be switched off and the animal allowed to breathe oxygen for a few minutes until the anaesthetic gas has been exhaled. Injectable agents, once they are given, have to be metabolised by the liver and excreted by the kidneys. This process can be prolonged, and recovery from injectable anaesthetics usually takes longer than for inhaled agents. This increases the risk of hypothermia or dehydration developing. With some of the barbiturate drugs, return to consciousness is rapid because the drug is redistributed away from the CNS into other body tissues (such as fat), due to their high lipid solubility. However, much drug is still present in the body and there is the potential for the animal to relapse into unconsciousness if the drug re-circulates into the CNS, which can occur in animals with little body fat. Some injectable drugs have specific reversal agents, the administration of which will lead to a return to consciousness within minutes. However if the half-life of the reversal agent is shorter than the anaesthetic agent, the animal will relapse into a sedated state unless repeat doses are given. Reversal agents can also be used to reverse any respiratory depression, which develops in the post-operative period. Some injectable agents are 'ultra-short acting', and are metabolised very quickly. Use of these newer drugs has overcome some of the problems previously associated with injectable agents.

## Injectable agents in laboratory species

The small size of many of the laboratory species and the problems of restraint in others means that injectable agents are most frequently given via the intramuscular (i.m.) or i.p. routes. These routes require a large total dose of the drug to be given. Drugs are usually administered as a single bolus, so it is essential to weigh the animal first, as a 'guesstimate' of the weight is likely to be wildly inaccurate and result in over- or under-dosing the animal. It is, therefore, important that drugs used in laboratory species have a wide safety margin, are non-irritant, and can be administered in a small volume through a small needle. Most anaesthetics will pass easily through a 25-gauge needle, and the smallest gauge practicable for the species should be used. Local anaesthetic cream (such as EMLA) can be used to desensitise the skin to block any acute pain caused by the placement of larger needles or cannulae or even for simple venepuncture in nervous animals.

Absorption from i.p., s.c. or i.m. injections can be slow, as it depends on the blood flow to the site, so induction can be slow. Recovery is also slow, and the residual effects of the drug can persist for long periods. There is also a time lag between the injection of the drug and deepening of anaesthesia, so if these agents are used for long procedures, good monitoring of the depth of anaesthesia is essential, in order that top-up injections can be given in good time. *It is not acceptable to give a further dose by injection as the animal starts to wake up*; i.v. injections allow dosing to be adjusted according to the individual animal's response, so there is less likelihood of over- or under-dosing. They have many advantages in terms of control of depth of anaesthesia and can be given by constant infusion to avoid the anaesthetic depth varying widely though the course of the procedure. It is worthwhile developing the skill required for giving i.v. injections. They can be given using needles and syringes, butterfly needles, or over-the-needle cannulae, the last of which can be maintained in a vein for long periods. To facilitate venepuncture in nervous animals, local anaesthetic cream can be applied 30–60 min beforehand, to desensitise the skin (EMLA cream, Astra Pharmaceuticals).

## Choice of anaesthetic agent

The quality of anaesthesia produced by the different agents varies considerably. Many of the injectable agents produce poor analgesia, and are insufficient for major surgery. The addition of a low level of a volatile agent can improve the level of analgesia. Therefore, before choosing an anaesthetic regime, the nature of the procedure should be considered. Many injectable agents are available.

### Propofol

This is a substituted phenol, which is administered i.v. slowly. Too rapid administration may induce apnoea. It acts rapidly, inducing anaesthesia smoothly without excitatory side effects. It is ultra-short acting, and recovery is rapid and smooth. It can be used by continuous infusion for prolonged anaesthesia. It can be used safely in cats, dogs, monkeys, pigs and rabbits, and can be combined with a wide range of premedicants, analgesics and inhaled agents.

### Saffan

This is a mixture of steroids, alphaxolone and alphadolone. It was first used as an anaesthetic for cats, but is now used in almost all domestic species except dogs. There is a component in the mixture (cremophor EL), which causes histamine release in dogs, and can cause anaphylaxis. Saffan is given i.v. in cats, rats, rabbits, sheep, goats, pigs and primates. In rabbits however, analgesia is poor, and these are best given an alternative agent. I.m. or i.p. injections produce variable results, and large volumes of the drug are required, which limits its use in these sites.

An i.v. injection rapidly results in anaesthesia and muscle relaxation is good, but there is some depression of the cardiovascular and respiratory centres. There may be some trembling, paddling or even convulsions on recovery, and oedema of the paws and ears may develop. Overall though, it has five features that make it popular as an anaesthetic agent:

- it has a high therapeutic index
- it does not accumulate in the body
- recovery of consciousness and appetite is rapid after administration ceases
- there is little respiratory depression but muscle relaxation is good
- it is not irritant, if given outside a vein.

Saffan can be used for short-term anaesthesia, for induction followed by maintenance with an inhaled agent, or for long-term anaesthesia by intermittent injections or continuous infusion.

## Ketamine

This is a non-competitive *N*-methyl-D-aspartate (NDMA)-receptor antagonist, which can be given by i.m. or i.v. injection. It circulates rapidly and produces analgesia but little muscle relaxation. There is an apparent lack of awareness of the surroundings, and analgesia varies with the species. The corneal reflex is lost very early with ketamine, and in long procedures it is necessary to protect the eye with a bland ophthalmic ointment. The laryngeal and pharyngeal reflexes are maintained, but there is an increase in salivary secretions, which could cause airway obstruction, so it is often used with a drying agent, such as atropine. There is good maintenance of blood pressure under ketamine sedation. In rodents, the dose required to produce light surgical anaesthesia with ketamine alone causes severe respiratory depression. When given alone it does not produce adequate anaesthesia for surgery, but it can be combined with xylazine, medctomidine, diazepam, midazolam or Saffan to produce good general anaesthesia in many species (sheep, cat, primate, pig, rabbit and hamster). It is the agent of choice for sedation of Old World Monkeys. Using ketamine in combination with other agents also avoids side effects, such as muscle tremors.

## Narcotic analgesics (opioid analgesics)

**Fentanyl**   Fentanyl is a potent analgesic that lasts for 15–20 min. In rats, dogs and primates, it has sedative effects; but in mice, cats and horses, it causes excitement. Respiratory depression can be marked, and facilities for IPPV should be available. It is useful in neuroleptanalgesia, or as a component of balanced anaesthetic regimes.

**Alfentanil**   Alfentanil is less potent than fentanyl, but the onset of activity is more rapid. Respiratory depression is marked. It is used in combinations, to increase analgesia in animals anaesthetised with other agents, or as a premedicant to reduce the amount of induction agent required.

**Sufentanil**   Sufentanil is 10 times more potent than fentanyl, but has not yet been extensively used in laboratory animals.

## Neuroleptanalgesics

Combinations of opioid analgesics and sedatives are used to provide neuroleptanalgesia, which is similar, but not equal to, a light plane of anaesthesia. The animal no longer responds to surroundings or to pain but is not totally unconscious. Neuroleptanalgesics produce some respiratory depression, and poor muscle relaxation, but when combined with a benzodiazepine these limitations are markedly reduced and a state of neuroleptanaesthesia may be produced under which surgical procedures may be carried out. So, combinations of fentanyl/fluanisone with midazolam, or diazepam can be used to provide good anaesthesia for rodents and rabbits. Midazolam is particularly useful since it is water soluble and can, therefore, be administered in the same syringe as the fentanyl/fluanisone. It can also be diluted with sterile water for accurate dosing in small rodents.

The actions of the opioid component of neuroleptanalgesics can be reversed by the use of narcotic antagonists (such as naloxone) or partial agonists (such as *buprenorphine*, *butorphanol* or *nalbuphine*), which will also provide post-operative analgesia. Naloxone reverses analgesia as well as any side effects (such as respiratory depression), so it must not be used unless surgery has been completed and adequate analgesia provided by some other means. Reversal is not always required, as most neuroleptanalgesics will wear off by themselves, but anaesthesia will be prolonged resulting in hypercapnia and hypothermia.

## Medetomidine and atipamezole

Medetomidine can be given by i.v., i.m. or s.c. injection. When used as a sedative, the animal must be left undisturbed for 10–15 min after administration for the drug to reach maximum effect, preferably in a quiet environment, as they may still react to noise. Medetomidine does not induce general anaesthesia when used alone, but is excellent when used in combinations. It reduces the requirement for halothane by about 70%, and can be used with fentanyl/fluanisone to produce good anaesthesia and analgesia. It may also be used successfully with ketamine in many species. The great advantage of medetomidine is that it can be reversed very rapidly with atipamezole, and if it is used in combinations with neuroleptanalgesics, buprenorphine or nalbuphine can be used as a partial antagonist for fentanyl, combining rapid recovery with the provision of analgesia.

## Barbiturates

**Pentobarbitone**    Pentobarbitone is a barbiturate which depresses the CNS, and produces marked cardiovascular and respiratory depression. It is weakly analgesic, and, therefore, very large doses must be given before pain perception is reduced. This means that it has a low therapeutic index: the lethal dose is only slightly above the clinical dose. After i.v. injections, pentobarbitone takes a long time to cross the blood–brain barrier into the CNS, so onset of anaesthesia is slow. Injections must, therefore, be given very slowly, to allow anaesthesia to deepen to its full extent before giving extra doses. If it is given carefully, safety can be improved, but if it is given i.p.

as a single bolus, it has a poor safety margin, and mortality can be high. Recovery from pentobarbitone anaesthesia is slow, and may be associated with convulsive movements and paddling. Pentobarbitone is best used at low doses to induce anaesthesia with an inhaled agent used to provide analgesia, or for terminal anaesthesia. In concentrated form, pentobarbitone is used for euthanasia.

**Thiopentone**   Thiopentone is a thiobarbiturate, which must be injected i.v., as it is very irritant if given perivascularly. It acts rapidly after injection, inducing anaesthesia almost immediately, and should be given carefully to avoid overdosage. It takes several days to be broken down by the liver, but anaesthesia is of short duration because thiopentone is absorbed by the body fat, and taken away from the CNS. Therefore, the duration and depth of anaesthesia produced with thiopentone depends on the amount of drug injected, the speed of the injection, and the rate of absorption by the body fat. It should be used with extreme care in animals with low body fat levels. It is not suitable for repeated injections for maintenance, as it builds up in the body causing prolonged anaesthesia. It tends to produce apnoea on induction, muscle relaxation is poor, and it is poorly analgesic. To improve analgesia, thiopentone should be given after premedication with a suitable analgesic, such as buprenorphine, and anaesthesia supplemented with an inhaled agent or opiate analgesic.

## Combination techniques

Using several anaesthetics together can overcome many of the disadvantages encountered when using the agents individually. For example, administering sedatives prior to induction with an inhaled agent, or inducing anaesthesia with an injectable agent, reduces the stress otherwise caused by induction with inhaled agents. Some injectable agents produce little analgesia alone, and addition of a low concentration of an inhaled agent is a safe way of providing this. Similarly, when using an inhaled agent as the major component of an anaesthetic regime, the concentration that is required to produce surgical anaesthesia can be reduced by administering a potent analgesic (such as fentanyl). During prolonged procedures this supplementation can be given intermittently during periods of major surgical stimulation. Induction of anaesthetic can be carried out using injectable combinations, such as ketamine, medetomidine and butorphanol, which is a particularly useful combination for use in wild animals.

The aim of these *balanced anaesthetic* regimens is to minimise the interference to the animal's physiology caused by the drugs, and to enable recovery to be smooth, rapid and pain free. Factors that may be taken into consideration when choosing an inhalational anaesthetic or an i.p. injection are outlined in Figure 7.9.

## Non-recovery anaesthesia

The same pre- and intra-operative care should be given to animals undergoing terminal procedures as to those which will recover. In fact, as terminal procedures are more likely to involve invasive techniques the animal will require more care. Some anaesthetics are only suitable for non-recovery procedures, for example pentobarbitone, which is poorly analgesic and associated with high mortality.

| | i.p. Injectable | Inhalational |
|---|---|---|
| Equipment required | Minimal | Considerable |
| Handling required | Considerable | Minimal |
| Induction and recovery speed | Slow | Rapid |
| Predictability | Moderate | High |
| Encumbrance during surgery | None | Moderate |
| Depth adjustment during maintenance | Difficult | Easy |
| Safety margin | Moderate | High |

Disadvantages (shaded)
Advantages (unshaded)

**Figure 7.9**   Choice of general anaesthetic.

## Long-term anaesthesia

Long-term anaesthesia may be achieved with intermittent injections. Inevitably, the plane of anaesthesia varies markedly. If the top up is not administered in time, the animal may experience pain, so good anaesthetic monitoring is essential. One of the best methods is to administer an anaesthetic i.v. by continuous infusion (e.g. Saffan, propofol or fentanyl/midazolam). Short-acting agents enable the plasma concentration and depth of anaesthesia to be adjusted quickly, and recovery is likely to be rapid. Many different types of infusion pump are now available to facilitate administration. Long-term anaesthesia can also be achieved by the use of inhaled agents for maintenance, after induction with inhaled or injectable agents.

## Local anaesthesia

Local anaesthetics act directly on nerves to block the conduction of impulses thus eliminating pain and other sensations. Local anaesthesia can be achieved by two methods.

### Topical application

This can be useful for anaesthetising sensitive areas. For the cornea and conjunctiva, drops (Ophthaine) are utilised; for the larynx, an aerosol may be used prior to intubation to prevent laryngospasm (Intubeaze) or on the skin, 'EMLA' cream is used prior to placement of i.v. cannulae. Ethyl chloride spray, which acts by cooling, is widely used to desensitise the tail tip in mice before amputation for DNA analysis.

### Infiltration of the skin and underlying tissues

This method is useful for minor techniques, such as skin biopsies or suturing minor wounds. It is administered using small syringes with very fine needles. This method can be very useful for provision of post-operative analgesia although care must be taken that the use of preparations with adrenaline does not delay wound healing. It may be used around the site of skin incisions for laparotomy in ruminants.

## *Regional anaesthesia*

This is the use of injectable local anaesthetic to desensitise a nerve or a number of nerves supplying a particular area. The use of nerve blocks for regional anaesthesia requires a detailed knowledge of anatomy and specific training in the techniques. The technique can be used for specific nerve blocks, such as the pudendal nerve for work in the pudendal region, the cornual nerve block for dehorning or foot blocks using specific nerves to regions of the feet in horses.

### *Paravertebral anaesthesia*

This is the blocking of several lumbar spinal nerves as they emerge from the vertebral column to produce desensitisation of the flank. This method is useful in ruminants.

### *Epidural anaesthesia*

The injection of local anaesthetic into the CSF filled space between the dura mater and the wall of the vertebral canal produces desensitisation of the region posterior to the site and is known as epidural anaesthesia. This is a useful technique to provide anaesthesia of the pelvic region in cattle and sheep, and may be used post-operatively to provide continuing analgesia.

Although local anaesthetics may be very successfully used in the post-operative period as an adjunct to other methods of pain control; in order to produce adequate restraint of animals used in most laboratory procedures and to reduce stress, it is usually preferable to use general anaesthetics for procedures.

Whatever method of anaesthesia is selected, high standards of patient care are essential, if meaningful research data are to be obtained and animal welfare is to be maintained. When designing your experiment and considering the anaesthetic protocol, ask your named veterinary surgeon (NVS) for advice on the most appropriate method.

For doses of anaesthetic agents for each species, see Section 2.

## ANAESTHETIC MANAGEMENT

All anaesthetic drugs will, if given in sufficient quantity, cause death. On the other hand, if insufficient is given, the animal will feel pain. To prevent these two extremes from occurring, care must be taken in the maintenance of *respiratory function*, *circulatory function* and *body temperature*, and in monitoring the *depth of anaesthesia*.

## Depth of anaesthesia

Anaesthesia cannot be described simply as awake, asleep or dead. Historically, it has been described as having four stages, with stage three (surgical anaesthesia) being divided into three planes. This classification was devised in man for use with a single volatile anaesthetic, and relies on assessment of cardiovascular and respiratory signs. In animals, with different species and for balanced anaesthetic regimes using combin-ations of drugs, this becomes unworkable. There exists a spectrum of levels of consciousness/depth of anaesthesia and it is essential to know where in that spectrum the animal is at any time.

The animal should be monitored frequently, at least every 5 min, or more often if stability has not been established, so that the anaesthetist knows exactly what depth of anaesthesia the animal has reached. More than one sign should be monitored. The depth cannot be judged from one sign alone, in isolation from the rest of the animal. The different combinations of drugs used and the nature of the procedure should be borne in mind, as these will affect the depth of anaesthesia.

There must be maintenance of adequate tissue oxygenation and removal of waste carbon dioxide. The amount of oxygen reaching the tissues depends on several factors as demonstrated by the oxygen flux equation:

$$O_2 \text{ available} = Q \times \text{arterial saturation } (\%) \times \text{Hb} \times K$$

where $Q$ is cardiac output (depends on the efficacy of the heart) in ml/min, arterial saturation (of the blood) depends on efficacy of the lungs, Hb is the haemoglobin level (g/ml) and $K$ is the constant, equal to 1.36.

Minor changes to one part of the equation may have little effect, but if there are changes in several parts, the overall effect is magnified. Health problems can affect any or all parts of the equation, leading to a reduction in the quantity of oxygen available to the tissues. As general anaesthesia will reduce both cardiac output and lung efficiency, the combined effects of disease and anaesthesia can cause a severe reduction in tissue oxygen levels leading to hypoxia or even death.

It must be ensured that sufficient depth of analgesia has been reached to prevent the animal perceiving pain, and that consciousness has been lost to a sufficient degree to prevent distress. This can only be judged by the presence or absence of certain reflexes, and by assessment of vital functions. The pedal withdrawal reflex is the most commonly used reflex, also pinching the tail or ear. The responses are abolished if surgical anaesthesia has been reached, but they give no indication if the anaesthesia is too deep. In this state, the animal may be in danger of dying from respiratory and cardiovascular failure. The signs are development of a fixed, staring eye, slow shallow breathing, or deep gasping breaths, blue coloration of the mucous membranes and a fall in blood pressure. *Monitoring of the vital signs will detect these changes early on, and enable action to be taken to prevent deterioration.*

## *Respiration*

This is easily monitored, and assessments should be made of the *rate*, *depth* and *pattern* of breathing. This is done by watching the movement of the chest wall, or reservoir bag, or in larger animals by the use of an oesophageal stethoscope. It is wise to use an apnoea alarm, even if using a mechanical ventilator, as these can be accidentally disconnected very easily. The effectiveness of pulmonary gas exchange can be assessed by the *colour of the mucous membranes*, and of blood being shed at the site of surgery. Virtually all anaesthetics cause some respiratory depression, leading to hypoxia and hypercapnia. Hypoxia may be indicated if the colour of blood or mucous membranes changes, but hypercapnia is not. Providing the animal with oxygen intra-operatively helps to prevent the development of hypoxia. Carbon dioxide concentration can be assessed by measuring the end-tidal $CO_2$, or by direct arterial blood-gas analysis. Transcutaneous $O_2$- and $CO_2$-monitoring equipment can be used in some species.

The respiratory rate usually falls during anaesthesia, and a fall of up to 50% from the normal is acceptable. If the rate continues to drop, there may be a problem. If the animal is not breathing, it is not necessarily too deeply anaesthetised. It may be too light, and holding its breath, which demonstrates the need to monitor more than one variable. Apnoea on induction of anaesthetic is common, particularly with the use of certain anaesthetic agents. If there is genuine apnoea, first ensure that the airway is unobstructed. The oropharynx may be blocked with mucus or blood particularly in very small animals, or the endotracheal tube may be kinked. Make sure that the thoracic movements are not restricted by the position of the animal, or by limbs being tied down too tightly. Check that undue pressure is not being placed on the chest wall by over-enthusiastic use of retractors, or by the use of the animal as an arm rest.

Respiration can be stimulated by moving the endotracheal tube, artificial ventilation, needle stimulation of the nasal philtrum or by respiratory stimulants (such as doxapram). Respiratory depression due to neuroleptanalgesic combinations can be reversed with naloxone, and medetomidine can be reversed with atipamezole, but only if surgery has been completed. In most instances, it is advantageous for the animal to be intubated, or in non-recovery cases for a tracheotomy to be performed, to facilitate intermittant positive pressure ventilation (IPPV). Even if IPPV is not required, this enables a clear airway to be maintained.

## *Cardiovascular signs*

The simplest method of monitoring is to assess the rate, rhythm and quality of the *pulse*, using a superficial artery depending on the species. An oesophageal stethoscope will indicate heart rate and rhythm, and *capillary refill time* indicates tissue perfusion. This can be tested by applying pressure briefly to a mucous membrane to blanch it, then measuring how long it takes for the pink colour to return. It should take less than 2–3 s.

Cardiac failure may occur dramatically as cardiac arrest, but more usually it is gradual in onset, and monitoring can prevent a disaster. Some anaesthetics cause a fall in cardiac output, and hypotension. Hypoxia and hypercapnia, resulting from respiratory depression, cause cardiac dysrhythmias. Loss of blood or body fluids can cause hypovolaemic shock and cardiac arrest. Blood loss commonly causes death in small rodents because a small loss represents a high proportion of the animals' total blood volume. This problem can be minimised if careful attention is paid to surgical technique. Use of a blood donor is a potentially useful technique in large species. Transfusion reactions are rarely encountered with an initial transfusion, and never if an animal of the same inbred strain is used.

A secure venous line should be established for infusion of fluids for circulatory support. This allows easy administration of analgesics and anaesthetics, and facilitates dosing with stimulant drugs in case of an emergency. An electrocardiogram (ECG) will give an indication of cardiac function, but it only indicates the electrical activity of the heart. It is possible to have a normal ECG with a cardiac output of zero for a short while. A pulse oximeter will indicate the blood oxygenation level and the pulse rate.

## Body temperature

It is essential to monitor this, but particularly in small animals. All anaesthetics affect thermoregulation, and an animal's body temperature will fall unless measures are taken to prevent this. The fall is exacerbated by the flow of cold air from the anaesthetic machine, shaving the animal, use of cold skin preps, placing on a cold operating table, exposing viscera during surgery and administering cold fluids. Smaller animals have a larger surface area to volume ratio, so are particularly susceptible to heat loss. Animals smaller than 1 kg in weight will require extra heating to avoid a drop in body temperature.

Temperature can be monitored using a rectal or oesophageal probe, and core temperature can be compared with skin surface temperature. The difference should be less than 2–3°C. Alternatively, the temperature can be monitored by simply feeling the animals' paws and ears. Heat loss can be minimised by insulation, with cotton wool, Vetbed, foil or bubble packing. Additional heating can be provided with heat lamps or heating blankets (see Chapter 8). Care must be taken not to burn the animal, and a thermostatically controlled heating pad is the best solution. If fluids are to be given, these should be warmed first. A bag of i.v. fluid can easily be warmed to body temperature by immersing it in warm water, or using an instant heat pouch.

It is important to ensure that measures to prevent hypothermia are continued throughout the recovery period. This can be achieved in small animals by using incubators. For adults, the temperature should be 25–30°C, and for neonates 35–37°C. Bedding also helps provide insulation (e.g. Vetbed, tissue paper). Sawdust should not be used as this will stick to the animal's nose and mouth, or to wound surfaces. Hypothermia is the commonest cause of mortality in small rodents or slow recovery in other species, so monitoring of body temperature and taking steps to prevent hypothermia are vitally important.

## Ocular signs

These can be useful in some circumstances but are variable indicators of the depth of anaesthesia. The palpebral reflex is lost at variable times depending on the species. In rodents it is hard to assess, and in rabbits it may not be lost until anaesthesia is very deep. If ketamine is used, the reflex is abolished very early. The corneal reflex is lost later and may be seen when drops are applied to moisturise the cornea.

Observation of the position of the eyeball, the degree of pupillary dilatation, and whether nystagmus is occurring are all useful indicators once experience is gained with one species and a particular anaesthetic regime.

## Equipment monitoring

Aside from monitoring vital signs, it is useful to monitor the *continued function of the anaesthetic delivery system*. Infusion pumps and anaesthetic machines should be fitted with alarms, which sound when the machines fail, or are empty. Also personnel carrying out prolonged procedures may become fatigued, and steps should be taken to prevent this. Records should be kept of the measurements as this enables adverse trends to be easily spotted and corrective action taken. It also allows a series of anaesthetics to be compared. Overall, anaesthetic monitoring depends on watching the animal very closely and writing down the measurements of the vital signs so as to be able to detect adverse trends and take appropriate action as soon as a problem is detected. An example of an anaesthetic record chart is shown at Figure 7.10. It is important to constantly *refine* the anaesthetic protocol as well as other parts of the experimental procedure to take into account developments in this field.

## Anaesthetic emergencies

If an animal goes into circulatory arrest, during or after an anaesthetic, and the cerebral circulation is not restored within 3 min, irreversible brain damage will occur. In order to maintain tissue oxygen levels, blood must first contain sufficient oxygen, and second, circulate properly to and from the tissues.

PIL holder . . . . . . . . . . . . . . . . . . . . . . . . . PPL No . . . . . . . . . . . . . . . . . . . . . . . . Date . . . . . . . . . . . . . . . . . . . . . . .

Species/strain . . . . . . . . . . . . . . . . . . . . . . Age . . . . . . . . . . . . . . . . . . . . . . . . . . . Sex . . . . . . . . . . . . . . . . . . . . . . . . . . .

Procedure . . . . . . . . . . . . . . . . . . . . . . . . . . . . . . . . . . . . . . . . . . . . . . . . . . . . . . . . . . . . . . . . . . . . . . . . . . . . . . . .

**Pre-Op details**

Temp . . . . . . . . . . . . . . . . . . . . . . . . °C  Pulse . . . . . . . . . . . . . . . . . . . . . . . ./min  Resp . . . . . . . . . . . . . . . . . . . . . ./min

Eating . . . . . . . . . . . . . . . . . . . . . . . . . Behaviour . . . . . . . . . . . . . . . . . . . . . . . . . . . . . (0 = normal; 4 = grossly abnormal)

Weight . . . . . . . . . . . . . . . . . . . . . . . Risk . . . . . . . . . . . . . . . . . . . . . . . . . . . . . . . . . . . . . . . . (0 = low; 4 = high)

| Time | | | | | | | | | | | | | | | | | | | |
|------|--|--|--|--|--|--|--|--|--|--|--|--|--|--|--|--|--|--|--|
| 300 | | | | | | | | | | | | | | | | | | | |
| 280 | | | | | | | | | | | | | | | | | | | |
| 260 | | | | | | | | | | | | | | | | | | | |
| 240 | | | | | | | | | | | | | | | | | | | |
| 220 | | | | | | | | | | | | | | | | | | | |
| 200 | | | | | | | | | | | | | | | | | | | |
| 180 | | | | | | | | | | | | | | | | | | | |
| 160 | | | | | | | | | | | | | | | | | | | |
| 140 | | | | | | | | | | | | | | | | | | | |
| 120 | | | | | | | | | | | | | | | | | | | |
| 100 | | | | | | | | | | | | | | | | | | | |
| 80 | | | | | | | | | | | | | | | | | | | |
| 60 | | | | | | | | | | | | | | | | | | | |
| 40 | | | | | | | | | | | | | | | | | | | |
| 20 | | | | | | | | | | | | | | | | | | | |

● Pulse   ○ Respiration   x Blood pressure

| Drugs given | | | | | | | | | | | | | | | | | | Total dose |
|-------------|--|--|--|--|--|--|--|--|--|--|--|--|--|--|--|--|--|------------|
| 1 | | | | | | | | | | | | | | | | | | |
| 2 | | | | | | | | | | | | | | | | | | |
| 3 | | | | | | | | | | | | | | | | | | |

Recovery . . . . . . . . . . . . . . . . . . . . . . . . . . . . . . . . . . . . . . . . . . . . . . . . . . . . . . . . . . . . . . . . . . . . . . . . . . . . . . . . . . . . . . . . . .

Post operative care instructions . . . . . . . . . . . . . . . . . . . . . . . . . . . . . . . . . . . . . . . . . . . . . . . . . . . . . . . . . . . . . . . . . . . . .

**Figure 7.10**   Record of general anaesthetic.

Therefore, monitoring and resuscitation attempts are directed towards:

- A for airway
- B for breathing and
- C for circulation, in that order.

The development of hypothermia should be considered whenever recovery from anaesthetic is slow, particularly in small animals in which it is a serious problem. It may be caused by reduced heat production or increased heat loss. Little can be done to increase heat production. To reduce heat loss, the fur should not be wetted excessively and dry drapes should be used to minimise evaporative losses. The environment should be warm, and ideally the operating table should be heated. A water blanket kept at 38°C is best. Fluids to be administered should first be heated to 38°C. Shivering to increase heat production results in an increase in oxygen demand; therefore, oxygen should be given to the hypothermic animal.

## MUSCLE RELAXATION IN ANAESTHESIA

Relaxation is part of the triad of anaesthesia (narcosis, analgesia and relaxation). The aim is to relax muscles to facilitate access to body cavities and to allow limbs to be moved easily. This reduces any damage caused to the muscles by using excess traction when trying to overcome muscle tone.

During anaesthesia, the abolition of muscle tone can be brought about in three ways:

1. The anaesthetic agents themselves, by acting on the CNS, decrease activity in the ventral horn cells of the spinal cord and produce relaxation of the muscles. The degree of relaxation will vary depending on the individual agent or the combination of agents used, for example, ketamine produces very little relaxation on its own but there will be good relaxation if it is used in combination with medetomidine or benzodiazepines.
2. Peripherally acting local analgesics can be injected into a muscle mass or around nerves to isolate the muscle from nervous input and produce relaxation.
3. Relaxation may be produced by the use of neuromuscular blocking agents.

*The use of neuromuscular blocking agents is strictly controlled under the ASPA. Specific permission must be obtained from the Secretary of State at the Home Office and it must be clearly written into the Project Licence. Guidelines on the use of neuromuscular blocking agents are available on the Home Office website.*

### Monitoring anaesthesia under neuromuscular blocking agents

Neuromuscular blockers have no narcotic or analgesic effects. Their administration abolishes all ability to respond to pain but does not abolish the ability to feel pain. It is essential to ensure complete unconsciousness of all animals to which they are administered. Many of the normal reflexes used to judge the depth of anaesthesia are abolished with neuromuscular blockers (e.g. palpebral reflex, pedal withdrawal reflex) so other methods need to be employed to monitor the depth of anaesthesia under these conditions. Commonly used parameters are as follows:

- Blood pressure.
- Heart rate.
- Twitching of muscles in response to surgical stimulation indicates that the depth of anaesthesia or neuromuscular block is inadequate.
- Electroencephalogram (EEG) is sometimes used to monitor the depth of anaesthesia in experimental animals. However, the interpretation of the EEG is often open to question and there is not always direct correlation with the level of narcosis. The reliability of this method is currently a matter of some discussion. It is perhaps relevant that monitoring of the EEG is not routinely used as the sole method of measuring the depth of narcosis in human clinical practice.

It is essential to use an endotracheal tube when using neuromuscular blockers to maintain the airway and because relaxation of the oesophagus can result in regurgitation. An endotracheal tube facilitates IPPV and prevents air from being forced into the stomach and intestines during forced breathing. To measure the degree of neuromuscular blockade, two features are studied:

1. The use of peripheral nerve stimulation to determine muscle response (so-called 'train of four response').
2. Clinical monitoring for the presence or absence of respiratory efforts in the anaesthetised animal. The intercostal muscles and the diaphragm are generally the last muscles to become paralysed by neuromuscular blockers and the first to recover. However, monitoring these alone is inadequate to monitor the depth of anaesthesia.

## Neuromuscular blocking agents

Sometimes simply called muscle relaxants, these produce paralysis of the skeletal muscles by blocking transmission of impulses from nerve endings across the neuromuscular junction (NMJ). There are two main types of neuromuscular blocking agents: the depolarising agents/blockers and the non-depolarising agents/blockers.

### Depolarising agents

These act by mimicking the action of the normal transmitter (acetylcholine, ACh) at the NMJ. As a result, these agents cause initial generalised muscle twitches, followed by complete skeletal paralysis. The main example of a depolarising blocker is suxamethonium. Depolarising blockers are usually short acting and are allowed to wear off naturally. Anticholinesterases should not be used with depolarising blockers as they simply serve to increase the depolarisation at the NMJ prolonging the block.

### Non-depolarising agents

These are sometimes called competitive blockers since they work by competing with ACh for its receptors at the NMJ. By limiting the number of molecules of ACh which can bind to the muscle membrane, they reduce the degree of depolarisation of the membrane in response to nerve impulses arriving at the NMJ. Examples of non-depolarising blockers are pancuronium, rocuronium, mivacurium, alcuronium, atracurium, vecuronium and gallamine. The effects of competitive blockers can be reversed by the administration of anticholinesterase drugs, such as neostigmine, edrophonium or pyridostigmine, which block the activity of enzymes that break down ACh. These drugs increase the quantity of ACh present at the NMJ, displacing the neuromuscular blocker and returning the function of the NMJ to normal.

## A GUIDE TO ANAESTHETICS/ANALGESICS AND RELATED DRUGS*

| Drug name | Trade name | Manufacturers |
|---|---|---|
| Acepromazine | ACP | Novartis Animal Health |
| Alfentanil | Rapifen | Janssen-Cilag |
| Alphaxalone/ alphadolone | Saffan | Schering-Plough Animal Health |
| Atipamezole | Antisedan | Pfizer |
| Atracurium | Tracrium | GlaxoSmithKline |
| Atropine | Atrocare | Animalcare |
| Azaperone | Stresnil | Janssen Animal Health |
| Bupivicaine | Marcain | AstraZeneca |
| Buprenorphine | Vetergesic | Animalcare |
|  | Temgesic | Schering-Plough |
| Butorphanol | Torbugesic | Fort Dodge Animal Health |
|  | Torbutrol | Fort Dodge Animal Health |
| Carprofen | Rimadyl | Pfizer |
| Diazepam | Valium | Roche |
| Doxapram | Dopram V | Fort Dodge Animal Health |
| Etomidate | Hypnomidate | Janssen-Cilag |
| Ethyl chloride | Cryogesic | Acorus |
| Fentanyl | Sublimaze | Janssen-Cilag |
| Fentanyl/ fluanisone | Hypnorm | Janssen Animal Health |
| Flunixin | Finadyne | Schering-Plough Animal Health |
| Gallamine | Flaxedil | Concord |
| Glycopyrronium | Robinul | Anpharm |
| Halothane | Fluothane | Schering-Plough Animal Health |
|  | Halothane-Vet | Merial Animal Health |
|  | Vetothane | Virbac |
| Isoflurane | Isocare | Animalcare |
|  | Isofane | Novartis Animal Health |
|  | Isoflo | Schering-Plough Animal Health |
|  | Isoflurane Vet | Merial Animal Health |
|  | Vetflurane | Virbac |
| Ketamine | Ketaset | Fort Dodge Animal Health |
|  | Vetalar | Pharmacia Animal Health |
| Ketoprofen | Ketofen | Merial Animal Health |
| Lignocaine | Intubeaze | Arnolds Veterinary Products |
| Lignocaine with adrenaline | Lignavet Plus | Novartis Animal Health |
|  | Lignadrin | Vetoquinol, UK |
|  | Lignol | Arnolds Veterinary Products |
|  | Locaine | Animalcare |
|  | Locovetic | Bimeda |
| Lignocaine with prilocaine | EMLA | AstraZeneca |
| Medetomidine | Domitor | Pfizer |
| Meclofenamic acid | Arquel V | Pharmacia Animal Health |
| Meloxicam | Metacam | Boehringer Ingelheim |
| Mepivacaine | Intra-Epicaine | Arnolds Veterinary Products |
| Morphine | Morphine | Non-proprietary |
| Nalbuphine | Nubain | BMS |
| Naloxone | Narcan | BMS |
| Neostigmine with glycopyrronium | Robinul neostigmine | Anpharm |
| Pancuronium | Pavulon | Organon |
| Pentazocine | Fortral | Sterwin |

*Drug trade names and manufacturers tend to change. This listing is a guide only.

| Pentobarbitone 200 mg/ml (for euthanasia) | Dolethal | Vetoquinol |
| | Euthatal | Merial Animal Health |
| | Lethobarb | Fort Dodge Animal Health |
| | Pentoject | Animalcare |
| Pethidine | Pethidine | Arnolds Veterinary Products |
| | Pamergan | Martindale |
| Phenylbutazone | Equipalazone | Arnolds Veterinary Products |
| | Phenogel | Fort Dodge Animal Health |
| | Phenycare | Animalcare |
| | Pro-Dynam | Leo Laboratories |
| Piroxicam | Feldene | Pfizer |
| Prilocaine | Citanest | AstraZeneca |
| Procaine | Willcain | Arnold Veterinary Products |
| Propofol | Rapinovet | Schering-Plough Animal Health |
| Romifidine | Sedivet | Boehringer Ingelheim |
| Sufentanil | Sufenta | Janssen |
| Suxamethonium | Anectine | GlaxoSmithKline |
| Thiopentone | Intraval Sodium | Merial Animal Health |
| | Thiovet | Novartis Animal Health |
| Tolfenamic acid | Tolfedine | Vetoquinol, UK |
| Vecuronium | Norcuron | Organon |
| Xylazine | Chanazine | Chanelle Animal Health |
| | Xylazine | Millpledge |
| | Xylacare | Animalcare |
| | Rompun | Bayer |

# FURTHER INFORMATION

Alexander, D.J. and Clark, G.C. (1980). A simple method of oral endotracheal intubation in rabbits. *Laboratory Animal Science* 30, 871–73.

Conlon, K.C., Corbally, M.T., Bading, J.R. and Brennan, M.F. (1990). Atraumatic endotracheal intubation in small rabbits. *Laboratory Animal Science* 40, 221–22.

Davies, A., Dallak, M. and Moores, C. (1996). Oral endotracheal intubation of rabbits (*Oryctolagus cuniculus*). *Laboratory Animals* 30, 182–83.

Flecknell, P.A. (1996). *Laboratory Animal Anaesthesia* (2nd edn). Academic Press, London.

Green, C.H., Knight, J., Precious, S. and Simpkin, S. (1981). Ketamine alone and combined with diazepam or xylazine in laboratory animals: a 10 year experience. *Laboratory Animals* 15(2), 163–70.

Hall, L.W. and Clarke, K.W. (1991). *Veterinary Anaesthesia* (9th edn). Ballière Tindall, London.

Hendenqvist, P., Roughan, J.V., Antunes, L., Orr, H. and Flecknell, P.A. (2001). Induction of anaesthesia with desflurane and isoflurane in the rabbit. *Laboratory Animals* 35, 172–79.

Hendenqvist, P., Roughan, J.V., Orr, H. and Antunes, L. (2001). Assessment of ketamine/medetomidine anaesthesia in the New Zealand White rabbit. *Veterinary Anaesthesia and Analgesia* 28, 18–25.

Kohn, D.F., Wixson, S.F., White, W. and Benson, J.G. (1997). *Anaesthesia and Analgesia in Laboratory Animals*. New York Academic Press.

Lumb, W.V. and Jones, W.E. (1984). *Veterinary Anaesthesia*. Lea and Febiger, Philadelphia.

Osofsky and Hirch (2000). Chemical restraint of endangered mammals for conservation purposes: a practical primer. *Oryx* 34, 27–33.

Short, C.E. (ed.) (1987). *Principles and Practice of Veterinary Anaesthesia*. Williams and Wilkins, Baltimore; pp. 28–46.

Soulsby, Lord and Morton D. (2000). Pain: its nature and management in man and animals. *International Congress and Symposium*, Series 246, Royal Society of Medicine Press.

Smith, A.C. and Swindle, M.M. (1994). *Research Animal Anaesthesia*. Analgesia and Surgery Scientists Centre for Animal Welfare.

Vickers, M.D., Schnieden, H. and Wood-Smith, F.G. (1984). *Drugs in Anaesthetic Practice*. Butterworths, Sevenoaks.

# Chapter 8

# Management of pain, suffering, distress and lasting harm

By carrying out work under the Animal (Scientific Procedures) Act 1986 (ASPA) you are, by definition, doing something that has 'the potential to cause pain, suffering, distress or lasting harm (P, S, D or LH)'. Under the Act, 'P, S, D & LH' are to be interpreted in their widest sense, to include death, disease, injury, physiological and psychological stress, significant discomfort or any disturbance to normal health. Section 19b vi of the project licence should outline the steps that will be taken to prevent, or minimise, this suffering, as required by Section 5.5 of the ASPA and standard condition 6 of the project licence. Animals do not suffer simply because they are being used in experimental procedures; this is a myth promoted by anti-vivisectionsists. However, they do all have the *potential* to suffer and it is the responsibility of the licensees working with the animal to ensure this is prevented or controlled. In many experiments, it can be prevented altogether; in others, some degree of suffering may be justified by the cost–benefit analysis and this will be minimised by the use of scoring systems, such as described in Chapter 4. In considering the prevention of P, S, D or LH, it is first necessary to consider the ways in which these states might arise. It is not simply a question of considering surgical pain, there are many other ways that the animal may be adversely affected.

The management of P, S, D and LH can be divided into three phases: first it has to be recognised, then quantified and then alleviated. The first two of these phases are dealt with in Chapter 4. The alleviation can be divided into first, animal care and second, the use of analgesic drugs (see Figure 8.1). The standards of animal care and husbandry must be as high as possible to ensure that the animals do not needlessly suffer from an inability

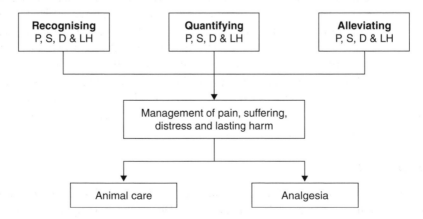

**Figure 8.1** Management of distress.

to express their normal behavioural repertoire (see Chapter 6). It may be that the addition of some specific changes to the husbandry regimes will be appropriate to prevent certain types of suffering. For example, animals used as a model of arthritic disease, that may potentially suffer joint stiffness, will benefit from the provision of softer, deeper bedding to lie on, and food and water supplies being provided nearby instead of having to climb on a food hopper to reach them. Monitoring parameters such as body weight or individual food and water consumption helps provide an assessment of progress.

## ANIMAL CARE: MANAGEMENT OF DISTRESS

### Fluid balance

It is vitally important to maintain fluid balance and support the circulation. Swabs can be weighed to estimate the loss of blood during surgery, but blood also seeps into drapes and body cavities and this blood loss may pass unnoticed. Plasma loss occurs by exudation from tissues and into the peritoneal cavity during prolonged abdominal surgery. The extracellular fluid is depleted by evaporation from the respiratory tract, exposed viscera and wounds. In a normal animal, loss of 15–20% of circulating blood volume will cause signs of hypovolaemic shock. In an anaesthetised animal, many of the mechanisms that normally maintain physiological stability are depressed, so losses which are less severe than 15% can have serious consequences.

In addition to these losses, the animal may not drink for 12–24 h post-operatively. Fluids *must* be given to replace the losses and to cover the period when intake is low. Only isotonic solutions should be given for fluid replacement. The requirement is *40–80 ml/kg/24 h*, and this is best given orally if the animal is conscious and can swallow. Depending on the species, the fluid can be offered as a drink or administered orally via syringe, gavage tube or stomach tube. Alternatively, moist food can be offered, such as mashes to large animals or 'Transgel' (Charles River Ltd.) or reconstituted fruit jelly to rodents. For some species, it is advisable to use convalescent diets in the immediate post-operative period. Pedigree Petfoods and Hills Pet Products both make convalescent diets for dogs and cats. Rats will also take 'Lectade' rehydration therapy very readily. The subcutaneous route provides a rapid and practical route for fluid therapy for the small animal weighing less than 7 kg, but this provides a way for administering fluids over a short-time period only. Intravenous fluids are the best means of fluid therapy for the severely dehydrated, hypotensive animal. It allows a controlled delivery rate to meet the changing needs of the animal. It requires the insertion of an intravenous cannula under sterile technique and the sterile maintenance of the intravenous delivery system (see Chapter 9). Intra-osseous fluid therapy can be used if the intravenous approach is impossible. The selection of needle size (18–23 gauge) will depend on the animal's size. The preferred sites for needle insertion are wing of the ilium, proximal femur and tibial crest, but care must be taken to avoid trauma to growth plates.

### *Fluid selection*

Isotonic fluids contain the same osmolality as the extracellular fluids. Commonly used isotonic solutions include 0.9% (normal) saline, lactated Ringer's (Hartmann's solution), Ringer's, acetated Ringer's and 4% dextrose in 0.18% saline (glucosaline).

Lactated Ringer's solution is a polyionic, isotonic solution. Each litre of lactated Ringer's solution is superior to isotonic saline because its electrolyte concentration is similar to that of blood. In addition, the lactate will be converted to bicarbonate by the animal's liver, if it is required to correct acid–base balance. Lactated Ringer's solution is commonly used as a routine rehydrating and maintenance solution, as a plasma space volume expander in the treatment of shock, and as the fluid of choice in the acidotic animal. As the bicarbonate derived from the lactate can propagate alkalemia, this solution should not be used if the animal has metabolic or respiratory alkalosis. The uses and restrictions of acetated Ringer's solution are similar to those for lactated Ringer's. However the acetated solution is not recommended for treating ketoacidosis because the acetate can serve as a substrate for the production of increased levels of aceto-acetate. 'Physiologic', 0.9% saline is also isotonic and commonly used for rehydration. Dextrose 4% in 0.18% saline is nearly isotonic and is a useful maintenance solution.

Hypotonic solutions have an osmolality that is less than blood and extracellular fluid. The most commonly used product is 5% dextrose solution. Dextrose in water should never be the sole intravenous fluid in animals receiving maintenance therapy because of the electrolyte depletion states that can result, namely hyponatraemia, hypochloraemia, hypokalaemia and hypomagnesaemia. In addition, this solution should not be administered subcutaneously because extracellular electrolytes will tend to diffuse into the area. When this occurs, the reduction of plasma solute can lower the circulating blood volume and result in hypotension. Dextrose 5% solution should not be given to correct extracellular volume depletion because two-thirds of the volume will enter the intracellular space, thereby failing to appropriately expand the plasma space.

Hypertonic solutions have a greater osmolality than blood and extracellular fluid. The most common type is dextrose 5% in 0.9% saline. It can be used as a partial maintenance solution once the animal is completely rehydrated, or for emergency correction of hypovolemia in a normally hydrated animal. Its administration should be restricted to the intravenous route. This solution should not be used in a dehydrated animal because it will promote cellular dehydration and intensify the hypovolaemia by stimulating a diuresis.

## *Fluid volume replacement*

The animal's fluid needs can be divided into

- rehydration
- maintenance.

For all practical purposes, the amount needed to correct dehydration deficits can be assessed from the degree of skin turgor, pulse rate and pulse quality. The degrees of dehydration range from 5% to 10% according to the magnitude of severity. Skin turgor assessment in the obese animal might be an unreliable index because the adipose tissue maintains its elasticity despite negative water balance. The older animal will normally show a decrease in skin elasticity, thereby giving a misleading impression of marked dehydration that might not actually exist. To clarify matters where the physical assessment of dehydration is equivocal, presence of an elevated packed cell volume will assist. Care must be taken, while interpreting these clinicopathological parameters in that an anaemic animal with hypoproteinaemia might reveal 'normal' laboratory values, while it is dehydrated.

The determination of the fluid volume needed to correct dehydration is made using the following formula:

Volume (ml) of fluid needed = % Dehydration × Body weight (kg) × 1000

The maintenance volume is the amount normally required over a 24-h period in a euhydrated animal. Taking the insensible fluid loss into consideration, *the 24-h maintenance volume of most species is approximately 40 ml/kg*. The total 24-h fluid requirement for the dehydrated animal, therefore, amounts to the sum of the dehydration plus the maintenance and incidental loss volumes.

## Monitoring physiological function

Provided that the animal does not have renal disease, if it is producing urine its mean arterial blood pressure is likely to be greater than 70 mmHg. Therefore, this is a useful guide to the adequacy of fluid therapy. It is not necessary to catheterise the bladder to monitor urine output, simply weighing the bedding should give an accurate estimation of urinary losses, provided there is no concurrent vomiting and diarrhoea. (An increase in weight of 30 g indicates an addition of 30 ml of urine.) Reduced urine output may be due to dehydration, urinary tract injury or pain.

If the animal fails to defaecate, this may be due to absence of faeces, or paralytic ileus, which occurs if the bowels are handled excessively during surgery or with certain anaesthetic agents. Careful surgical and anaesthetic techniques are important to avoid this. Sometimes the animal is constipated, and this may be corrected by the administration of a suitable enema.

Monitoring of body weight or individual food and water consumption helps provide an assessment of recovery from surgery. In order to avoid digestive disturbances, it is beneficial to wean the animal on to a suitable convalescent diet *before* the surgery.

The animal's position must be considered carefully. If the animal is restrained in one position for a prolonged time, ensure that ties are not too tight, and that bony areas are padded to prevent pressure sores. In animals anaesthetised for a long period, and those in which ketamine has been used, the cornea must be prevented from drying by the use of a bland ophthalmic ointment or drops of false tears, such as hypromellose eye drops or viscotears liquid gel. Good sterility and surgical technique (see Chapter 10) will go a long way towards reducing post-operative problems, and reducing the need for high doses of analgesics or the use of antibiotics.

The amount of individual attention given to the animal during the post-operative period depends on the species. Companion animals react well to personal contact, whereas rodents or rabbits may be stressed by it. For procedures where it is anticipated the animal will require close monitoring post-operatively, it is advisable to habituate it to handling and nursing procedures before surgery is carried out. The design of the recovery area should take account of the species and their individual needs. The noise level, light intensity and temperature should be appropriate. The ambient light level should be fairly low for the animal's comfort, but capable of being raised to a brighter level in order to be able to examine the animal satisfactorily. If dealing with rodents, consider the ultrasound range, which may cause distress. Animals prefer a familiar environment, and may or may not prefer the presence of other animals, depending on how they were housed before surgery. Companionship must be balanced with the risk of bullying and cannibalism. The stocking density must be kept low, so recovering animals do not have to climb over each other to reach food and water. The caging and bedding must provide warmth and comfort, and keep the animal clean and dry. Some bedding materials, such as sawdust, may stick to the animal's eyes, nose and mouth and to the wound. Shredded paper is also unsuitable, as many animals will just push this to one side and end up lying directly on the floor of a plastic cage, in a pool of urine and faeces. Advantage should be taken of bedding materials, such as artificial sheepskin (Vetbed), which is absorbent, keeps the skin dry, and is comfortable if the animal is lying in one place for a long time. Grid floors should be avoided in recovery cages, as they are uncomfortable. Appropriate use of well applied bandages and pressure pads can help control pain in limbs and around the head.

The animal must be frequently observed, and the findings recorded, together with any drugs administered. The record chart should be easily available. An example of a post-operative record chart is shown in Figure 8.2 and it can be adapted to the individual needs of the procedure and combined with an appropriate welfare assessment scoring system (see Chapter 4).

## MANAGEMENT OF PAIN

Pain is unnecessary in the majority of scientific procedures, since with modern treatments it can be largely controlled. An appropriate pain management strategy should form part of the anaesthetic protocol and all animals should receive post-operative pain assessment, and additional analgesics administered if they are needed. Following their administration, the animal *must* be reassessed to ensure that the pain has been adequately controlled. On some occasions, one type of analgesic may be contraindicated, but it is most unlikely that no suitable analgesic will be available. It is important to remember that pain produces physiological changes that alter the rate of recovery from surgical procedures, and these changes may affect the experiment as well as the animal's welfare. The assessment of pain is discussed in Chapter 4.

As well as considering whether pain may be present, it is also important to consider whether the animal might be suffering 'distress' (see Chapter 4). A cold wet environment, without any suitable bedding material, is likely to cause distress to many animal species, and states of physiological imbalance, such as dehydration caused by inadequate fluid therapy, would not be referred to as painful, but could cause distress. It is important to recognise that pain can have an emotional component, and in man, both the intensity of pain as reported by the patient, and the requirement for analgesics to control pain are increased by factors such as fear and apprehension.

Pain can be alleviated by the systemic use of centrally or peripherally acting analgesics, by the use of local anaesthetics, and in the larger animals, by the application of supporting bandages to protect and immobilise damaged tissues. The particular type of treatment chosen will depend on the species, the nature of the pain, its cause, and its estimated severity and duration; but whatever treatment is chosen, the aim will be to reduce the discomfort to the animal as much as possible.

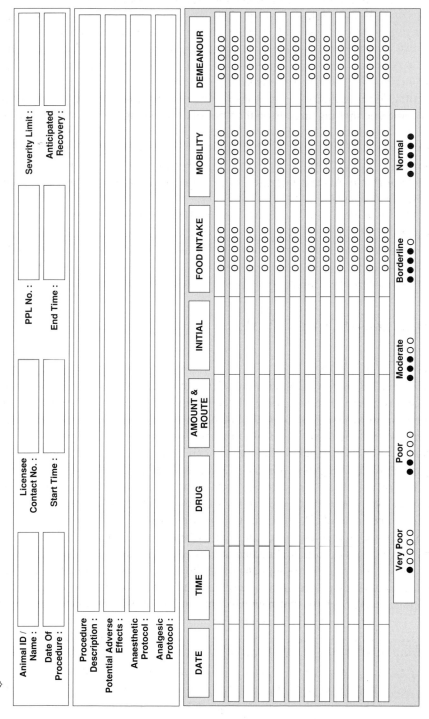

**Figure 8.2**   Post-operative record.

Experience in animals and controlled trials in man have shown that analgesics are most effective in controlling post-operative pain, if they are administered *before* pain is experienced. It is, therefore, preferable to administer analgesics either as part of the pre-anaesthetic medication, or intra-operatively before pain is perceived by the animal, as part of the balanced anaesthetic regime (see Chapter 7).

In man, it has been demonstrated that more effective pain relief is provided by the technique of administering opioids by continuous infusion rather than by intermittent dosing. This approach can be used in animals by adding opioids to intravenous fluids administered via a giving set, but there can be practical difficulties. If analgesics have been given as part of the balanced anaesthetic regime, they will control pain before it is experienced, and if extra doses are required they may be administered by constant intravenous infusion, subcutaneous or intramuscular injection, or orally. If the animal is eating and drinking normally, they may be administered with food, which reduces the disturbance caused by giving injections, and any associated stress caused to the animal. Rats will take analgesic drugs mixed into a cube of jelly, and it has been found that the preferred flavours are the berry fruits.

Whatever pain relief is given, reassessment of the animal a short time afterwards is vital to ensure that the required analgesic is actually working. In laboratory species, analgesics will usually be given by the subcutaneous, intramuscular or oral routes, and an appropriate amount of time should be allowed between the administration of the analgesic and reassessment of the animal's condition.

## Use of opioids to control pain

If pain is assessed to be moderate or severe, opioids are the drugs usually required to produce pain relief. A wide variety of different opioids are available, but the duration of action of most of them is under 4 h. However, buprenorphine has been shown to have a longer duration of action of 6–12 h in some species.

*Buprenorphine is usually the opioid analgesic of choice in laboratory animal species.*

Some researchers have expressed concern about the wide range of effects that opioids have, which are unrelated to their analgesic action. These potential side effects should not, however, be used as an excuse for withholding pain relief. The most serious consequence of overdose with opioids in man is respiratory depression. This may occasionally be seen in animals given very high doses of morphine or pethidine, or if potent agonists such as fentanyl or alfentanil are administered, and can be alleviated by the use of doxapram. Significant respiratory depression rarely occurs following the use of mixed agonist/antagonist drugs, such as buprenorphine, nalbuphine and butorphanol.

## The use of non-steroidal anti-inflammatory drugs

These compounds are very useful in the management of pain in animals, and may also be used in circumstances when the use of opioids is contraindicated. As a result of tissue injury, the enzyme phospholipase $A_2$ is activated and this leads to the detachment of arachidonic acid from cell membranes, which acts as a substrate for two enzymes, namely cyclo-oxygenase and lipo-oxygenase. The cyclo-oxygenase acts to form the eicosanoids, which include many important inflammatory mediators/modulators, such as $PGE_2$ and $PGI_2$. The analgesic, antipyretic and anti-inflammatory actions of the classical non-steroidal anti-inflammatory drugs (NSAIDs) are caused by the inhibition of cyclo-oxygenase. Lipo-oxygenase acts on arachidonic acid to form other derivatives including the leukotriene group of compounds. From Figure 8.3, it can be seen that the corticosteroids with anti-inflammatory activity act in the same biochemical pathway, but more proximally than the classical NSAIDs, and, therefore, have a wider spectrum of activity as they will inhibit both cyclo-oxygenase and lipo-oxygenase, although the mode of action is indirect via the induction of lipocortins, which have anti-phospholipase $A_2$ activity. There is, therefore, a latent period before the onset of clinical activity and, because the steroids exert their anti-inflammatory activity by other means apart from the inhibition of phospholipase $A_2$, there are more varied side effects. The use of compounds, which will exert their effects directly on both the lipo-oxygenase and cyclo-oxygenase, will have obvious advantages since they will inhibit the production of both groups of inflammatory mediators.

As well as therapeutic activity, some NSAIDs may have side effects, which include gastrointestinal ulceration, nephrotoxicity, hepatotoxicity, blood dyscrasias, urticaria and teratogenic effects. The newer NSAIDs, such as carprofen and meloxicam, are useful alternatives to opioids in the control of even quite severe post-operative pain. These are long lasting and carprofen and meloxicam do not produce gastrointestinal ulceration as readily, unlike some of the other non-steroidals. Ketoprofen is 15 times more potent than phenylbutazone and 30 times more potent than aspirin. Following

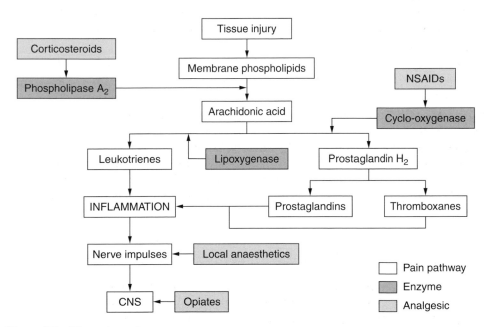

**Figure 8.3** The pain pathway.

intravenous injection, there is activity within 2 h, which reaches a peak at 12 h and is still present at 24 h. Care must be taken with the use of flunixin during the immediate post-operative period or during surgery due to potential nephrotoxicity. The predisposition to the various side effects depends on many factors including species, drug formulation, age, diet and *stress*. Good experimental design and good animal management can control most of these factors.

## Local anaesthetics

The use of agents such as xylocaine, lignocaine or bupivacaine should also be considered for controlling pain. They may be applied topically, infiltrated locally around a wound, or infiltrated around a major sensory nerve supplying a specific area of the body for regional anaesthesia. In some circumstances, this can provide a good method of post-operative pain control. Local analgesics can also be used pre-operatively, for example EMLA cream can be applied over the site of venepuncture to remove sensation from the area and make implantation of catheters or needles into the vein much easier.

## POST-OPERATIVE CARE

All of the parameters monitored during surgery (see anaesthetic monitoring, Chapter 7) should continue to be monitored in the immediate post-operative period. Some special attention will be required post-operatively, so it is preferable to have a specific recovery area where individual nursing care may be given. Emergency drugs and equipment should be available. Warmth and comfort should continue to be provided. Hypothermia is potentially a very serious problem, particularly in small animals. The recovery area should be warmer than the normal animal accommodation. To prevent post-operative hypothermia, extra heat may need to be supplied, with care being taken not to burn the animal's skin. Electronic heat pads are available with thermostats linked to the animal's body temperature. Reusable instant heat pouches provide heat anywhere without the need for electricity. The pouch must be placed within an insulating bag to prevent excess heat reaching the animal. These can also be used for warming fluids prior to injection. Respiratory depression frequently develops post-operatively, but it often goes unnoticed, resulting in death. Respiration must be monitored and treatments given as required. If depression continues, a continuous infusion of the drug doxapram may be needed. Supplementary oxygen should be available.

## Control of infection

Animals in the post-operative period are always at an increased risk of infection, due to the presence of indwelling catheters, with invasive surgical procedures and this factor is often combined with the presence of virulent organisms in the environment. Drugs like the corticosteroids and chemotherapeutics will also specifically reduce the animals' tolerance to infection. Emphasis should always be placed on caring for the animal in a way that minimises contamination; the animal and its immediate environment should be clean. All indwelling catheters should receive proper care and maintenance (see Chapter 9). All procedures should be completed under strict aseptic conditions, using only sterilised equipment. All fluids administered to the animal should be sterile and all fluids being collected continually from the animal should be collected in sterile containers that are completely closed to the atmosphere. All administration and collection apparatus should be changed at least at 48-h intervals. Recumbent animals should be turned every 3 h and convalescing animals should be encouraged to ambulate early to minimise the accumulation of respiratory secretions in the lower lung, which can predispose to pneumonia.

All personnel should wash their hands regularly between animal handling, and soiled clothing should be changed immediately. Floors, treatment tables and cages should be scrubbed regularly with water and appropriate disinfectant solutions.

The use of antibiotics in post-operative care is controversial. Obviously, they are indicated if the animal has an overt infection. However, they do predispose to overgrowth of resistant organisms and fungi. They should certainly not be used to overcome inadequate post-operative care or surgical techniques. If animals are receiving high doses of corticosteroids for longer than 48 h, antibiotics should be given under the direction of the Named Veterinary Surgeon.

## Wound dressings

Bandages may be used to protect traumatised skin, prevent infection, promote healing or immobilise areas, and reduce pain. The type of bandage required depends on the purpose of the dressing. In general, bandages should have at least three layers. The layer adjacent to the wound may be a non-stick dressing (e.g. Rondopad, Millpledge), which allows exudates to pass through into the next layer, or an occlusive dressing, which prevents the passage of fluid into the next layer, keeping the wound moist. The latter is useful for large contaminated wounds and for promoting epithelialisation. Haemostatic dressings such as calcium alginate dressings (e.g. C-Stat, Millpledge) promote haemostasis, and antibiotic impregnated gauze promotes granulation, while reducing infection. The second layer of padding, which is applied under casts, around extremities or over pressure points, should be a layer of absorbent material, such as Ortho-Band or Soffban (Millpledge). Cotton wool is not suitable, as it tends to bunch up and create areas of increased pressure. The third layer of conforming bandage will support the area. If sufficient padding has been applied, it should eliminate the possibility of bandaging too tightly and will be well tolerated by the animal. Examples of conforming bandage are Knit-Fix or Knit-Firm. The final layer is either a cohesive bandage (e.g. Co-Ripwrap, Co-Flex), which is a conforming bandage covered in latex, such that it clings to itself but not to the animals' skin or fur. These are easy to apply, air permeable, comfortable and easy to remove. An alternative, which is being used less nowadays, is the adhesive bandage (e.g. Bandesive, E-Bans, Elastoplast, Treatplast), but these may be useful for awkwardly positioned bandages to hold the dressing in place.

## ADDITIONAL CONSIDERATIONS IN PAIN MANAGEMENT

The use of analgesics should be included not only with the anaesthetic regime but also with the overall plan of the animal's care. It has been shown in man that the provision of effective analgesia will reduce the time taken for post-operative recovery. Surgery should be planned for a time in the day and a day in the week, when there will be adequate number of staff available to provide an adequate level of observation of the animal. Good post-operative care is essential for the animal's welfare and for good scientific practice; and the responsibility for that care of the animal lies with the licensee since, in the standard conditions under which personal licences are granted, 'the personal licensee must take effective precautions, including the appropriate use of sedatives, tranquilisers, analgesics or anaesthetics, to prevent or reduce to the minimum level consistent with the aims of the procedure any pain, suffering, distress or discomfort caused to the animals used.'

## FURTHER INFORMATION

Beynen, A.C., Baumans, V., Bertens, A.P.M.G., Haas, J.W.M., Van Hellemond, K.K., Van Herck, H., Peters, M.A.W., Stafleu, F.R. and Van Tintelen, G. (1988). Assessment of discomfort in rats with hepatomegaly. *Laboratory Animals* 22, 320–25.

Beynen, A.C., Baumans, V., Bertens, A.P.M.G., Havenaar, R., Hesp, A.P.M. and Van Zutphen, L.F.M. (1987). Assessment of discomfort in gallstone-bearing mice: a practical example of the problems encountered in an attempt to recognise discomfort in laboratory animals. *Laboratory Animals* 21, 35–42.

Costa, P. (1996). Neuro-behavioural tests in welfare assessment of transgenic animals. *Harmonization of Laboratory Animal Husbandry: 6th FELASA Symposium*, 19–21 June 1996, Basel, Switzerland.

Dyson, D.H. (1990). Update on butorphanol tartrate: use in small animals. *Canadian Veterinary Journal* 31, 120–21.

FELASA working group on pain and distress (1994). Pain and distress in laboratory rodents and lagomorphs. *Laboratory Animals* 28, 97–112.

Flecknell, P.A. (1984). The relief of pain in laboratory animals. *Laboratory Animals* 18, 147–60.

Flecknell, P.A. (1991). Anaesthesia and post-operative care of small mammals. *In Practice* 13, 180–89.

Flecknell, P.A. (1994). Refinement of animal use – assessment and alleviation of pain and distress. *Laboratory Animals* 28, 222–31.

Flecknell, P.A., Roughan, J.V. and Stewart, R. (1999). Use of oral buprenorphine ('buprenorphine jello') for postoperative analgesia in rats – a clinical trial. *Laboratory Animals* 33, 169–74.

Jablonski, P. and Howden, B.O. (2002). Oral buprenorphine and aspirin analgesia in rats undergoing liver transplantation. *Laboratory Animals* 36, 134–43.

Jenkins, W.L. (1987). Pharmacologic aspects of analgesic drugs in animals: an overview. *Journal of the American Veterinary Medical Association* 191, 1231–40.

Kitchell, R.L., Erikson, H.H. and Karstens, E. (1983). *Animal Pain*. American Physiological Society, Bethesda.

Lees, P., May, S.A. and McKellar, Q.A. (1991). Pharmacology and therapeutics of non-steroidal anti-inflammatory drugs in the dog and cat. 1. General pharmacology. *Journal of Small Animal Practice* 32, 183–93.

McKellar, Q.A., May, S.A. and Lees, P. (1991). Pharmacology and therapeutics of non-steroidal anti-inflammatory drugs in the dog and cat. 2. Individual agents. *Journal of Small Animal Practice* 32, 225–35.

Michell, A.R., Bywater, R.J., Clarke, K.W., Hall, L.W. and Waterman, A.E. (1989). *Veterinary Fluid Therapy*. Blackwell Scientific Publications, Oxford.

Orlans, F.B. (1996). Invasiveness scales for animal pain and distress. *Lab Animal* June 1996, 23–25.

Otterness, I.G. and Gans, D.H. (1988). Non-steroidal anti-inflammatory drugs: an analysis of the relationship between laboratory animal and clinical doses, including species scaling. *Journal of Pharmaceutical Science* 77, 790–95.

Pekow, C. (1992). Buprenorphine jell-o recipe for rodent analgesia. *Synapse* 25, 35.

Shaw, K. *et al.* (1988). Analgesic and anaesthetic applications of butorphanol in veterinary practice. In *Proceedings, Western Veterinary Conference*, Las Vegas, Nevada. Vet Learning Systems Inc., Philadelphia.

Smith and Nephew Website: http://wound.smith-nephew.com/

Soulsby, Lord and Morton, D. (2000). Pain: its nature and management in man and animals. *International Congress and Symposium*, Series 246, Royal Society of Medicine Press.

Strub, K.M., Aeppll, L. and Müller, R.K.M. (1982). Pharmacological properties of carprofen. *European Journal of Rheumatology and Inflammation* 5, 478–87.

# Chapter 9
# Conduct of minor procedures

Whatever the procedure to be done, the first step is to check the paperwork and ensure that the necessary authorities under the Animals (Scientific Procedures) Act 1986 (ASPA) have been granted. You *must* check the following:

1. The *project licence* – is what you intend to do clearly described in Section 19b?
2. Your *personal licence* – is the technique you are going to use clearly set out in Section 15?
3. The *certificate of designation* – is the place where you intend to do this listed on the certificate of designation with the appropriate purposes?

*Only* when you have checked those should you proceed.

When carrying out any procedure on an animal, however minor, the following points should be considered:

- *Restraint* of the animals. Good restraint depends on skilled handling technique and may require the use of suitable equipment and/or drugs. If the latter are necessary, then some knowledge of anaesthesia is required (see Chapter 7) to cover the groups of anaesthetic compounds, their means of delivery, anaesthetic monitoring and patient support.
- Most minor procedures involve the administration of a substance so the *pharmacokinetics of the compound in the particular species and suitable techniques for the administration of substances* must be considered.
- Finally, since many procedures require the *collection of blood samples* the technique for sampling must be considered.

The procedures will in themselves have some effects on the animal, and it is essential to minimise any distress caused. This section gives *guidelines* on safe volumes and sites for administration and withdrawal of substances.

## ADMINISTRATION OF SUBSTANCES

### Introduction to pharmacokinetics

#### Administration and absorption

Substances may be administered to laboratory animals orally, or by intravenous (i.v.), intradermal (i.d.), intraperitoneal (i.p.) or subcutaneous injection, per rectum, or by injection directly into other body parts such as joints or parts of the gastrointestinal system. The substances may act locally or may act throughout the body or at single target systems after absorption into the bloodstream. The rate at which administered

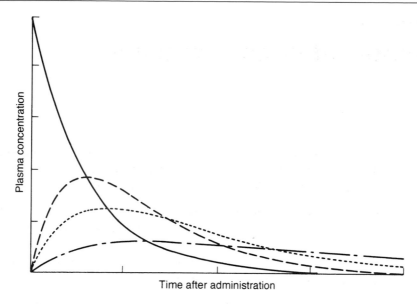

**Figure 9.1**  Graph to show plasma concentration of typical compound following different routes of administration. (—) Intravenous; (– –) intramuscular; (-----) intraperitoneal; (— · —) oral.

compounds are absorbed into the bloodstream depends on the site of administration (Figure 9.1), the nature of the compound, and the manner in which it is presented.

Compounds that are given i.v. reach a high blood concentration immediately. This then tails off as the compound is eliminated, for example, by the liver and kidneys, or redistributed, for example, by absorption into fat. Compounds given by other routes are absorbed at rates depending on the blood flow to the site, and the solubility of the compound in the tissue fluids. Muscles have a good blood supply, so substances administered intramuscularly (i.m.) are absorbed more quickly than those given subcutaneously, as the subcutis has a poorer blood supply. Compounds that are highly soluble in the tissue fluids will be absorbed quickly. Some injectable preparations are designed to have a long duration of action, and the active compound in these is mixed with a carrier of low solubility to slow down absorption into the bloodstream. With orally administered compounds, absorption tends to be slower, and takes place over a longer period.

Compounds that are given orally may be absorbed at various points in the gastrointestinal tract. Substances will only be absorbed across the gut wall if they are lipid soluble. Some compounds are designed to be absorbed locally in the large bowel, and are insoluble unless they are activated by enzymes during passage through the stomach and small intestines. The absorption of other compounds may be affected by pH. Compounds that are ionised are not lipid soluble and will only be absorbed if a specific carrier exists to transport them across the gut wall into the blood. Basic or alkaline compounds are likely to be fully ionised in the acid environment of the stomach, and will be poorly absorbed. However, once in the small intestine, the higher pH will reduce the level of ionisation and increase the absorption. The reverse is true for acidic compounds.

For solids, the particle size affects the rate of absorption, because the surface area relative to volume increases as particle size decreases, presenting more of the compound for solubilisation and absorption. Intestinal passage time will vary depending on the species and on whether or not the animal has been food deprived prior to the administration.

Another factor which complicates oral administration is the *first pass effect*. All substances absorbed in the stomach or intestine, have to pass through the liver before reaching the systemic circulation. This may result in the metabolism of some or all of the compound to active or inactive products, reducing the amount of the original compound which reaches the circulating blood volume. Many compounds induce the liver to produce enzymes, which metabolise them, thereby increasing the first pass effect with repeated dosing. Alternatively, there may be some *enterohepatic recycling*, in which the compound is conjugated and secreted into bile, and therefore, passed back into the intestine without reaching the systemic circulation.

These factors affect the *bioavailability* of substances administered orally, which is essentially the difference between the amount of an oral dose which reaches the bloodstream compared with an equivalent i.v. dose. However, even if the bioavailability is high, it does not necessarily mean that the blood concentration reaches the peak seen immediately after an i.v. dose. Many compounds are absorbed very slowly after oral administration, and may never reach high levels in the blood even if the bioavailability is high.

## *Distribution*

Where and how compounds are distributed within the body also depends on the blood flow to the site and the solubility of the compound in the tissue fluids. There are some special cases however. For example, compounds will only enter the central nervous system (CNS) if they can cross the blood–brain barrier. Lipid soluble compounds will accumulate in fatty tissues, even if the blood supply is poor. This phenomenon can be used to ensure rapid elimination of lipid soluble drugs from the CNS by redistribution to fat (see thiopentone in anaesthetics, Chapter 7). Drugs will also tend to accumulate at sites of metabolism or excretion, such as the liver and kidneys. In pregnant animals, the fetus is separated from the mother by the placenta so only certain compounds will enter the fetus. Some compounds may accumulate in the fetus and some may accumulate in specific tissues, such as the kidney. Compounds will generally be secreted into milk if they can cross the lipid membrane in the mammary gland. Milk is slightly more acidic than blood, so basic compounds tend to accumulate in milk because they ionise after having crossed the lipid barrier and cannot then return to the blood.

These factors that affect the absorption and distribution of administered compounds define the *pharmacokinetics* of the compound, and should be studied prior to administration to ensure that the compound is being given in the most effective way.

## Administration volumes

The volume of any substance given must be as small as is practicable for the procedure, and will be limited ultimately by the size of the animal (Table 9.1). If fluids are to

**Table 9.1** Administration volumes for laboratory species.

| Species | Reference weight | Intravenous or intra-arterial (ml) | Intra-peritoneal (ml) | Intra-muscular (ml/site) | Sub-cutaneous (ml/site) | Oral (ml) | Intra-dermal (µl/site) |
|---|---|---|---|---|---|---|---|
| Mouse | 20 g | 0.2 | 1–2 | 0.05 | 0.5[a] | 0.4 | 100 |
| Rat | 250 g | 1 | 2–4 | 0.1 | 1–2[a] | 5 | 100 |
| Hamster | 120 g | 0.3 | 2–3 | 0.1 | 0.5–1* | 3 | 100 |
| Guinea-pig | 500 g | 1 | 5–7 | 0.1 | 1–2* | 5 | 100 |
| Rabbit | 2 kg | 4 | 10–15 | 0.25 | 1–3* | 10 | 100 |
| Ferret | 750 g | 1–3 | 5–10 | 0.2 | 1–2* | 5 | – |
| Cat | 3 kg | 2–5 | 15–30 | 0.5 | 5–15[a] | 3 | – |
| Dog | 12 kg[b] | 10–15 | 60–120 | 2 | 15–30* | 50 | 100 |
| Fowl | 2.5 kg | 3–5 | 10–15 | 0.25 | 1–2 | – | – |
| Rhesus | 5 kg | 5–10 | 50–100 | 1 | 5–10[a] | 5–20 | 100 |

Note: The figures in this table have been calculated for the 'average' size animal for that species, for ease of reference. Adjust as necessary for the actual weight of the individual.
*Maximum of four sites.
[a]Maximum of two to four sites.
[b]Beagle.

be administered by infusion, the flow rate should be as low as possible, and the infusion given over as short a time as possible. However, if too much fluid is given too rapidly, the circulation may become overloaded, causing pulmonary oedema. If the administration is slower, excess fluid can be cleared by the kidneys. The maintenance requirement for fluid is approximately 40 ml/kg per 24 h in normal animals and care should be taken not to exceed this unless there are deficiencies to replace.

## Administration techniques

Injections should be performed using aseptic techniques, as for blood sampling. It is important to use equipment appropriate for the species (see Tables 9.2a and b). For example, injections in small rodents should be given with 25 or 27 G needles. For rabbits, guinea pigs and cats, 23 or 25 G needles are best, and for dogs 21 G needles are adequate. For farm animals, needles larger than 21 G may be used. The viscosity of the substance also affects the size of needle used. Thick, viscous liquids may not pass through narrow gauge needles. Intradermal injections are performed with 25–27 G needles. To minimise the distress caused to animals during administration of substances, they must be carefully and expertly handled, and given a sedative or short acting general anaesthetic, if required.

### Subcutaneous injections

For most species, subcutaneous injections can be given into the scruff of the neck (Figure 9.2). A fold of skin is lifted using the thumb and first two fingers of one hand, and the needle is passed through the skin at the base of the fold parallel to the body, to avoid penetrating deeper tissues. Subcutaneous injections are rarely painful, unless the substance being injected causes stinging.

**Table 9.2a**    Suggested hypodermic needle sizes for laboratory animals.

| Species | Intraperitoneal | Intramuscular | Intravenous | Subcutaneous |
|---|---|---|---|---|
| Mouse | 27 | 27 | 27–28 | 25 |
| Rat | 23–25 | 25 | 25–27 | 25 |
| Hamster | 23–25 | 25 | 25–27 | 25 |
| Gerbil | 27 | 27 | 27–28 | 25 |
| Guinea-pig | 21–25 | 25 | 25–27 | 23–25 |
| Rabbit | 21–23 | 23–25 | 23–25 | 21–25 |
| Ferret | 21–23 | 23–25 | 21–25 | 21–23 |
| Cat | 21–23 | 23 | 21–25 | 21–23 |
| Dog | 21–23 | 21–23 | 21–23 | 21–23 |
| Rhesus | 21–23 | 23–25 | 21–25 | 21–25 |
| Sheep | 19–21 | 21 | 19–21 | 19–21 |

**Table 9.2b**    Recommended cannulae sizes for laboratory animals.

| Species | Site | Gauge | Length |
|---|---|---|---|
| Rats | Tail vein | 24–25 | 12–19 mm (1/2–3/4 in.) |
| Rabbit | Ear vein | 24 | 19 mm (3/4 in.) |
| Dog | Cephalic or jugular vein | 20–21* | 25–40 mm (1–11/2 in.) |
| Cat | Cephalic or jugular vein | 22–23 | 25 mm (1 in.) |
| Rhesus | Cephalic or saphenous vein | 21–24 | 19–25 mm (3/4–1 in.) |
| Pig | Ear vein | 21–23 | 25–40 mm (1–11/2 in.) |
| Sheep/goat | Jugular vein | 19–21 | 40 mm (11/2 in.) |
| Cattle/horses | Jugular vein | 19–21 | 40 mm (11/2 in.) |

*Depends on breed and age. For puppies, a 23 or 25 G cannula can be used.

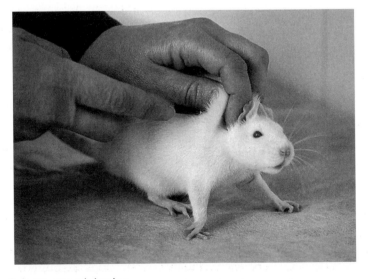

**Figure 9.2**    Subcutaneous injection.

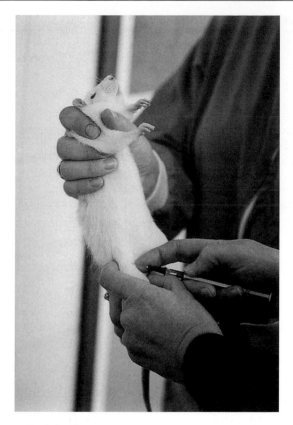

**Figure 9.3**    Intramuscular injection.

In rabbits, subcutaneous injections can also be given over the flank, provided that care is taken with adjuvants, because if there is an adjuvant reaction in the skin over the respiratory muscles this can cause pain on breathing. In sheep and goats fluid can be given under the skin over the ribs. For pigs, small volumes can be injected into the skin behind the ear, or into the fold between the leg and the abdomen. Pigs have much subcutaneous fat, and injections given elsewhere are likely to enter the fat, where absorption will be particularly slow due to the poor blood supply.

## Intramuscular injections

Intramuscular injections are frequently painful, due to the distension of muscle fibres, which occurs, and therefore, good restraint is required. They are usually given into the muscles of the thigh. Larger volumes or irritant compounds should be injected into the quadriceps group on the front of the thigh. The muscle can be immobilised with one hand while injecting with the other. Injections can be given into the caudal thigh muscles, but as the sciatic nerve runs through these muscles, irritant compounds should not be given here or damage may be caused to the nerve. In rodents, the quadriceps feels like a small peanut on the front of the thigh, and can be immobilised with the thumb and forefinger of one hand while injecting with the other (Figure 9.3).

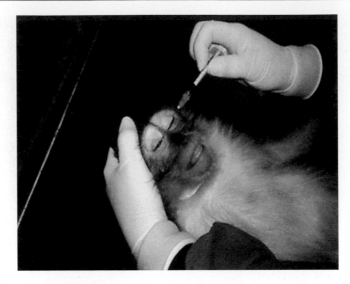

**Figure 9.4**   Intradermal injection used for tuberculin testing in a macaque.

In dogs and cats, injections can be given with care into the muscles on each side of the spine, and in large animals the gluteal muscles are used. In adult pigs, injections are given into the neck muscles, but a long needle is required to penetrate the fat layer. Piglets can be injected by lifting them by one hindleg and injecting into the caudal thigh muscle on that side. Fowl are given i.m. injections into the pectoral muscles. After the injection, the site should be massaged to disperse the dose.

## Intravenous injection

Intravenous injections may be given into the cephalic veins of dogs, cats, primates, and ferrets (see Figure 9.7b). In rats and mice, the lateral tail vein is used. Rats can also be given injections into the dorsal metatarsal vein. The hindlimb is held in extension, and the vein raised by occluding it at the stifle joint. The jugular vein can be used in dogs, cats, hamsters and ferrets (see Figure 9.8), and is the method of choice in ruminants and horses. The ear veins are used in guinea pigs and pigs. Fowl can be injected via the brachial vein.

## Intradermal injections

Intradermal injections for most species can be given in the same area as subcutaneous injections. For tuberculin testing in primates, the skin of the upper eyelid is often used (Figure 9.4).

## Intraperitoneal injections

Intraperitoneal injections in rodents are given in the lower left or right quadrant of the abdomen as there are no vital organs in this area. The quadrants are demarcated

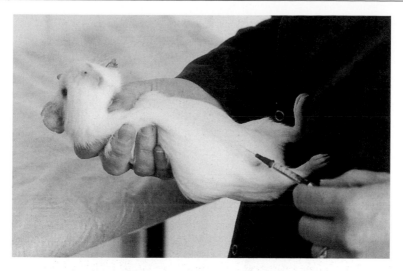

**Figure 9.5**    Intraperitoneal injection.

by the midline and a line perpendicular to it passing through the umbilicus. The animal should be held either by an assistant or in one hand on its back, upright, so that it is comfortable and securely supported. The needle is angled at 45° to the skin and no resistance should be encountered to the passage of the needle (Figure 9.5).

## Oral administration

Substances may be given orally by inclusion in the diet or drinking water. These methods have the disadvantages that it is impossible to be sure that the animal has had the entire dose, and in some species it will lead to the animal refusing to eat and drink. With ad lib feeding, or if there is an increase in metabolic rate, the animal may overeat and thus ingest an overdose of the drug. In mice particularly, adding drugs to the water tends to lead to dehydration, because the mouse avoids drinking it, and this can lead to a rapid deterioration in the condition of the mouse, especially if the compounds have been given for therapeutic reasons. If the watering system is automated, it is impossible to give compounds in this way. To overcome these problems, gastric intubation or gavage may be employed (Figure 9.6). Flexible catheters or stainless steel needles with rounded tips are used. The animal is restrained with its neck extended, and the needle or catheter passed gently down the oesophagus. Care must be taken not to damage the oesophagus, or to put the needle into the trachea. The needle or catheter can usually be observed passing down the oesophagus on the left side of the neck. Damage to the catheter from chewing can be avoided by using an oral speculum, or by using a flexible nasogastric or pharyngostomy tube instead. The animal may or may not need to be starved prior to administering the compound, depending on the nature of the compound and the particular project.

For dogs and cats, tablets may be administered orally in the conscious animal by placing one hand over the top of the head, placing the thumb at the commissure of the lips on one side and the fingers at the other, and tilting the head back. This will

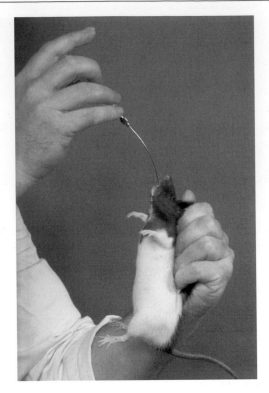

**Figure 9.6**    Gavage in the rat.

cause the mouth to open slightly. The tablet can be held between the thumb and fore-finger of the other hand, and the middle finger used to open the mouth. The tablet can then be placed onto the tongue as far back as possible, to stimulate the swallowing reflex.

## LEGAL CATEGORIES AND RESTRICTIONS GOVERNING THE USE OF DRUGS USED IN EXPERIMENTAL ANIMALS

The Medicines (Restrictions on the Administration of Veterinary Medicinal Products) Regulations 1994 prevent the administration of a veterinary medicine to an animal without a marketing authorisation (a product licence) for the indication and species. Exceptions may be made in the absence of a licensed product (the cascade principle). In the UK, prescription of veterinary medicines is primarily the responsibility of registered veterinary surgeons. Personal licence holders under the ASPA who are authorised to perform anaesthesia and surgery in research animals and who do not hold veterinary qualifications must obtain and administer drugs under the direction of a veterinary surgeon. A pharmacist may only supply licensed medicines for use in animals under the direction or prescription of a veterinary surgeon. Medical practitioners may not legally prescribe medicines for use in animals.

The cascade for prescribing veterinary medicines where no product for the species or indication has a marketing authorisation (off label prescribing) is as follows:

No veterinary-licensed product exists for a condition in a particular species?

(1) use a veterinary medicinal product licensed for use in another animal species or another condition in the same species;

(2) if no product as described in (1) exists, a human-licensed product; or ...

(3) if no product as described in (2) exists, a product prepared extemporaneously by an authorised person in accordance with a veterinary prescription.

## Legal classifications of veterinary medicines (Medicines Act 1968)

| | |
|---|---|
| General sales list | GSL |
| Pharmacy medicines | P |
| Pharmacy and merchants list medicines | PML |
| Prescription-only medicines | POM |
| Controlled drugs (Misuse of Drugs Regulations 1985 amended 2002) | CD (Schedules 1–5). |

## Storage and record keeping

All drugs must be stored appropriately to ensure that they maintain their full activity. Some must be kept in a refrigerator at 2–5°C, some need to be kept away from light, some should not be kept in plastic bottles. The data sheet supplied with the drug will specify the requirements.

It is good practice to keep a record of all drugs held and used, it is a legal requirement to keep records of purchase and use of all controlled drugs listed in Schedules 1–3 of the Misuse of Drugs Regulations.

## REMOVAL OF BLOOD

### Causes of stress

The removal of blood from an animal is a procedure with three potentially stressful components.

- Handling and restraining the animal is stressful. To minimise the distress caused, the licensee should be familiar with humane methods of handling and restraint (see Section 2 for species-specific information), and should consider using an appropriate sedative or anaesthetic (see Chapter 7). Many animals can be trained to accept the handling required to take blood samples, such as cats, dogs, rabbits, pigs and primates (see Figure 15.5), and although this takes time, it is worthwhile.

- Venepuncture causes some minor pain and discomfort, whatever the site, and requires considerable skill. The expertise required to carry this out successfully must be gained first by watching others, then by practising on cadavers or models such as the KOKEN rat simulator, and then by carrying out the technique oneself, once a licence has been granted, under direct supervision.

- The removal of blood causes physiological responses, the magnitude of which depend on the volume of blood removed (as a percentage of the total), and the speed of withdrawal. The rapid removal of large quantities of blood will cause the animal to go into hypovolaemic shock, and may even cause death. The percentage blood loss required to cause hypovolaemic shock varies with the speed of withdrawal, whether or not fluid is replaced concurrently, and the psychophysiological state of the animal at the time. Chronic slow haemorrhage is tolerated better than acute blood loss, and placid animals tolerate greater losses than nervous ones, again indicating the need for competent handling and training of the animals.

Stress responses in the animal result in the release of hormones and other substances to counteract the stress, which can cause anomalous experimental results. It is essential to minimise the stress caused to an animal when removing blood from the humane viewpoint, and also to ensure good scientific practice. The experimental technique should be refined such that the quantity of blood removed is minimised. This is particularly important in small mammals, such as mice, where the blood volume is small and sample volume is critical. The withdrawal of blood from any vessel requires skill in handling the animal and in manipulating the equipment. The person taking the samples should be fully familiar with the chosen technique, and have all the equipment ready before starting. You are advised to consult the BVA/FRAME/ RSPCA/UFAW (1993) working group report on the removal of blood from laboratory mammals and birds.

## Quality of samples

To achieve meaningful results, any samples taken must be of good quality, and be preserved in the best possible manner. If the sampling technique is poor, blood may clot or haemolyse rendering results invalid. To avoid these problems, samples must be taken skillfully, and treated appropriately thereafter.

Blood may be collected using syringes and hypodermic or butterfly needles, through indwelling cannulae, with double ended needles and evacuated tubes (e.g. 'Vacutainers'), or in very small species by incision of a vein using a sterile lancet or scalpel blade. The latter however is not best practice, as inadvertent movement can result in the severing of an appendage. If needles are used, the needle should be as large as is practicable for the species. This allows blood to flow faster, reducing the likelihood of clotting, and also causes less damage to the red cells, reducing the possibility of haemolysis.

Thought should be given to the desirability of using anticoagulants. Different anti-clotting agents are suitable for different purposes:

- *No anticoagulant*: Blood clots, and serum can be removed after centrifugation.
- *Lithium heparin*: This is the anticoagulant of choice for most biochemical assays. The yield of plasma from heparinised blood is greater than the yield of serum from clotted blood, which may make heparin a good choice for collecting blood for harvesting antibodies. Sodium heparin is sometimes used if preservation of the white cells is required.
- *Potassium EDTA (ethylene diamine tetra-acetic acid)*: This is used for haematological analyses.
- *Oxalate/fluoride*: This is used for blood glucose determination.

Several other anticoagulants are available, for example, for collecting blood for transfusions or for analysis of clotting factors. After collection into anticoagulant, the blood should be mixed thoroughly by *rolling*, not by shaking as this can damage the cells and lead to haemolysis.

It is preferable for samples to be submitted fresh for analysis. If this is impossible, samples may need to be refrigerated or deep frozen. For some enzyme determinations, degeneration of the enzyme renders analysis useless if performed more than a few hours after blood collection. It is advisable to determine the exact requirements of the laboratory protocol prior to sample collection.

## Venepuncture technique

### Restraint

When taking samples, the animal should be gently restrained by an experienced handler who is known to the animal. Chemical restraint is generally only required if the technique involves more than a pinprick, for example, for tail tip amputation, or in primates if the animals are not trained or are under quarantine restrictions.

### Site and location of the vein

It is important to be certain of the location of the vein, either by visualising it or palpating its course, and to have it immobilised, before piercing the skin. The handler may be required to raise the vein, by occluding the venous drainage proximal to the site of venepuncture. This must be performed correctly, or withdrawal of blood will be difficult. If unsure of the position of the vein, venepuncture should not be attempted. The use of a quick release tourniquet greatly facilitates blood sampling in some species and vasodilating agents may be used in other species (e.g. 'Vasolate', IMS) (Figure 9.7).

### Preparation of the site

Blood should be collected using an aseptic technique. The area should be clipped to remove hair if necessary, then cleaned. The use of warm water with or without

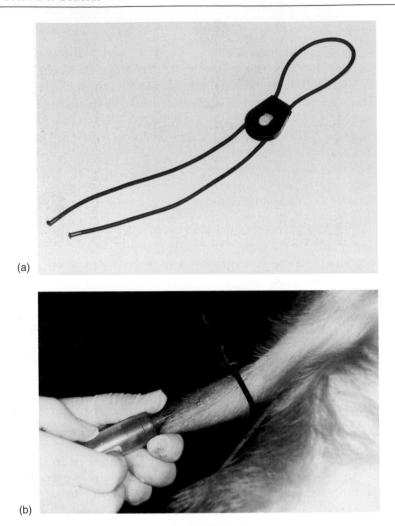

(a)

(b)

**Figure 9.7**   (a) Quick release tourniquet and (b) tourniquet in use.

disinfectant will help dilate superficial veins as well as cleansing the skin. After cleansing, the skin can be swabbed with 70% ethanol or disinfectant. In some species, it may be advantageous to apply local anaesthetic cream (e.g. 'EMLA', Astra Pharmaceuticals) to the site 30–60 min before venepuncture to prevent any discomfort in such animals as the cat, dog, rabbit, or pig.

## Taking the sample

For needle venepuncture, the needle should be held bevel uppermost and directed through the skin following the course of the vein. This should be completed in one movement. Once in the lumen of the vein, as determined by the presence of blood in the needle hub, the needle should be advanced parallel to the skin up to the hub, so that the body of the needle is in the lumen of the vein. The needle may be bent at an

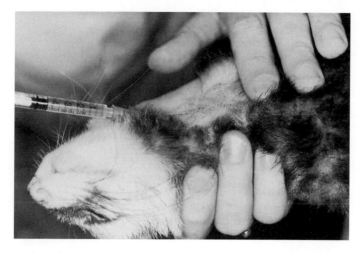

**Figure 9.8**  Jugular venepuncture in the ferret, note the needle has been bent at an angle to the hub to facilitate location in the vein.

angle if required to facilitate location in the vein, for example, in the jugular vein in the ferret (see Figure 9.8).

A similar method can be used for butterfly needles and over-the-needle cannulae (Figure 9.9). These can be used in almost all species, except possibly mice. Choose the largest, longest cannula, which will pass into the vein. Before inserting a cannula, make sure you have all the necessary equipment to hand. Clip the fur from a wide area over the vein, and clean the skin using a suitable antibacterial cleanser such as chlorhexidine. Iodine-based preparations may also be used but are less persistent. Raise and immobilise the vein (an assistant may be required for this), remove the bung from the stylet which runs through the cannula and insert it through the skin until the tip is in the lumen of the vessel and blood is seen in the hub of the stylet. For thick-skinned animals, it may be worth making a tiny skin incision first, using the bevelled edge of a needle or a no 11 scalpel blade, to facilitate passing the cannula through the skin. The cannula can then be advanced into the vein while retaining the stylet: this prevents the stylet from lacerating the vein as it advances up the vessel, and also the stylet blocks the lumen of the cannula so blood may only be withdrawn once the stylet is removed. Flexible cannulae are less traumatic to the tissues than needles, and are therefore less painful to insert and more suitable for long-term cannulation.

Veins will collapse around the needle if attempts are made to withdraw the blood too quickly, so patience is required, particularly with small mammals. For these species, blood can be allowed to drip from a needle or flexible cannula placed in the vein. A syringe may be attached and gentle suction applied for larger animals. Evacuated tubes can be used if the vein diameter allows it. These are quick and easy to use, but can increase the likelihood of haemolysis as blood cells can become damaged by the rapid passage into the low-pressure container. In mice a very satisfactory method of collection of small blood samples is the saphenous vein puncture technique described by Hem *et al.* (1998) (see http://www.uib.no/vivariet/mou_blood/Blood_coll_mice_.html). The vein is punctured using 23 or 25 G needle, a drop of blood

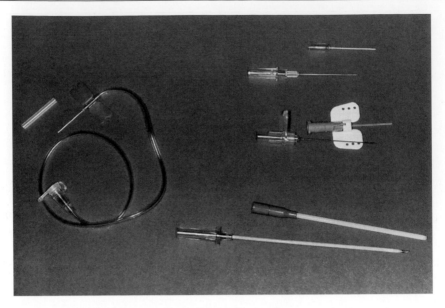

**Figure 9.9**   Over-the-needle cannulae and butterfly needle.

forms at the puncture site and can be collected into a micro-capillary tube. The scab that forms at the site can be gently rubbed off to enable serial samples to be collected from the same puncture site. After taking samples, gentle pressure should be applied to the site of venepuncture for 30–60 s to prevent haemorrhage.

### Potential sequelae

Haemorrhage may occur from the punctured vein. If this occurs, pressure should be applied until the haemorrhage ceases. Dressings are available which if applied to a wound will accelerate haemostasis (e.g. Kaltostat). Bruising may occur if the vein bleeds under the skin. Pressure should be applied as above, and the site rechecked after 30 min. If the bruised area continues to spread, advice should be sought from the Named Veterinary Surgeon. The occurrence of thrombosis or phlebitis following venepuncture indicates poor technique. The method should be reviewed and advice sought from the Named Veterinary Surgeon.

### Sample volume

The volume of the sample taken is determined by the requirements of the experiment, and by the safe limit which can be withdrawn without causing distress to the animal. In general, as small a volume as possible should be taken. Not more than 10 per cent of the blood volume should be removed at one time, and less than 15 per cent of the blood volume should be removed in any 30-day period. Animals are considered to have 70 ml blood per kg bodyweight, but this varies with the species (see Tables 9.3a–c). Maximum limits of volume and frequency of sampling will normally be stipulated on the project licence.

**Table 9.3a**    Practical blood sampling volumes for small laboratory species.

| Species | Reference weight | Blood volume (ml/kg) | Total blood volume, normal adult (ml) | | Safe volume of single bleed (ml)* | | Bleed out volume (ml) | |
|---|---|---|---|---|---|---|---|---|
| Mouse | 18–40 g | 58.5 | Male | 1.5–2.4 | | 0.1–0.2 | Male | 0.8–1.4 |
| | | | Female | 1.0–2.4 | | | Female | 0.6–1.4 |
| Rat | 250–500 g | 54–70 | Male | 29–33 | Male | 2.9–3.3 | Male | 13–15 |
| | | | Female | 16–19 | Female | 1.6–1.9 | Female | 7.5–9 |
| Hamster | 85–150 g | 78 | Male | 6.3–9.7 | Male | 0.6–0.9 | Male | 2.9–4.5 |
| | | | Female | 7.1–11.2 | Female | 0.7–1.1 | Female | 3.3–5.2 |
| Gerbil | 55–100 g | 66–78 | Male | 4.5–7 | Male | 0.4–0.7 | Male | 2.2–3.5 |
| | | | Female | 3.8–6 | Female | 0.4–0.6 | Female | 1.9–2.9 |
| Guinea pig | 700–1200 g | 69–75 | Male | 59–84 | Male | 6–8 | Male | 29–42 |
| | | | Female | 48–63 | Female | 5–6 | Female | 24–31 |
| Rabbit | 1–6 kg | 57–65 | 58.5–585 | | 5–50 | | 31–310 | |
| Ferret | 600–2000 g | 70 | 42–140 | | 4–14 | | 21–70 | |

*A single bleed of 10% of the blood volume averages 7 ml/kg.

**Table 9.3b**    Practical blood sampling volumes for laboratory primates.

| Species | Blood volume (ml/kg) | Total blood volume normal adult (ml) | | Safe volume of single bleed (ml)* | |
|---|---|---|---|---|---|
| Marmoset | 60–70 | 21–24.5 | | 2.1–2.4 | |
| Rhesus | 55–80 | Male | 420–770 | Male | 42–77 |
| | | Female | 280–630 | Female | 28–63 |
| Cynomolgus | 50–96 | Male | 280–560 | Male | 28–56 |
| | | Female | 140–420 | Female | 14–42 |

*Single bleed of 10% of blood volume.

**Table 9.3c**    Practical blood sampling volumes for larger domestic species.

| Species | Blood volume (ml/kg) | Total blood volume Normal adult (ml) | Safe volume Single bleed (ml)* |
|---|---|---|---|
| Dog | 70–110† | 900–1170[a] | 90–110 |
| Cat | 47–65 | 140–200 | 14–20 |
| Pig – Large white | 56–69 | 13,200–15,000 | 1320–1500 |
| Pig – Yucatan | 56–69 | 4200–4800 | 420–480 |
| Sheep | 58–64 | 4060–4480 | 400–450 |
| Goat | 57–90 | 3990–6300 | 400–630 |
| Cattle | 60 | 27,000–36,000[b] | 2700–3600 |
| Horse | 75 | 33,750–45,000[b] | 3375–4500 |

*Single bleed of 10% of blood volume.
†Much breed variation.
[a]Beagle.
[b]Assumes adult weight 450–600 kg.

## *Methods of venepuncture*

### *Rodents*

For most rodents saphenous vein puncture is the most satisfactory site for obtaining small quantities of blood (see Hem *et al.* 1998). For those rodents with tails, this is a good site for obtaining rather larger quantities of blood. The lateral coccygeal or tail vein may be easily visualised. Warming the tail first increases the blood flow to the site and makes sample collection easier. Blood samples may be obtained by incising the skin over the vein using a sterile lancet and collecting the blood into a plain or anti-coagulant coated capillary tube, or allowing it to drip into a container. Scalpel blades are not recommended as they can easily slip causing damage to the tail. Larger samples can be obtained from rats by placing a 23–26 G flexible cannula or butterfly needle into the tail vein and allowing blood to drip into a collection pot or applying gentle suction with a syringe. If a butterfly needle is used, the plastic tube should be shortened to prevent clotting within it.

Amputation of the tail tip to obtain a sample of mixed arterial and venous blood can be carried out on rats, mice, and gerbils, but must be done under general anaesthetic (BVA/FRAME/RSPCA/UFAW, 1993), gaseous anaesthesia using isoflurane being ideal for such a procedure. In mice, this does not appear to involve the removal of any vertebrae, which it does in rats. This should be performed only once in rats, or a maximum of twice in mice.

Large samples can be obtained from rats and gerbils via jugular venepuncture. The vein is raised on one side of the neck by applying pressure at the thoracic inlet, and a needle placed through the skin and into the vein pointing towards the head.

For animals with no tails, such as guinea pigs and hamsters, it is possible to obtain tiny samples from the ear veins. A technique has been described for cannulating the lateral saphenous vein in the hindlimb of guinea pigs under general anaesthesia for repeated sampling (Nau and Schunck, 1993).

For terminal sampling it is acceptable to perform cardiac puncture, which must be done under general anaesthesia. There are many potentially harmful sequelae to this procedure, such as cardiac tamponade, and it should be done under terminal anaesthesia. The heart may be reached by placing the animal on its right side and piercing the left ventricle through the chest wall at the sixth intercostal space, one third of the way up, to obtain arterial blood, or by piercing the right ventricle with the animal on its left side for venous blood. Alternatively, the animal may be placed on its back, and the heart reached by passing the needle under the sternum and through the diaphragm. Jugular venepuncture, although possible, is extremely difficult in these animals.

Collection of blood from the orbital venous sinus can have severe consequences for the animal, and although it has been used for bleeding rats and tail-less animals, it is not recommended for sampling with recovery.

### *Rabbits*

Blood can be collected relatively easily from the marginal ear vein using an over-the-needle cannula or butterfly needle. A peripheral vasodilator may be applied to the skin over the vein, (e.g. 'Vasolate', IMS), 5–10 min before blood collection. Once the vein is engorged, the cannula is inserted and blood can be collected by allowing it to drip into a pot. After collection, the vasodilator is wiped off and pressure applied until the bleeding ceases. Haemostatic dressings can be applied as discussed earlier in this chapter. Bleeding from the central ear artery is possible, but can result in the formation of large haematomata, which can cause damage to the ear or even necrosis.

## Ferrets

For tiny quantities of blood, for example, for an Aleutian disease test, a toenail can be clipped and a drop of blood collected into a capillary tube. For moderate sized samples the saphenous or tail veins can be used, while larger quantities can be collected from the jugular vein. The fur on the neck needs to be well clipped, and the vein raised by placing a thumb over the jugular groove in the thoracic inlet. Blood is collected by inserting a needle up the vein towards the head, or down towards the thoracic inlet. Collection is facilitated by bending the needle to an angle of 30° prior to penetrating the skin. Pressure on the vein in the thoracic inlet is maintained until the blood has been collected (see Figure 9.8).

## Primates

The best method of blood withdrawal in primates is to use the femoral vein, in the groin. This can be used for Old World Monkeys and New World Monkeys. The needle is inserted in the femoral triangle, slightly medial to the femoral pulse, pointing towards the head. For larger Old World Monkeys, the cephalic vein on the top of the foreleg below the elbow can be used, as for cats and dogs. The jugular vein can be used as an alternative route. The micro-capillary tube method can be used to collect small samples from the heel of primates without anaesthetic after they have been trained to accept minimal restraint (see Figure 15.7). Marmosets may also be bled from the coccygeal vein.

## Dogs and cats

These can be bled from the jugular vein. A handler places their right arm over the body of the animal to hold the forelegs. The elbow is used to hold the body of the animal to the body of the handler (Figure 9.10). The left hand is placed under the chin to raise the head. The person collecting the blood raises the vein by placing a thumb in the jugular groove at the thoracic inlet. The cephalic vein can also be used.

## Ruminants and horses

For sheep, goats, cattle and horses the jugular vein is used. The vein can be visualised by clipping hair or wool from over the jugular groove. The vein is raised by applying firm pressure to the base of the jugular groove. The needle is advanced through the skin up towards the head (Figure 9.11). Cattle can also be bled from the ventral coccygeal vein.

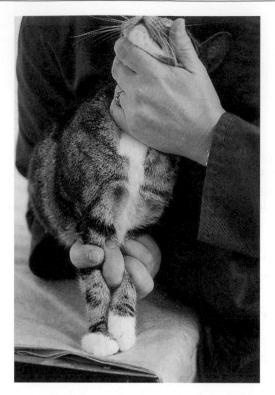

**Figure 9.10**    Holding a cat for jugular venepuncture.

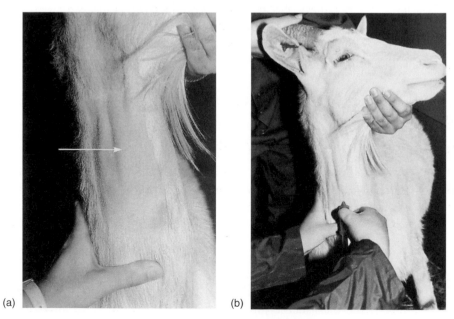

(a)                                    (b)

**Figure 9.11**    (a) Visualising the jugular vein in the goat and (b) jugular venepuncture in the goat.

*Pigs*

These are probably the most difficult animals to bleed. For small volumes in large pigs, an ear vein can be used. For larger volumes, the anterior vena cava is used. A long needle is inserted in the thoracic inlet, and angled slightly upwards and medially to enter the anterior vena cava.

*Birds*

The brachial (alar or wing) vein is usually used for blood sampling in birds. It can be visualised as it crosses the elbow by plucking the feathers over the medial surface of the wing. Samples should be removed slowly to prevent the vein collapsing. Pressure is generally not applied after venepuncture in birds as this can promote haematoma formation.

The right jugular vein can also be used. It is found between the feathers on the dorsolateral surface of the neck. It can be raised by applying pressure at the base of the neck. Haematomata rarely form after jugular venepuncture.

## RECORD KEEPING (SEE ALSO CHAPTER 2)

Standard condition 11 to a personal licence states 'It is the responsibility of a personal licensee to ensure that all cages, pens or other enclosures are clearly labelled.', and Standard condition 21 to a personal licence states 'The personal licensee shall maintain a record of all animals on which procedures have been carried out, including details of supervision and declarations of competence by the project licence holder as appropriate. This record shall be retained for at least 5 years and shall, on request, be submitted to the Secretary of State or made available to an Inspector.'

It cannot be overstated how important it is to keep excellent, clear records of all work done under ASPA. For details on records required by the project licence holder to make the annual returns, see Chapter 11.

## INDWELLING CANNULAE, ARTERIAL LOOPS AND FISTULAE

### Placement and maintenance of indwelling cannulae

Indwelling vascular cannulae can be maintained for prolonged periods if cared for properly. Butterfly needles may be used, but flexible plastic cannulae are better as butterfly needles may lacerate the vein if there is any movement. Cannulae may be implanted surgically, or passed into a superficial vein by puncture of the skin, as for needle venepuncture. Percutaneous insertions are associated with fewer complications. Cannulae can be placed in a major vessel, or into a minor one with the tip passing into a major vessel. Cannulae placed in the jugular vein should not enter the right atrium, or arrhythmias may be caused. The cannula may be tunnelled through the subcutis to exit the skin at a distant site (e.g. over the back) to reduce interference from the animal and the risk of ascending infection. Such cannulae should not kink or pull out when the animal moves. Once the cannula is in place, it should be capped using an injection bung (which is capable of being pierced several times or easily removed) or a three-way tap, and sutured or bandaged to the skin. To prevent clotting in the cannula, it should be flushed with heparinised saline or another anticoagulant after placement, and between sampling or administering compounds. A concentration of 10–15 units heparin per ml saline is adequate. If there is a three-way tap or multiple sampling port on the end, this is made much easier as the anticoagulant delivery and sampling/administrating systems may be attached at the same time. Exit sites are potential sources of infection and irritation, and must be inspected at least once daily. The skin around the cannula should be cleaned every 24 h, checked for signs of inflammation, and a suitable antibiotic–antifungal ointment applied before redressing.

Maintenance of cannulae for repeated administration is easier than for repeated withdrawal, as blood clots on the end of the cannula tend to allow administration but act as valves preventing withdrawal. Wipe the injection port with spirit prior to injection, and keep the ports of three-way taps capped. Substances to be given through the cannula must be sterile, and fluid-giving sets must be changed every 48 h.

## Withdrawal of blood

When withdrawing blood from a cannula, the first sample taken each time should be discarded, as it will contain anticoagulant and be diluted. After sampling, the cannula should be flushed with a calculated amount of anticoagulant: enough to fill the cannula, but not to enter the bloodstream.

## Long-term cannulation

Long-term cannulae are usually implanted surgically, which must be done under aseptic conditions and requires considerable skill. Cannulae will last longer if placed with the flow of blood, and may be maintained for prolonged periods provided the flow of fluid is not interrupted and the cannula is flushed frequently with a suitable anticoagulant such as heparin. In young animals, room must be left so the cannula is not pulled out as the animal grows, and in all animals movement can be a problem. The strategic positioning of lengths of flexible tubing attached to the cannula can reduce the likelihood of it being dislodged by movement.

Cannulae can be kept patent for more than 3 or 4 weeks in small animals, and longer in large animals. The period can be increased if the animal is restrained, but this results in distress to the animal and is best avoided.

Cannulae need to be of a suitable inert material, which will not cause any irritation, and be strong enough to withstand kinking and occlusion due to movement or tightening of ligatures. Polypropylene cannulae are strong, but silicone rubber causes less tissue reaction. The two can be combined by placing a silicone rubber cannula over a polypropylene one, or by coating a polypropylene cannula with silicone rubber.

## Removal of cannulae

After removal, haemostasis can be achieved by applying pressure to the vessel for several minutes, or by ligating the vessel with a suitable suture material (see Chapter 10).

## Potential sequelae

If cannulae are maintained for longer than 24–48 h, blockages due to thrombi can become a serious problem. Thrombi may embolise and travel to distant sites, and will be filtered out in a capillary bed depending on the site of the cannula. Emboli originating from jugular catheters, for example, will travel through the right heart and be trapped in the capillary beds of the lungs, whereas emboli from arterial cannulae lodge in end organs such as the brain, kidney, or muscles.

# Arterial sampling and arterial loops

Arterial sampling allows very large samples to be taken rapidly. Often, the carotid artery is used, but the central ear artery can be used in rabbits, or the femoral artery in many other species.

## Needle puncture

Good restraint is essential when taking samples with a needle as accidental movement can result in laceration of the artery and profuse haemorrhage. Once the needle is in the artery, the high blood pressure will normally force the plunger in the syringe back. Firm pressure should be applied to the site for 2–5 min afterwards to prevent haematoma formation.

## Arterial cannulae

When introducing arterial cannulae, the artery should be clamped with atraumatic vascular clamps, as otherwise there will be haemorrhage as soon as the artery is punctured. Cannulae should be placed in the direction of the flow of blood. There is a greater potential for thrombi to cause problems in arterial cannulae than venous ones, as thrombi may embolise and cause infarctions in distant sites such as the renal artery.

## Arterial loops

This method involves bringing an artery into a subcutaneous position for easy sampling. This has to be done surgically, and is technically difficult. This must first be practised on cadavers and then performed under very close supervision.

# Maintenance of fistulae

A fistula is an artificial passage created between two hollow organs, or between a hollow organ and the outside. For example, ruminal fistulae may be created to study the physiology of the rumen in sheep, goats and cattle, or for the treatment of bloat. Fistulae are created surgically under general anaesthetic. An incision is made in the skin overlying the organ, and the organ is brought up to the surface. An incision is made in the wall of the organ, and the skin edges are sutured to the cut edges of the organ. Aftercare involves checking and cleaning daily to prevent early closure, or damage to the skin around the fistula from exudation of serum or organ contents. At the end of the experiment, the fistula may be closed surgically, or allowed to heal over by second intention healing.

## MISCELLANEOUS METHODS OF ADMINISTRATION AND SAMPLING

### Administration

#### *Footpad/tail base injection*

Substances such as Freund's Complete Adjuvant (FCA) may be injected into the footpad or tail base of rodents to induce localised or generalised arthritis respectively. Animals with arthritis must be given soft bedding, and may be provided with food and water in a gel placed adjacent to the bed to avoid the necessity for them to walk around. Social animals should be kept in groups but at a low stocking density so they do not have to climb over each other to reach food or water.

#### *Nebulisation/administration into the respiratory tract*

Some liquids may be nebulised into tiny particles for administration into the respiratory tract. This may be necessary for some drugs and vaccines. The compound is given in a spray, which is inhaled, or in some cases absorbed through the skin. The spray may be administered to the entire body, or just to the nose.

#### *Instillation into eyes*

Compounds for topical ocular administration must be non-irritant, or there may be discomfort, lacrimation, and corneal damage, with scarring in the long term.

#### *Intracerebral injection*

This technique is used to deliver pharmacological agents to the CNS either where the blood–brain barrier must be crossed, or to avoid direct systemic effects. The route may be used in neonatal and adult rodents and neonatal chicks. In neonatal rodents and chicks use a small bore, low volume (less than 0.5 ml) plastic syringe with a 27 G needle. Draw the inoculum into the syringe and check smooth operation of the plunger before picking up the animal. Mice, rats and chicks should be no more than 3 days of age. Neonatal animals require very careful, gentle handling and it is essential to gain experience in handling them before starting procedures. To perform the procedure, hold the animal gently but firmly. It is easiest to do this by resting it on an absorbent pad on a firm surface with the dorsal surface of the animal held uppermost between the gloved thumb and forefinger. Insert the tip of the needle into the brain, usually from the front, at an angle of 45°, in the area of the anterior cranial fontanelle and gently depress the plunger of the syringe to expel the dose. Practise minimal depression of syringe plungers using fragile inanimate objects (such as artificial sponges), which mimic the texture and the pressure needed to expel fluids. Return the animal to its mother, check for adverse effects after 1 h (to avoid too much immediate disturbance) and monitor closely at least once per day post-injection for adverse effects of the technique or the inoculum. Occasionally, the mother rejects the young when they are returned to her. If there is blood leaking from the injection site she may eat them.

There is debate over whether the use of anaesthesia for animals of this age would be appropriate, since this in itself can cause distress which has to be balanced against the stress of intracerebral injection. However, modern anaesthetics can be given safely by competent personnel. The perception of pain in neonatal animals has been the subject of considerable investigation and advance in the last few years. See Chapter 4 for more detail on assessing the condition of neonatal rodents. The non-use of anaesthesia in very young animals is very outdated.

In adult rodents a stereotaxic frame is needed to ensure that there is no lateral movement of the needle, which would cause trauma. Anaesthesia is essential for this, as is aseptic technique and sterile material. Injection volumes should not exceed 2% of brain volume and should always be given slowly enough to avoid increasing cerebrospinal fluid pressure. Penetration of the ventricle is readily assessed by the sudden reduction of back pressure in the injection line. Chronic placement of cannulae allows injections, or continuous intraventricular infusion, without need for repeated anaesthesia.

Alternative methods of obtaining the results required should always be considered before using this route. The procedure is not easy to perform and the most common adverse effects result from clumsy technique since incorrect placement of the needle can kill the animal. Substances with high protein content may also cause the death of the animal, so check the protein content of the substance to be administered and avoid the intra-cerebral route if this is high. Any animal showing unexpected neural deficits, for example, ataxis or paralysis, within the first 24–36 h should be killed as this is most likely to be due to faulty technique.

## *Intra-articular injection*

Injections into joints *must* be carried out under aseptic conditions to avoid causing septic arthritis. Compounds may be administered by this route for experimental or therapeutic reasons, or samples of joint fluid may be taken for analysis. It is essential to be certain of the anatomy of the joint and its synovial capsule before penetrating the skin, so as to be certain of entering the correct part of the joint. The procedure should be practised on cadavers first.

## *Per rectum*

Enemas may be given to empty the rectum before bowel surgery or radiography, or fluids and some drugs may be given into the rectum or distal colon. Substances may be given via a flexible rubber or polythene tube, or a rigid sigmoidoscope. Whichever method is used, it is essential that the instrument is well lubricated and inserted very gently.

## *Transcutaneous administration*

Delivery of drugs and vaccines via the transcutaneous route is becoming increasingly common in experimental studies with the advent of devices specifically designed for this purpose. Such devices deliver either micro-particulate formulations travelling at high velocity, or liquid formulations coupled to a delivery system designed to breach the outer layer of the skin (stratum corneum).

Depending on the species and site of administration, light anaesthesia or sedation may be required to allow site preparation and/or administration of the test material. Animals with dense fur such as rodents and rabbits should have the administration site clipped and shaved to remove as much hair as possible. Animals such as the pig may only require close clipping in order to remove course hairs. For the actual administration, the device or delivery system should be positioned so that it is in close contact with the skin, usually perpendicular to the skin's surface.

Following delivery, the site can be monitored for dermal responses including erythema and oedema using assessment criteria such as the modified Draize score.

# Sampling

## *Urine*

Urine may be collected as it is voided naturally in all species, or by using various techniques. A metabolism cage, in which all the animal's waste products can be collected, can be used in all species, and in rodents this is the only reliable method for obtaining a sample. For larger species, urine may be expressed manually (e.g. cats), collected by using a urethral catheter if the urethra is wide enough (e.g. rabbits and larger species), or withdrawn by cystocentesis under aseptic conditions. With the latter method, the skin over the lower abdomen is clipped and cleaned as for surgery, the full bladder is immobilised with one hand and a sterile needle of a suitable gauge (see Table 9.2a) inserted through the body wall into the bladder.

Urinary catheters may be maintained in situ for prolonged periods, either after surgical implantation (in which the catheter may be channelled to exit the skin at a distant site as for venous cannulae), or passing into the urethra. Urinary catheters predispose to cystitis and urethritis, so particular care must be taken when maintaining them for prolonged periods, and they should not be kept in place for any longer than necessary. Clean the prepuce or vulva prior to insertion of the catheter using an antibacterial cleanser. Use a soft, flexible, sterile catheter and lubricate it before insertion. The catheter should not be introduced too far into the bladder or there will be trauma to the bladder wall, and it can be sutured in place to prevent movement. It is important to avoid urine scald, by collecting the urine into a bag, or by ensuring meticulous cleanliness around the end of the catheter and protecting the skin with petroleum jelly or a similar barrier. It is also important to prevent infection from tracking up the catheter into the urinary tract. If using a collecting bag, make sure urine always drains out of the bladder. Clean the vulva or prepuce around the catheter daily with antibacterial cleanser, and the catheter can be flushed with sterile saline or dilute chlorhexidine if necessary. Do not flush antibiotic solutions into the bladder, since this may predispose to resistant infections. The urine can be monitored bacteriologically, and antibiotics given systemically if appropriate.

## *Faeces*

Faeces may be collected after being voided naturally, by using an enema, or by using a rectal swab. A metabolism cage can be used, and in rodents again this is the most reliable method. Enemas may be given to collect large quantities of faeces, or swabs may be used for small samples, for example, for bacteriology. It is essential that anything passed into the rectum is inserted gently.

In rodents and rabbits, which are coprophagic, hard faeces can be collected as above, but to collect soft faeces, which are normally eaten straight from the anus, restraining devices must be used.

## *Semen*

Semen can be collected from the larger animals in a number of ways. In cattle and horses, a teaser female can be used to excite the male, and an artificial vagina used to collect the semen. In rams and larger primates, electroejaculation is usually used. A probe is inserted gently into the rectum, and an electric current stimulates the nerves to the genitals resulting in ejaculation. In dogs, digital manipulation can be used, with or without the presence of a bitch in season. Semen collection in rodents may require the surgical removal of the seminal vesicles prior to collection to prevent the semen clotting.

## *Milk*

The mammary glands of ruminants and horses are served by teats, whereas those of the smaller animals have nipples. Teats are larger, with one or two orifices from which milk can be expressed, and the udders of these species are large enough to permit the taking of large samples. At peak lactation, up to 17 l of milk may be withdrawn twice daily from a Friesian cow. Nipples have several orifices from which milk flows, and small samples can be collected from these.

Milk can be expressed by grasping the nipple or teat at its base and gently pulling towards the tip. In newly parturient females, injections of oxytocin may increase the release of milk.

To collect milk samples from mice: Separate the pups from the mother and keep them warm for about 3 h prior to milking. Give 1–10 IU of oxytocin about 30 min prior to a short acting anaesthetic (isoflurane/O$_2$) and milking. Day 10–12 of lactation is the highest in milk production and milking at around this time should yield the most milk (see www.mp.ucdavis.edu/tgmice/milk/momilk.html).

## POLYCLONAL ANTIBODY PRODUCTION IN LABORATORY ANIMALS

Antibodies are used in a huge variety of studies, ranging from medical research to archaeological and forensic enquiries. There are methods of producing some types of antibodies *in vitro*, but if these are impossible they are manufactured by injecting the appropriate antigen into an animal. The choice of species for antibody production is important. Ideally, the recipient should be a diverse species from the donor of the antigen to ensure a maximal immune response. Rabbits are good for making antibodies to other mammals. Chickens are good for raising antibodies to mammalian proteins, and some antibody is passed into the egg yolk and can be harvested non-invasively. Rats are good for creating IgE antibodies, and farm animal species are useful if large volumes of serum are required.

The route of injection affects the efficacy of the immunisation. Ideally, the antigen should be distributed to the widest area and the largest number of lymph nodes possible. Intradermal inoculation is the most effective route for soluble antigens without adjuvant, but tends to produce the most local reaction. For other routes, the relative efficacies are:

$$i.d. > i.p. > s.c. > i.m. > i.v.$$

Particulate antigens and those with adjuvant may be given effectively by the s.c. or i.p. route.

## Polyclonal antibody production using adjuvants

Production of antibody may be achieved by injection of the required antigen into an animal, in combination with a suitable adjuvant. Adjuvants stimulate the immune system to produce the appropriate class of antibody, by prolonging exposure of the antigen to the immune system, and promoting phagocytosis and antigen processing. They may also act as immunostimulators or immunomodifiers, activating immune cells directly, altering the balance of the immune cells, or activating complement.

There are a wide range of adjuvants available such as Titermax, aluminium hydroxide and muramyl dipeptide. Freund's Complete Adjuvant (FCA) uses paraffin oil to produce the depot effect and killed mycobacteria to stimulate macrophage responses and antigen processing. Unfortunately, this adjuvant often produces severe inflammatory reactions, such as tissue swelling, necrosis, abscessation and sloughing and there are many better alternatives now available.

## Principles for protocols of minimal severity

These notes, reproduced from the Home Office, provide information appropriate to protocols of minimal severity for raising antibodies using living animals. Where protocols of greater severity can be justified in a project licence application, consideration will be given on a case by case basis for licence authority to cover such procedures.

### *Primary immunisation*

It may be necessary to combine the antigen with an adjuvant in order to enhance the antibody response. A range of adjuvants are available; one should be chosen which will stimulate antibodies of the desired affinity, avidity, titre and class, with minimal

**Table 9.4**  Recommended injection volumes for immunisations.

| Route | Species | Volume of single dose (ml) | Volume of maximum total dose (ml)* |
|---|---|---|---|
| Intradermal | Rabbit | 0.05–0.1 | 0.4 |
| Intramuscular | Rabbit | 0.1–0.25 | 0.5 |
| Subcutaneous | Guinea-pig | <0.25 | <1 |
| | Mouse | <0.1 | <0.2 |
| | Rabbit | 0.1–0.25 | 1.0 |
| | Rat | <0.2 | <0.4 |
| | Sheep and goats | <0.25 | <1 |

*In rabbits, guinea pigs, sheep and goats a maximum of four sites should be used, and in rats and mice a maximum of two sites should be used.

local tissue damage. Some adjuvants, such as FCA, cause significant local reactions and should be used as set out below. No adjuvants should be used via the i.v. route, although antigen in PBS may be given i.v., usually as the final booster inoculation. The i.d. route should be avoided when adjuvants are used.

When a significant local reaction is expected, such as with FCA, the antigen/adjuvant mixture should be given subcutaneously in areas of loose skin and doses should not exceed 0.1 ml at each of two sites in mice, 0.2 ml at each of two sites in rats and 0.25 ml at each of four sites in guinea-pigs, rabbits, sheep, goats and equids. FCA should never be used on more than one occasion in the same animal. Stable emulsions should be used with no more that 50% FCA mixed with antigen in aqueous solution. FCA should not be used in horses or other equids. The i.m. route may be used in chickens and should not exceed 0.1 ml in each of four sites. For recommended injection volumes, see Table 9.4.

## Boosting

In order to raise or maintain the antibody titre it may be necessary to administer the antigen on one or more further occasions. These 'boosters' should conform to the principles set out for primary immunisation, but must not include FCA, and should be no more in number than required to achieve and maintain the required titre. Animals that fail to respond within four 'boosts' should be withdrawn from the protocol.

## Sampling

Superficial blood vessels are usually adequate for blood collection during monitoring of antibody titre in all species. No more than 15% of total blood volume (TBV) should be taken over any 4-week period and usually no more than 10% TBV should be removed as a single collection. The TBV of laboratory animal species averages 65 ml/kg. Consideration should be given to the use of local or general anaesthesia as appropriate for the species.

## Harvesting

It is recommended that when the antibody titre has reached a plateau, rodents and rabbits should be bled out under terminal general anaesthesia. The serum can then be separated, divided into aliquots and deep frozen. Eggs should be collected during a laying season, but moulting must not be induced. Where serial harvesting is appropriate, the volume of blood collected should be limited as set out above, unless special arrangements such as haematological monitoring can be included in the licence authority.

## Additional points to note

Foot pad immunisation in rodents should only be performed if study of the draining lymph node in isolation is required. If this is necessary, only one foot should be immunised per animal, and soft bedding should be provided. The tail base of rodents can be used to induce polyarthritis. With the i.d. route, the depot effect produced by the adjuvant is prolonged. The antigen is protected from degradation and is undispersed, remaining exposed to the immune system for longer. Large non-painful granulomas with ulceration of the skin may develop, which may become painful abscesses if traumatised by the animal or if the injection is not sterile. The severity of any reaction to i.d. injections varies with the injection volume. Subcutaneous injections are easier and produce fewer granulomas. However, with subcutaneous administration, the adjuvant may track ventrally, producing fistulous tracts and firm linear lesions distant from the injection site. With i.m. injections, although any lesions developing are not readily detectable, they will be particularly painful when the muscles are used, for example, for respiration or locomotion. Therefore, subcutaneous administration is preferable, although care must be taken not to inadvertently give the injection i.d. or i.m. Strict adherence to sterile technique when giving the injection is essential, in order to reduce the occurrence of bacterial infections. The skin should be clipped of fur and swabbed with alcohol before the injection, and a new sterile syringe and needle must be used. Any adjuvant-induced granulomas are composed mainly of macrophages and lymphocytes, and are non-painful. The introduction of bacteria causes an infiltration of polymorphonuclear leucocytes, which tends to be painful. This pain predisposes to self-mutilation by the animal.

## Injection volumes

The initial immunisation should not exceed the recommendations in Table 9.4. They should be given at intervals such that complete recovery from one injection is allowed before the next is given. A period of 30–45 days is adequate for this. Ideally, the antibody titre should be monitored, and booster injections given as this begins to decline.

## ANIMAL MODELS

There are a number of specific animal models of diseases, such as osteoporosis, atherosclerosis, neurodegenerative diseases and various models of infectious agents. For a good review, see Registry of Comparative Pathology Symposium 1997 Animal Models of Human Disease for the 21st Century.

# EQUIPMENT FOR CARRYING OUT MINOR PROCEDURES

The performance of any scientific procedure will be facilitated if the correct equipment is available. Think carefully about the procedure that you are going to do, and make sure that you have all the necessary equipment ready.

## Blood collection and intravenous administration of substances

Before attempting i.v. injections on a live animal, it is desirable to gain practical experience on a cadaver or a model, in order to develop the necessary skills. The KOKEN rat (B&K Universal Ltd) is an anatomically correct model rat with lifelike tail veins on which i.v. injections and blood sampling can be practised. It is also possible to practise gavage and endotracheal intubation using this model. Simple models for practising i.v. injections may also be made by covering soft rubber cannulae with plastic, and other types of injection can be practised using soft toys or even oranges.

### *Over-the-needle cannulae*

Flexible over-the-needle cannulae (see Figure 9.9) can be obtained in a variety of sizes to suit the species and the intended site of administration or withdrawal. They are easily inserted into the superficial veins of most species, and once in situ they do not lacerate the vein if the animal moves. For recommended sizes see Table 9.2b.

### *Evacuated blood collection tubes*

These are tubes with a rubber seal on one end which contain a partial vacuum (e.g. 'Vacutainers', Becton Dickinson, and 'Wexvac' tubes or 'Monovettes', Sarstedt). Double ended needles and a special holder are required to use evacuated tubes. The needle is screwed into the holder, with one end of the needle just touching the rubber seal of the tube without penetrating it. The other end of the needle is placed into the vein, and the tube advanced until the needle penetrates the seal. The vacuum in the tube sucks blood into the tube. If the tube is advanced too soon, then air will be sucked into the tube and the vacuum will be lost. Once the tube is full, no more blood is sucked in. The tube should be taken out of the holder as the needle is withdrawn from the animal. Evacuated tubes are quick and easy to use, but are only useful if the vein is large enough to allow rapid flow of blood. Occasionally, the rapid passage into the evacuated tube will damage the red blood cells and result in haemolysis. Evacuated tubes are available with or without anticoagulant: if anticoagulant is required, mix it with the blood by rolling the tube, not shaking it as this can damage the cells (Figure 9.12).

### *Butterfly needles*

These are needles with a long flexible tube attached, with a fitting on the end for syringes (see Figure 9.9). They are useful because a syringe can be attached at some distance from the animal, and the needle can be taped in place in a vein using the wings. They can be used for administration of substances and withdrawal of blood.

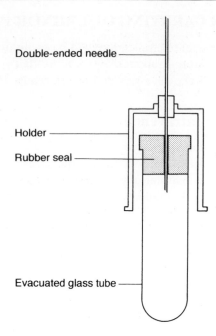

Double-ended needle

Holder

Rubber seal

Evacuated glass tube

**Figure 9.12**   Vacutainer.

## *Tourniquets*

When performing i.v. injections or withdrawing blood from some superficial veins, such as the cephalic, jugular or saphenous veins, the vein must be raised in order for a needle to enter it. This can be done by an assistant, placing their thumb over the vein proximal to the site of venepuncture, but this can be awkward, and it is often easier to use a tourniquet. These occlude the venous drainage, raising the vein, and usually have quick release mechanisms so they can be removed rapidly (see Figure 9.7, 'Vetourni-quet', Animalcare).

## *Vasodilating agents*

For some smaller species, for example, rabbits and rats, collecting blood can be facili-tated by applying vasodilators to a superficial vein to engorge it and increase the blood flow. Warm water has some effect, but there are safe chemical agents available, which cause vasodilation within 5–10 min after application, and which can be wiped off once the blood has been collected. An example is d-limonene oil ('Vasolate', IMS). Note that xylene is carcinogenic and its use is not recommended.

## FURTHER INFORMATION

Adjuvants and antibody production (1995). *Institute of Laboratory Animal Resources Journal* 37, 3.
BVA/FRAME/RSPCA/UFAW (1993). Joint working group on refinement. Removal of blood from laboratory mammals and birds. *Laboratory Animals* 27, 1–22.

Draize, J.H., Woodard, G. and Calvery, H.O. (1944). Methods for the study of irritation and toxicity of substances applied topically to the skin and mucous membranes. *Journal of Pharmacology and Experimental Therapeutics* 82, 377–90.

ECVAM Workshop report 23 (1997). Monoclonal antibody production ATLA 25, 121–137.

Hem, A., Smith, A.J. and Solberg, P. (1998). Saphenous vein puncture for blood sampling of the mouse, rat, hamster, gerbil, guineapig, ferret and mink. *Laboratory Animals* 32, 364–68.

Home Office (2000). Antibody production: principles for protocols of minimum severity: www.homeoffice.gov.uk

LASA Good Practice Guidelines Series 1 issue 1 Oct 1998 from LASA PO Box 3993 Tamworth Staffs.

McGuill, M.W. and Rowan, A.N. (1989). Biological effects of blood loss: implications for sampling volumes and techniques. *Institute of Laboratory Animal Resources News*, 31(4), 5–18.

Nau, R. and Schunck, O. (1993). Cannulation of the lateral saphenous vein – a rapid method to gain access to the circulation in anaesthetised guinea pigs. *Laboratory Animals* 27, 23–25.

O'Hagan, D. (ed.) (2000). *Vaccine Adjuvants – Preparation Methods and Research Protocols.* Humana Press.

Osebold, J.W. (1982). Mechanisms of action by immunological adjuvants. *Journal of the American Veterinary Medical Association* 181, 983–87.

Registry of Comparative Pathology Symposium (1997). Animal Models of Human Disease for the 21st Century. *Laboratory Animal Science* 48, 559–629.

United Kingdom Coordinating Committee on Cancer Research (1997). *Guidelines for the Welfare of Animals in Experimental Neoplasia.* UKCCCR, London.

# Chapter 10
# Introduction to surgery and suturing

Before starting to carry out any surgical procedure, make sure you know how to achieve the best results. Think carefully about the facilities that are available and whether they are adequate for what you wish to achieve. Ensure you are completely familiar with the anatomy of the species and the part that you will be working on, and practise by dissecting cadavers before obtaining your licence and attempting the procedure on a live animal.

## INTRODUCTION TO SURGICAL BIOLOGY

### Inflammation and wound healing

The mechanisms of wound healing need to be considered before performing surgical techniques, because good surgical technique relies on an understanding of the ways in which tissues respond to injury. Any injury to living animal tissues, whatever the cause, causes damage to cells. These damaged cells release mediators, which result in the accumulation of cells, including polymorphs and macrophages, and humoral factors such as antibodies at the site of injury. This process is known as *inflammation*. These cells and humoral factors begin the process of healing.

Inflammation produces several clinical features known as the cardinal signs of inflammation. These are as follows:

- *Heat* (*calor*). The affected area becomes warm to the touch.
- *Redness* (*rubor*). The tissue becomes red (non-pigmented areas) due to dilation of blood vessels.
- *Swelling* (*tumor*). The infiltration of cells and fluid causes the area to swell.
- *Pain* (*dolor*). Inflammatory mediators stimulate nerve endings to cause pain. Some analgesics work by blocking the release of these inflammatory mediators.
- *Loss of function* (*defunctor*). Voluntary or involuntary restriction of movement.

After injury, changes occur in the tissues which result in inflammation and begin healing. The sequence of events is as follows.

### *Inflammatory phase*

1. *Haemorrhage*. Bleeding from damaged blood vessels occurs and is then arrested by the aggregation of platelets and fibrin, which form a scab.
2. *Inflammation*. Mediators from damaged cells cause the influx of cells and humoral factors.
3. *Primary wound contraction*. Local fibroblast cells contract to reduce the area of the wound as much as possible.

## *Proliferation phase*

1. *Epithelial proliferation*. This begins within 12–24 h. The cells divide and migrate over the surface of the wound. A moist environment facilitates this.
2. *Granulation*. Fibroblasts and capillaries beneath the epithelium begin proliferating after approximately 36 h. They form granulation tissue, which is bright pink, firm, flat and resistant to infection. It fills in any defects in tissues and provides oxygen for the proliferating epithelium and surrounding parenchymal tissues. Granulation tissue will only form once inflammation has subsided and the area has been cleared of necrotic debris by macrophages.

It is normal for the epithelium to heal before granulation has filled in the defects in deeper tissues, leaving a concave surface. Granulation will continue beneath the surface until the surface is flat.

## *Maturation phase*

Local fibroblasts lay down collagen, and granulation tissue matures into fibrous tissue to form a scar. This area then undergoes secondary wound contraction or cicatrisation, which reduces the area of the scar, but can result in the restriction of movement or the occlusion of a hollow organ. Initially, old collagen at the wound edges softens before sufficient new collagen is laid down to increase wound strength after 5–7 days. Wound strength continues to increase for up to 2 years depending on the nature and site of the injury.

Remember that wound edges swell due to inflammation and weaken in the first few days post-trauma, so sutures must not be too tight or too close to the edge, or they will cut into the tissues in this period.

## Types of healing

There are several possible outcomes following healing, depending on the nature of the injury and the tissue type:

- *Resolution*. This occurs when there is minimal tissue damage. The inflammatory exudate and cells are resorbed with no tissue destruction or scarring, and the tissues return to normal.
- *Regeneration*. Areas of lost or damaged tissue are replaced by differentiation of surrounding tissues until the organ mass has returned to normal, with no permanent loss of function. There may be disruption to the architecture of the organ. Bone and liver heal this way.
- *Suppuration with tissue death*. If there is much tissue damage, areas of devitalised tissue undergo necrosis and liquefy, with or without the presence of infection. The purulent exudate formed is released by sloughing or tracking along lines of low resistance to the outside. The defect produced will eventually heal by granulation and scarring, once the exudate has been cleared.

- *Repair by fibrosis.* Lost tissues are replaced by fibrous tissues to form a scar. Scar tissue is non-functional, and tends to contract, which can lead to problems as outlined above.

Healing is affected by a number of factors, local and general, which are listed below.

## *Local*

- *Infection.* Bacteria consume oxygen, attract inflammatory cells and mediators, and inhibit epithelialisation and wound contraction.
- *Tension and pressure.* Excess tension or pressure interferes with nutrition of the wound edges.
- *Interference with blood supply.* A satisfactory blood supply is required for healing.
- *Presence of alien tissues.* For example, pieces of fat between skin edges or neoplastic cells in any wound prevent healing.
- *Persistent irritation.* Hair around the wound edges or interference from the animal or its cage mates may prevent healing.

## *General*

- *Age.* Healing tends to be slower in older animals.
- *Nutritional status.* Protein malnutrition in particular leads to poor healing.
- *Corticosteroid level.* These hormones are released during stress. They affect the function of phagocytic cells and reduce collagen formation.
- *Reduced tissue oxygen and intercurrent disease.* Diseases may reduce tissue oxygen, cause stress or affect nutrition, all of which affect healing. Regular health monitoring will ensure the animals are disease free.
- *Region of body and tissue type.* Different tissues have different blood supplies and, therefore, different oxygen levels. Tissues such as muscle and epithelium have good blood supplies and heal quickly, whereas fascia and connective tissues have poor blood supplies and heal slowly.

Many of these are under the control of the person performing the surgical procedure. The amount of pain, suppuration, fibrous tissue and scarring produced during a surgical procedure depends on the degree of tissue damage and inflammation produced. Good surgical techniques will result in minimal production of inflammation, infection and scarring. Luck is not a factor, and good techniques will produce good results.

## PRINCIPLES OF SURGERY

### Historical perspective

Prior to 1862, doctors performed surgery on animals and people without understanding the mechanisms of healing outlined above. The instruments were not sterilised, the patient's skin was not cleaned, and doctors did not wash their hands or their equipment. The central tenet of a 'good' doctor was a coat, which was so caked in blood and tissue fluid that it would stand up on its own. The major problem associated with surgery under those conditions was sepsis, and patients frequently died from infection. In 1862, Lister determined that there was a link between contamination of wounds and infection, and set about changing the way things were done. He advocated two things:

1. Removal of necrotic (dead) tissue and dirt from wounds.
2. Application of chemical disinfectants, such as carbonic acid, to the surgeon's hands and to the wounds.

This was the start of antiseptic surgery, which developed over several decades into the aseptic surgery, which is used today. Here, instead of trying to remove infection from wounds, it is prevented by ensuring good sterility of the operating room, the equipment, the surgeon and the patient/animal.

## Principles of asepsis

All possible sources of contamination or infection need to be removed from the surgical field prior to surgery, so as not to contaminate the wound. The main sources of contamination are

- the atmosphere
- the surgical team
- the instruments and equipment
- the skin of the animal.

### *The atmosphere*

The atmosphere of the operating room is the source of contamination which is most difficult to control. Dust and other airborne particles can settle in the wound, bringing bacteria with them. To reduce this problem, there must be less dust and less air movement. Operating rooms should remain uncluttered, with few fixtures and fittings where dust can collect, and they must be thoroughly cleaned and disinfected regularly. This is facilitated in a well-designed operating theatre in which there are few ledges or cupboards, and where all fittings are flush with the walls. Even non-recovery procedures depend on good surgery, which requires precision and clarity of thought, so all unnecessary clutter should be kept away and there must be adequate space for all the equipment and instruments, which you intend to use.

The best ventilation system is one which uses an input fan with a filter. This produces positive pressure in the room, and tends to push dust particles out of the room away from the animal. When people enter and leave dirt is brought in and stirred up, so as few people as possible should be allowed into the room. The operating room should not be used as a storeroom or a thoroughfare. The best way to maintain the operating room is to keep it as just that – an operating room and nothing else. Ideally, major surgery should be performed within a suite of rooms, each room having its own function:

- *The 'prep room'* is the area where animals should be prepared for surgery. They are brought to this room from the animal room/kennel, anaesthetised, clipped and cleaned. Only once they are ready, do they go through into the theatre.

- *The operating theatre* is used just for surgery. Care must be taken not to bring dust, dirt and hair through from the prep room.
- *A recovery area* should be provided where animals can be taken after surgery for intensive nursing care and observation, while recovering from anaesthetic. This room needs to be easily accessible for people, unlike the operating room.

The whole suite of rooms should be made with impervious floors, walls and ceilings to allow thorough cleaning and fumigation, if required.

It is also essential for the operating room to be equipped with a good, shadowless light source, to enable the surgeon to see what he is doing, a steady table with facilities to adjust the height and tilt, a chair which can also be adjusted, and for surgery on very small animals, or for microsurgery, a binocular microscope. An anglepoise lamp is not satisfactory, since it can produce excessive heat over a long period of time, and casts shadows, which make working difficult. For large animal surgery, there must be adequate equipment for lifting and moving an anaesthetised or recumbent animal, without injury to it or to the handler. The human hand is capable of very precise movements, but this skill is limited by the ability to see what is being done. Consider the use of optical assistance such as an operating microscope or binocular loupe for small-scale precision surgery, or even just regular sight tests and the wearing of appropriate spectacles. The operating table must be steady to allow precise movements and the height should be adjustable. Used in conjunction with an adjustable seat, this will assist the operator's comfort and precision, reducing fatigue and strain.

## *Preparation of instruments and equipment*

Sterilisation or disinfection of instruments and equipment is mandatory prior to surgery, and there are many simple ways to achieve sterility.

- *Sterilisation* is the removal or destruction of all living microbes, including spores.
- *Disinfection* is the removal or destruction of all living microbes, but excluding spores.

All disinfectants and sterilising agents act by denaturing proteins.

Drapes and swabs can be bought pre-sterilised in packs. They are more expensive this way, but much more convenient and remove the necessity for an autoclave.

After use, instruments must always be washed thoroughly. Cold water will facilitate the removal of blood, then hot water with detergent is used to remove grease, which acts as a barrier to the penetration of chemical and physical sterilising agents. Care must be taken to clean inside the joints and teeth of instruments where blood and tissue fluids collect. After sterilisation, instruments should be allowed to dry, to prevent rusting.

## Physical methods of sterilisation

Heat is the main physical method, either wet or dry:

1. *Boiling water.* Boiling at 100°C for 20 min will disinfect instruments, but will not kill spores. This method is not suitable for fabrics. Care must be taken that the instruments are allowed to cool before use or the animal's skin may be damaged.

2. *Autoclaves.* These utilise steam under pressure, and are considered to sterilise if used correctly. The time, pressure and temperature used vary with the material. Instruments are usually autoclaved at 121°C and 15 psi for 20 min. Autoclaves producing higher temperatures and pressures take less time. Rubber and some plastics can be autoclaved at lower temperatures, but take longer. The steam used in autoclaves penetrates through fabrics, so this method is useful for drapes, gowns, swabs and dressings.

   Items to be autoclaved may be free in the autoclave, or prepacked into autoclave bags made of plastic, paper or cloth. Such bags allow the penetration of steam but not microbes, and can be used for short-term storage of items after autoclaving.

   Several rules must be followed when using the autoclave:
   (a) Steam must first displace the air before the sterilisation cycle can begin. Some machines use a vacuum to remove the air.
   (b) Steam must be allowed to penetrate through to the items inside the machine. Wrappings must, therefore, be of suitable permeable material, specifically designed for use in autoclaves.
   (c) Fabrics must be folded loosely and not tightly packed or steam will not penetrate. If the autoclave is too full, it will not run efficiently.
   (d) Autoclave tape which changes colour placed on the outside of the pack to seal it, simply indicates that the pack has been exposed to steam; it does not provide assurance that the pack has been exposed to sufficient temperature for sufficient time. Indicators placed within the packaging should be used to check that sterility has been achieved.
   (e) Steam must be allowed to escape from the packaging after autoclaving, so the contents may dry out.

   Once they leave the autoclave, packets containing instruments have only a limited shelf-life during which they remain sterile. The date of autoclaving should, therefore, be written on each packet and old packets re-sterilised at intervals.

   Autoclaving is not suitable for catheters, endoscopes and delicate materials.
3. *Dry heat.* Hot air ovens held at 160°C for at least 1 h will sterilise items. This is only suitable for some metal and glass articles. The method is efficient at removing pathogens, but slow. It is useful because it does not cause corrosion of metals or pitting of glass, which can occur with repeated autoclaving. Also, instruments can be sterilised, coated with grease, as this does not prevent the object from being heated. It is used for sharp optical instruments, as it does not cause blunting. It is not suitable for fabrics and paper.
4. *Burning.* This is used for destruction of contaminated materials.
5. *Ionising radiation (gamma irradiation).* This is used commercially for sterilisation of needles, syringes, suture materials and delicate items. The method is very efficient, but not suitable for use in a standard operating theatre.
6. *Ultraviolet light.* This has very limited efficiency and cannot be recommended in a surgical environment.

### Chemical sterilisation

Chemical methods are less efficient than physical means, but are often used for delicate items. Instructions must be followed carefully for good results. Several factors must be taken into consideration before using chemical sterilising agents:

- Items to be sterilised must be very clean or the chemical will not penetrate. Many chemicals are inactivated by debris, such as blood.
- The method is slow, and sufficient time must be allowed for sterilisation to occur.
- Liquid sterilisers must be at the correct concentration. A higher concentration does not necessarily mean more efficient sterilisation.
- Most chemical agents are irritant, so all residues must be removed prior to use of the instrument.
- For gaseous agents, items must be dry and moisture free.

Chemical agents are often used as quick sterilising agents in field situations, where there is no access to an autoclave:

- *Ethanol.* Ethanol at 70% will disinfect instruments, but will not sterilise even after several days' immersion. Higher or lower concentrations are less effective.
- *Phenolics.* Chlorocresol may be used as a cold steriliser, combined with tri-ethanolamine as a cleansing agent; sodium formate as a descaler; and sodium citrate to prevent blood from clotting on the instruments. If instruments are cleaned of gross contamination, then immersed in it for 1–2 min, they will be disinfected. Aqueous or organic iodine preparations are also disinfectant. They corrode metals, but are useful in emergencies.
- *Quaternary ammonium compounds.* These are relatively non-toxic and non-irritant, such as chlorhexidine, which can be made up in 70% alcohol for emergency disinfection of instruments if items are placed in it for 3–4 min.
- *Glutaraldehyde.* This disinfects in 3–4 min, and sterilises in 12–24 h. It is useful for optical instruments.
- *Ethylene oxide.* This is a potent and effective way to sterilise items such as plastic disposables that will not withstand autoclaving, or delicate items such as electrical and optical equipment. It is inflammable and potentially explosive, so batteries should be removed first. Items are pre-sealed in packs and the ethylene oxide ampoule is opened within a sealed plastic liner and then left in a chamber with the items for a defined period of time. Items such as catheters require longer and a higher concentration. Items that are going to come into contact with animal tissue, particularly those that are to be implanted must have an adequate period for all traces of the ethylene oxide to be eliminated or there will be severe tissue reactions. Due regard must be paid to COSHH regulations on its use because of its toxicity and irritancy.

## Preparation of the animal

The body of the animal carries two sorts of contaminants:

- Resident commensal or symbiotic flora, which are hard to eliminate.
- Extraneous potential pathogens, which are easier to eliminate.

These bacteria feed on debris on the surface of the skin. Prior to surgery, mechanical cleansing is required to remove this debris. Animals covered with fur need to be clipped to allow cleansing of the skin. Ideally, this should be done 24 h before surgery, to allow any trauma to the skin to recover and to allow loose hair to fall off. If shaving is done immediately prior to an operation, care must be taken to remove any loose hair. Clippers are available with a variety of blades for different purposes. All-purpose blades can be used on most species, and there are special blades for coarse hair and for clipping sheep. Size 40 blades are general blades for surgical and laboratory use. Size 10 blades are useful for sensitive skin and in awkward areas. Clippers need to be maintained in good condition, or they stop clipping effectively. They should be brushed after each use, to remove the loose hair, and sprayed with a disinfecting lubricant spray. If this is not done, they start to pull the hair and can cut the skin, particularly in animals with delicate skin, such as rabbits, and around delicate areas, such as the nipple. Periodically, the blades need to be sharpened. An adequate area must be shaved to prevent contamination of the wound by adjacent fur, but too much fur removal will contribute to heat loss in smaller animals during and after surgery.

The animal must be appropriately positioned for surgery. Ensure that there is no restriction to respiration by extending the head and neck, and position the limbs such that they do not cross the chest. If limb ties are used, take care to ensure that they are not applied too tightly. There are a variety of commercial cradles available for positioning animals. Cheap animal positioning devices can be made from pieces of foam rubber or sand bags, which can be covered in washable material, and these also provide some insulation around the animal reducing heat loss. If the procedure is to be prolonged, bony areas should be padded to prevent pressure sores, bland ophthalmic ointment put into the eye to prevent corneal drying; and in ruminants, a stomach tube passed to prevent ruminal tympany.

There are three stages in preparation of the skin:

1. A wash to remove any gross debris, such as mud or faeces. Be sure to use a cleaning agent that is compatible with antiseptic agent you will be using.
2. An antiseptic wash, with a quaternary ammonium compound or an organic iodine preparation. These must be used at the recommended concentrations to avoid causing any tissue damage. Chlorhexidine is more effective and is to be preferred. It is particularly important with small laboratory animals to avoid hypothermia, so solutions used for preparation of the skin must be warm, and the fur must not be allowed to get overwet. Skin should be cleansed from the middle of the clipped area towards the outside, never the other way round, or this will drag dirt from the fur at the edge on to the skin where the incision will be.
3. A final skin prep of alcohol may be applied to the skin. Again, in small animals this may be omitted to prevent excess heat loss.

After the skin has been cleaned, sterile drapes are applied, by the surgeon, to cover all but the surgical field. Fabric or paper drapes may be used. Drapes must be dry, or they act as a wick drawing contamination up from beneath and onto the surgical site.

## *Preparation of the surgical team*

The bodies of the surgical team are potential sources of contamination of the wound. The resident population of bacteria and other microbes, which are found on the skin may be pathogenic if they penetrate into a wound, and the surgeon can spread infection from one animal to another on his hands. To prevent infection from being spread by the surgical team, the day's operations should be planned in advance so as to proceed in a logical order. Dirty operations and autopsies should not be done before clean surgery: do clean operations first, to reduce the risk of spread of infection between animals.

To control contamination from the skin of the surgeon, the body should be encased in sterile material. All people intending to enter the operating room should arrive clean, with washed hands and no jewellery. Surgeons should have short neatly trimmed fingernails to prevent harbouring contamination and to prevent injury to the animal. It is usual for all clothing including footwear to be either changed for 'scrub suits' used only in the theatre, or completely covered up. A cap and a face mask should be worn. Masks protect the animal from pathogens in the respiratory tract of the people in the room, and also protect the people from animal allergens and pathogens arising during the procedure. Once everyone in the operating room has changed into the appropriate clothing, the surgeon and those involved directly in the operation encase themselves in sterile material. For full aseptic technique, the following protocol should be used. For minor surgical procedures, less stringent precautions need to be taken and the protocol can be modified accordingly, but as a minimum, hands should be washed well with an antibacterial agent and sterile gloves worn. Not only do the gloves protect the animals, they also protect the surgeon from pathogens or allergens that may be carried by the animal.

1. *Scrubbing up*. A 5 min wash of hands and forearms removes many microbes from the skin. First, the hands and forearms, including the elbows, should be washed using antibacterial skin cleanser and running water. Quaternary ammonium compounds such as chlorhexidine have been found to be more effective at reducing the levels of skin bacteria than organic iodine preparations. The fingernails should be scrubbed, then the skin cleanser should be massaged well into hands and forearms and worked down to the elbows. The hands should always be held above the elbows to prevent dirty water from running down the arm on to clean areas. The wash is repeated at least twice. Having done the elbows, the hands and arms should be rinsed from hand to elbow.

    The next stage is the 1 min scrub. A sterile scrubbing brush is used to scrub the fingernails, fingers and palms with antibacterial skin cleanser for 1 min. Then the cleanser is massaged down the forearms, omitting the elbows.

    After rinsing, the final stage is to wash the hands and forearms again with antibacterial skin cleanser, without touching the elbows, then finally rinse with running water from hands to elbows. Hands may or may not be dried with sterile towels.

    After scrubbing up, the hands should always be held together in front of the body above the elbows, to prevent them from touching any non-sterile material and to prevent contamination running down the arm from the elbow.

2. *Gowning*. If sterile gowns are worn, they are autoclaved prior to use, and usually come in bags packed inside out. An assistant should open the bag without touching the contents, and the surgeon takes the gown by the collar and pulls it out of the bag. The gown is held up and shaken lightly; this should allow the surgeon to see the armholes. The surgeon puts the gown on without touching the outside of it, and the ties at the back are done up by an assistant. Once the surgeon has his

gown on, he is considered to be sterile and must not touch any non-sterile objects or personnel.

3. *Gloving*. Surgical gloves come in sterile packs, which are easily opened by an assistant without compromising sterility. The choice of glove will depend on personal preference, but should provide good sensitivity and be micro-roughened for good grip. Modern gloves are coated to provide extra comfort and yet are powder free and low in allergens (e.g. Marigold Suretech Biogel P). Sterile surgical gloves are packaged with the cuffs turned back, and the surgeon picks them up from the bottom of the cuff, so as not to touch the outside of the glove. For long procedures, surgeons sometimes wear two pairs of gloves.

## SURGICAL TECHNIQUES

It is important to perform surgical procedures competently, to cause the minimum amount of trauma to the tissue and facilitate rapid healing. Learn how to handle instruments correctly and to avoid damaging tissues by grasping them with excessive force or with inappropriate instruments. Cutting instruments must be kept sharp and crushing instruments must not be used on tissues that are to be left in situ. There are many different companies producing surgical instruments. Looking through their catalogues will help in the selection of appropriate instruments for the procedure you wish to carry out. Instruments must also be a suitable size for the species and area on which you are working. Good quality instruments are always worth the additional cost, and they must be looked after to ensure they remain in good condition. Surgical instruments must be used *only* for surgery.

Halstead's principles of surgery provide guidelines which will give good results if followed carefully. These are

1. handle tissues gently
2. ensure meticulous haemostasis
3. preserve the blood supply
4. ensure strict asepsis
5. apply minimal tension to tissues
6. ensure accurate tissue apposition (see suturing techniques)
7. obliterate any dead space.

Before starting any surgical procedure involving entry to a body cavity, it is important to count the number of swabs provided and the number of instruments, paying particular attention to the number of any small items, such as loose suture needles. Any additional swabs or other items provided during the procedure should also be noted in writing by an assistant; and when the wound is closed, it is important to check carefully that everything has been accounted for. Surgical procedures should always be kept as short as possible and care must be taken to stop tissues from drying out under the heat of the operating lights and from exposure to the air. Post-operative infection is often related to the length of the procedure. Tissues should be protected from drying by covering them with sterile gauze swabs soaked in warmed saline or by regular applications of warmed sterile saline directly onto the exposed viscera. Any surgical procedure consists of three components, namely the skin incision, the dissection of deeper tissues and haemostasis.

## Skin incision

For optimum healing the skin should be incised with minimum trauma, so usually the skin incision will be made using a sharp (i.e. new) scalpel blade. The scalpel should be held like a pen and the tissue cut with a firm single stroke. A scalpel causes minimal damage to the tissue, as it cuts without crushing. The skin should be tensed at right angles to the line of the incision to ensure that the incision is straight and divides the full thickness of the skin, but no deeper, in one stroke. Scissors can be used to cut skin; but since they exert a crushing action, they will cause more trauma and the crushed tissue will heal more slowly. Diathermy can also be used to incise tissues. This uses an electrical current and heat to cut and cauterise at the same time. Bleeding is minimal, but there is more trauma compared with a scalpel, so again the tissue will heal more slowly. Haemorrhage from the skin edge may consist of oozing from the capillaries and occasionally from small arteries and veins. Firm pressure from a sterile swab is usually sufficient to stop this oozing, although specific vessels may require arrest of haemorrhage with diathermy, ligatures or application of mosquito forceps. When applying the tips of haemostatic forceps to a bleeding point in the cut edge of the skin, it is essential to use the smallest possible forceps and to grasp only the vessel itself, not the full thickness of the skin. Skin is handled with fine rat-toothed forceps, which grip positively but with minimal trauma. If it is necessary to hold the skin flaps, then tissue forceps such as Allis or Lanes forceps should be used.

## Dissection of deeper tissues

*Subcutaneous tissues* can be separated using blunt dissection and then cut once clearly identified. Blunt dissection allows tissues to be separated without risk of damage to nerves and blood vessels. The points of round-ended scissors (e.g. Mayo scissors) are used to spread tissue and separate it atraumatically into its distinct layers, which can then be cut with the blades once vessels and nerves have been safely identified and isolated. Fingers are also useful for blunt dissection, as they feel structures such as a pulsing artery which may be hidden in fat layers. 'Paintbrushing' is a technique of blunt dissection that uses a sterile cotton bud or a gauze swab wrapped around the jaws of sponge-holding forceps to wipe away fatty connective tissue from structures, such as arteries. Fatty tissue may be held during procedures with fine-toothed forceps or Allis tissue-holding forceps. Avoid crushing fatty tissue, as it will be prone to liquefactive necrosis. Since it has a poor blood supply, it will heal slowly if damaged and will be at risk of infection.

*Fibrous connective tissue* is made up of a dense network of collagen and, therefore, needs to be divided by sharp dissection. However, due to the proximity of nerves and blood vessels, it must be done with care and scissors may be preferable to use of a scalpel. Toothed forceps or tissue-holding forceps are needed to handle this tough tissue.

*Muscle* is very vascular and will bleed profusely when incised. Surgical approaches, which avoid cutting muscles, are to be preferred, such as approaches through connective tissue or fascia (e.g. approaching the abdominal cavity via the linea alba). If an approach has to be through a muscle, then it is better to split the muscle longitudinally between the fibres rather than cut it transversely since this will not result in a significant loss of function once healing has occurred. For an incision into the abdominal cavity, other than midline, there are several muscle layers whose fibres run in different directions; these can be split in the corresponding directions to produce a gridiron incision. This will then close by the natural muscle action and heal much better than if muscles were transected.

Some tissues, such as a fatty liver, cannot be satisfactorily held with forceps at all because of the risk of damage and haemorrhage. If you are operating to remove tissue, and do not need to preserve it for histology or other examinations, it is possible to grasp it with larger and more powerful instruments. In general, try to hold the tissue that is to be discarded, and touch the tissue that is to be left in situ as little as possible. In order to avoid bruising, tearing and stretching of tissue, it is preferable to make a larger, rather than a smaller incision. Wounds heal from side to side, not from end to end and, therefore, a larger incision, which allows adequate vision, is always better and will not have any effect on the rate of healing. An incision made with sharp instruments with minimal handling of tissue and sutured appropriately will heal rapidly with minimum discomfort to the animal.

## Haemostasis

Haemostasis can be achieved by taking a swab and applying pressure to the bleeding vessel. When using swabs, always dab or press, never wipe as this will remove the clot and allow continued haemorrhage. For small vessels, a clot may form to seal the hole within a few minutes. If not, bleeding vessels can be picked up and crushed using suitable artery forceps, and then tied off with a simple ligature using a fine suture material, or sealed using diathermy, radiosurgery or cautery, all of which apply heat to the vessels to coagulate them. The most common haemostatic forceps used to grasp bleeding vessels are Spencer–Wells artery forceps or Kocher's forceps, and are particularly useful for picking up bleeding vessels which have retracted into tissue, such as fat. Large vessels require ligatures for secure haemostasis, although it may be possible to seal them effectively enough with diathermy to prevent retrograde haemorrhage from tissue which is about to be discarded. Metal clips can also be used, but they are expensive and require special instruments. Ligatures for haemostasis should be made of absorbable materials, such as Vicryl. The use of non-absorbable materials, such as nylon, can act as a focus for infection, which may lead to the formation of a discharging sinus or give rise to peritonitis, if used in the abdomen.

The amount of blood loss should be carefully monitored, as a very small volume is potentially very significant in a small animal. In larger animals, it is useful to weigh the swabs used to give an estimate of blood loss, so fluids can be infused at an appropriate rate. Whatever the size of the animal, good control of haemorrhage is always important in order to avoid post-operative swelling and to minimise surgical shock and risk to the animal. Artery forceps need to be in good condition with jaws that meet properly. To check the jaws, hold the instrument up to the light and look between the closed jaws for distortion or gaps.

## SURGICAL EQUIPMENT

When performing surgical procedures, the exact instruments required will depend on the nature of the procedure. A wide variety of surgical instruments and other equipment is available, and the licensee should consult the many catalogues published by instrument manufacturers to determine which equipment is suitable for their particular project. As a minimum, instruments will be needed for the three parts of the surgical procedure, namely incision, dissection and haemostasis, and for suturing the wound afterwards.

### Skin incision

#### Scalpel blades

Scalpel blades are available in a variety of shapes and sizes, which are designed for different purposes (Figure 10.1). They may come individually wrapped and pre-sterilised, or non-sterile in packs. Before use, they should be attached to a suitable scalpel handle. Fixed-blade scalpels are also available:

- Size 10 blades are all-purpose blades with a rounded cutting edge, which can be used for most surgical procedures.

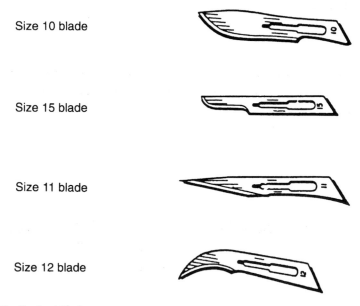

Size 10 blade

Size 15 blade

Size 11 blade

Size 12 blade

**Figure 10.1**    Scalpel blades.

- Size 15 blades are similar to size 10, but smaller and are useful all-purpose blades for fine work on small animals.
- Size 11 blades are pointed, with a straight blade, and are particularly useful for work involving fine cutting of connective tissue.
- Size 12 blades are curved with the cutting edge on the inside of the curve. They are useful for situations where the skin needs to be cut without damaging the structures beneath.

## *Diathermy*

Diathermy units use an electric current to cut the skin and coagulate blood vessels at the same time, or they can be used just for haemostasis. The animal needs to be in contact with an indifferent electrode, consisting of a large flexible metal plate, usually placed under the shaved abdomen. Good contact with the whole of the plate is required: if the plate is bent and the animal is only in contact over a few small areas, it is possible for these areas to become very hot and burn the animal. A small active electrode, consisting of a fine needle, fine forceps or a small metal loop, is used to cut the skin or coagulate vessels at the surgical site. A foot-operated pedal switches the current on and off.

## Deep dissection

### *Scissors*

The dissecting of deeper tissues may involve blunt or sharp dissection. Blunt dissection uses round-ended scissors, such as Mayo or Metzenbaum scissors (Figure 10.2) to separate tissues along natural cleavage planes. Metzenbaum scissors are fine scissors with long handles and rounded tips. The long handles allow the tip to be precisely controlled when operating.

### *Forceps*

Forceps are needed to hold tissues during dissection and when suturing. They are available in many different patterns. Blunt forceps are useful for holding delicate tissues, and rat-toothed forceps (Figure 10.3) are used for tough tissues such as skin and fascia, although they are more traumatic to use.

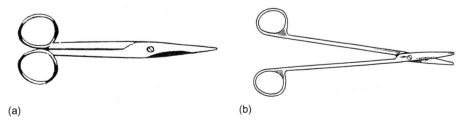

(a)                                         (b)

**Figure 10.2**   (a) Mayo and (b) Metzenbaum scissors.

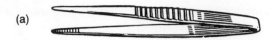

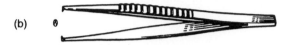

**Figure 10.3**    (a) Blunt and (b) rat-toothed forceps.

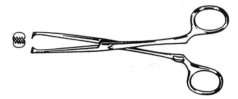

**Figure 10.4**    Allis tissue forceps.

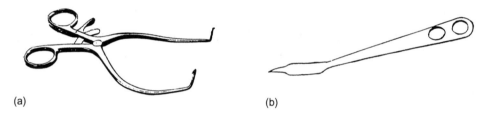

(a)                                                 (b)

**Figure 10.5**    (a) Gelpi and (b) Hohman retractors.

Allis tissue forceps are long forceps with small gripping jaws (Figure 10.4). They are useful for grasping pieces of tissue to hold them to one side temporarily, and cause relatively little trauma.

## Retractors

Retractors are used to improve surgical access and visibility, and to hold tissues to one side. They may or may not be self-retaining. Many different varieties of retractors are available. Gelpi retractors have small hooks on the end, which are inserted between the tissues to be separated. As the handles are pushed together, the hooks separate forcing the tissues apart and the ratchet holds the retractor open. Hohman retractors are designed for lifting bones in orthopaedic operations, and need to be held by an assistant (Figure 10.5).

## Atraumatic clamps

When performing vascular or intestinal surgery, it may be necessary to occlude a vessel or organ temporarily without causing damage. It is essential to use the correct

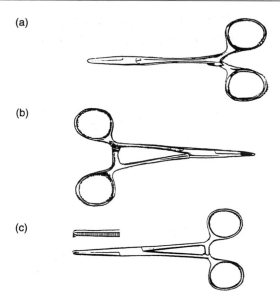

**Figure 10.6**    Artery forceps. (a) Spencer-Wells' forceps; (b) Dunhill's forceps; (c) Kocher's forceps.

atraumatic bowel or vascular clamp in these circumstances, which will occlude the lumen without causing damage to the wall of the vessel or intestine.

## Haemostasis

Good surgical technique should prevent excess bleeding from a surgical site; but if haemorrhage occurs, there are several ways to arrest it. Digital pressure for a few minutes is sufficient for most cases. Pressure bandages may be applied to the limbs or even to the trunk in larger animals, with care being taken not to make the bandage too tight. If a bleeding vessel can be identified, artery forceps can be used to clamp them (Figure 10.6), and they may then be ligated or sealed using diathermy. Spencer–Wells and Dunhill artery forceps are general-purpose haemostats. Halstead's mosquito forceps are very fine, and are useful in small animals and for delicate work. Kochers artery forceps combine a rat-toothed tip with crushing jaws, and are useful for grasping bleeding vessels deep within tissues.

## Needle holders

When suturing, needle holders may be needed to pass curved needles through skin and deeper tissues. Straight needles are usually held by hand. Needle holders come in many patterns (Figure 10.7). Gillies' needle holders combine a cutting blade with jaws to hold a needle, so separate scissors are unnecessary. However, they do not have a ratchet, so considerable digital pressure may be required to hold the needle if the tissue is tough. Right- and left-handed versions are available. Olsen–Hegar needle holders are like Gillies', but have a ratchet. Mayo needle holders are similar to Olsen Hegar's, but with

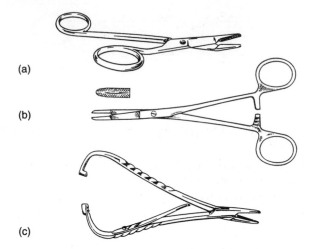

(a)

(b)

(c)

**Figure 10.7**   Needle holders. (a) Gillies' neddle holders; (b) Olsen-Hegar's needle holders; (c) MacPhail's needle holders.

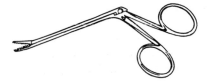

**Figure 10.8**   Crocodile forceps.

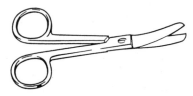

**Figure 10.9**   General-purpose scissors.

no cutting blade. MacPhail's needle holders have a unique handle that does not require the fingers and thumb to be placed through metal rings. Much practice is required to be competent with them, but they are comfortable to use for long periods of time, particularly for people with large hands.

## Other useful instruments

Crocodile forceps are long, fine instruments with small jaws, operated like scissors (Figure 10.8). They are particularly useful for retrieving material from deep within a cavity, and are often used for removing foreign bodies from the ear canal.

Blunt, curved flat scissors are useful general-purpose scissors (Figure 10.9). They are good for clipping fur from small areas, as the curved blades prevent the skin from

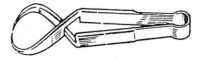

**Figure 10.10**    Towel clips.

being cut. They are also useful for cutting dressings, etc., as again the blunt tip prevents trauma to the skin.

Ophthalmic instruments such as enucleation scissors or corneal scissors are very fine and may be useful for procedures on mice and rats.

Towel clips are available in a variety of patterns (Figure 10.10). These are useful for holding drapes in place, so that surgical instruments and suture materials do not come into contact with non-sterile parts of the animal. Care must be taken in their use, however, since they have sharp teeth and can cause trauma if used incorrectly.

## PERIOPERATIVE ANTIBIOSIS AND POST-OPERATIVE WOUND INFECTIONS

Animals in the post-operative period are often at increased risk of infection. There may be indwelling cannulae, virulent organisms in the environment, or the animal may be receiving corticosteroids or other drugs, which affect the immune system. If aseptic techniques have been used and the animal is kept in a hygienic environment, there should be minimal need for antibiotic therapy after surgical procedures; but given that some wound contamination is likely, it may be wise to consider the judicious use of appropriate prophylactic antibiotics. Antibiotics are most effective if given before the bacteria enter the wound and multiply, so should be given either by intravenous injection 30 min before surgery, or by other routes 12 h beforehand. Prolonged courses after surgery or topical applications are unnecessary and ineffective, and inappropriate use of antibiotics predisposes to the development of resistant organisms and fungal growth. Antibiotic therapy should only be given after consultation with the Named Veterinary Surgeon.

Post-operative infections will be favoured by the following:

- A high level of *contamination* from dirty equipment, a dirty room, dirty hands and poorly cleaned wounds.
- *Injured tissues.* Poor surgical technique results in excessive bruising. Damaged tissues cannot fight infection well.
- *Bleeding.* Blood is a perfect medium for the growth of bacteria.
- *'Dead space'.* Pockets will be left between tissues after surgery (if wound closure is inadequate), where blood and serum can accumulate predisposing to infection.
- *Immunosuppression.* May be caused by drugs, for example corticosteroids, some inbred strains have reduced immunocompetence, and stress reduces the efficiency of the immune system.

These factors can all be controlled by the licensee. *Antibiotic cover is not a substitute for poor technique and inadequate hygiene.* There is a common belief that rats are in some way resistant to post-operative wound infections, and so much experimental rat surgery is performed under non-sterile conditions. Bradfield *et al.* (1992) have shown that, although the rat may not show clinical signs of infection, those with high wound bacterial counts show changes in behavioural, biochemical and histological parameters which may confound experimental data.

## Batch surgery

Rodent experimental surgery is frequently performed on batches of animals which live together and are microbiologically identical. The same principles of asepsis should still be applied and each animal should receive the same degree of care. However, for each batch the same set of instruments may be used without re-sterilising them in between. The use of a hot bead steriliser for cleaning the tips of instruments between animals is useful in this situation.

## SUTURING TECHNIQUES AND MATERIALS

When closing a wound, it is necessary to insert sutures in order to restore the anatomical structure of the tissues and support them during the healing process. Sutures are generally placed using needle holders and tissue forceps. Needle holders come in many patterns and sizes (see section on Surgical equipment), and the choice will depend largely on personal preference. Whichever one is chosen, it is essential to know how to hold it properly and how to manipulate it with dexterity. Practice is essential for good suturing technique. Inefficient use of the needle holders will lead to wasted time and poor suturing. The licensee should observe those who are skilled, and the technique should be practised. Skin simulators designed specifically for training may be used or freshly incised banana skins or foam rubber make good models for practice, as does the use of dead animals.

## Suture materials

There is a wide choice of both type and size of suture materials available. Suture materials can be described as

- *natural* or *synthetic*
- *absorbable* or *non-absorbable*
- *monofilament* or *braided*.

No one type is suitable for all situations. It is important to consider the nature and location of the tissues to be sutured, as different tissues have different healing rates. The peritoneum heals within a few days, skin takes 7–10 days, tendons can take a month or more, and fascia has only 70% of its original strength 9 months post-operatively. Absorbable suture materials are digested by body enzymes and will eventually dissolve. They are generally used in buried or visceral locations, although some can be used in skin if it is not possible to take them out at a later date (e.g. in a fractious or wild animal). Non-absorbable sutures are only used in skin from where they can be removed or in very specific situations where the continued presence of the material is required (e.g. in orthopaedic surgery). Until the mid-1970s, there was little choice of absorbable suture for the surgeon. It was difficult to sterilise sutures, and braided sutures gave rise to post-operative infections more easily than monofilaments. This is because fluids are drawn from the end of the suture into the knot and the tissue by capillary action. However, modern sutures are sterilised by the manufacturer and a better awareness of sterility reduces the risk of infection. Modern synthetic materials are far superior to the old natural products like catgut and silk, and they are the standard ones in use. Synthetic suture materials are stronger, more predictable and cause much less tissue reaction than natural materials.

## Absorbable sutures

### Natural origin

Catgut is a natural suture material made from the submucosa of sheep intestine or the serosa of bovine intestine. It is unpredictably absorbed and can be used in all tissue layers except those that require extended tissue holding. Since it is absorbed by the action of cells and enzymes, it actively promotes inflammation. It has been known to disappear in only 72 h, if implanted in patients with a high white cell count, with resultant wound breakdown.

### Synthetic origin

There are several modern synthetic suture materials available with different absorption times as shown in Figure 10.11.

Coated Vicryl (Polyglactin 910) is a synthetic absorbable braided suture which is absorbed by simple water hydrolysis and thus does not promote an inflammatory

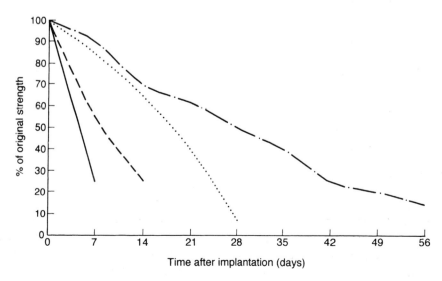

**Figure 10.11**   Tensile strength of synthetic absorbable suture materials. (——) Vicryl rapide; (– –) Monocryl; (• • •) Vicryl; (— - —) PDS.

response. It gives a predictable 21 days' support in tissue. Once its holding strength has gone, it is absorbed much more quickly from the tissue and this process is complete in 70 days. Vicryl is coated with polyglactin 370 and calcium stearate, which allow knots to be snugged down easily, and, therefore, provides more secure knotting. Synthetic absorbable sutures are stronger than catgut, and finer gauges can be used. A piece of Vicryl is as strong as a piece of catgut at least one or two gauges thicker, so less foreign material has to be used in the animal. Dexon is another example of a synthetic absorbable suture. It is a polyglycolic acid and its absorption is complete in 90–130 days.

Vicryl rapide is made from the same polymer as Vicryl, but changes to the manufacturing process mean that it provides just 66% of the initial strength of ordinary Vicryl, it loses its tensile strength more rapidly and it is absorbed in less time. It usually falls off or can be wiped away 7–10 days post-operatively. It provides short-term wound support with greatly increased comfort for the animal and is ideal for closure of skin and mucosa following minor surgery.

Monocryl is Poliglecaprone 25, a copolymer of 75% glycolide and 25% caprolactone. It is absorbed slightly more quickly than Vicryl, also by hydrolysis and also completely predictably. At 7 days post-implantation, there is about 55% of the original strength and 25% at 14 days. The great advantage of Monocryl is that it is monofilament, and so there is no problem with capillary action and it glides through tissue easily with no drag effect. Although it is monofilament, it is very supple and much easier to handle than other monofilament sutures and the knots are quite secure.

Polydioxanone (PDS) is a monofilament synthetic absorbable suture with high tensile strength, which provides wound support for more than 42 days. It has good handling and knotting properties.

## Non-absorbable sutures

### Natural origin

The natural non-absorbable materials are linen and silk. Both of these are multifilament: the linen is twisted and the silk is braided. Both give rise to an inflammatory reaction and have been superseded by more modern materials.

### Synthetic origin

The classic synthetic non-absorbable material is nylon (polyamide). This is available as monofilament or braided. Larger sizes of monofilament nylon can be difficult to tie. The braided form is also available with a sheathed coat, which improves handling and reduces capillarity. Nylon is commonly used as a skin closure material. It can be used as a buried suture, but can cause problems such as sinus formation. Prolene is monofilament polypropylene and is used in skin and as a buried suture. It is totally inert and causes no reaction when used in a buried location. It handles fairly well, and is used in areas where prolonged support is required. It is good for ophthalmic surgery and cardiovascular surgery because it flexes with the action of pulsatile tissue.

Stainless steel wire is available as a suture material and is used in special situations, such as orthopaedic surgery.

Staples may be used for wound closure for the skin layer. They are supplied presterilised inside a special applicator and are removed after 10 days with a purpose-made device. Removal can cause mild pain and may be resented by some animals. It is important to be accurate with the apposition of skin edges when using this technique. The main advantage of staples is their speed of application. *Michel clips* are applied using special applicator forceps and have to be sterilised before use. There is a tendency for them to be overcrimped, leading to tissue damage and necrosis which acts as a focus for wound infection. This overcrimping cannot occur with skin staples because of the design of the applicator and the staples, which allow for the normal post-operative tissue oedema that occurs in the first phase of wound healing, thus skin staples are to be preferred over the use of Michel clips.

## *Tissue adhesives*

*n-Butyl cyanoacrylate* adhesive ('Vetbond', 3M) can be used to bond tissue together. On contact with tissue and body fluids, it changes from a liquid to a solid state by rapid polymerisation and thus seals the wound. It can only be used on relatively small skin wounds, where there is no tension and when there is unlikely to be interference from the animal by excess grooming. It is most useful, not as a replacement for sutures but as a supplement to them, and will help to approximate wound edges between sutures. If used with staples, it should only be placed *between* the staples and not on them, or it may interfere with staple removal.

## Suture needles

Surgical needles either have eyes or are swaged on to the suture material in manufacture and are, therefore, eyeless (see Figure 10.12). This type of eyeless suture should be used in preference since only one thickness of the material has to be dragged through the tissue, and thus there is much less tissue damage, which improves wound healing. The surgeon has a new sharp needle each time, thus reducing tissue bruising and damage from use of blunt needles and it also eliminates the chore of cleaning and re-sterilising needles.

The needles are either straight or bent into shape as part of a circle (see Figure 10.13) and are measured in millimetres. The choice of needle shape will be governed by the accessibility of the tissue to be sutured, and the more confined the operative

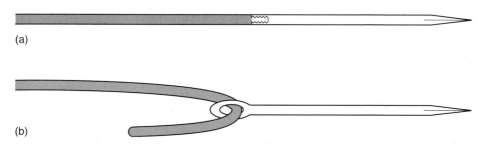

(a)

(b)

**Figure 10.12** Types of needle: (a) swaged-on needle and (b) eyed needle.

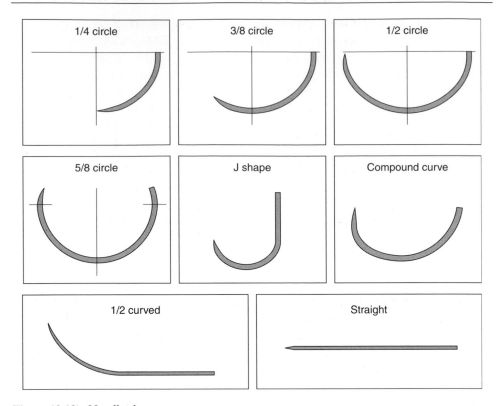

**Figure 10.13**   Needle shapes.

site, the greater the curvature that will be required, but control of the tip is more difficult. Generally, you should use the straightest needle you can. The basic shapes available are straight, 1/4 circle, 3/8 circle, 1/2 circle, 5/8 circle, half curved, J-needle and compound curve.

Needles may be round bodied, which are atraumatic, and are designed to separate tissues rather than to cut them. They are used in soft tissues such as bowel, internal organs and muscle, and as the needle passes through, the tissue closes tightly round the suture material forming a leak-proof suture line, which is obviously essential in intestinal and cardiovascular surgery.

Cutting needles are used in tough tissues, such as skin and fascia. Cutting needles leave triangular holes behind and should not be used in hollow organs as they encourage leakage of the contents.

Curved cutting needles may have the apex of the triangle on the inside of the curve, or the outside, in which case they are known as reverse cutting. With reverse cutting needles, the suture material is less likely to pull through the tissue, as the suture is not left sitting at an apex of the hole left in the tissues and there is increased strength of the needle and its resistance to bending (see Figure 10.14).

There are several other different types of cutting needles:

- *The tapercut needle* combines the initial penetration of a cutting needle with the minimum trauma of a round-bodied needle. The cutting point is only at the very tip.

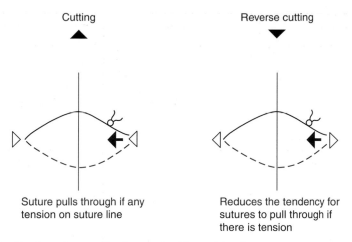

Cutting

Reverse cutting

Suture pulls through if any
tension on suture line

Reduces the tendency for
sutures to pull through if
there is tension

**Figure 10.14**   Cutting edge needles for use in skin and fascia.

- *P-needles* have a conventional or reverse cutting profile but have very sharp cutting edges to aid penetration of skin. The needle body has a square cross section, which improves resistance to bending and stability in the needle holder.
- *Slim blade needles* are for use in plastic and cosmetic surgery to leave minimal scarring from the suture line.
- *Prime needles* are the sharpest needles available. Ethicon describe them as 'specially designed for surgeons seeking excellence in skin closure'.
- *The trocar point needle* has a strong cutting head which merges into a robust round body for use in dense tissue.

There is also a range of special needles available for ophthalmic use.

## Sizes of suture

Sutures come in a variety of sizes, denoting the diameter of the material, in different precut lengths and even in different colours. In the metric system, the diameter is represented in tenths of a millimetre. A violet suture is much easier to see against a white rat's fur than a white suture and is thus easier to remove. The choice of appropriate sized material is governed by the nature of the tissues and the size of the animal. It is important to ensure adequate tensile strength, while remembering that using too thick a suture material will impair healing.

## Packaging

Modern sutures are supplied pre-sterilised in a double-layered pack, usually in boxes of 12. The outer envelope has a clear window through which the inner foil pack can be seen and gives the following information (see Figure 10.15):

- type of suture material
- gauge of material

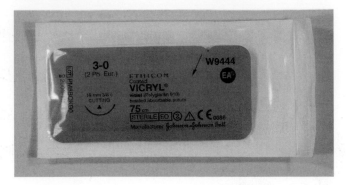

**Figure 10.15**    The suture pack.

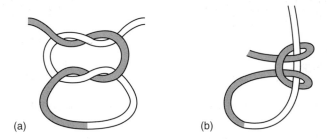

(a)                                         (b)

**Figure 10.16**    The basic surgical knot. (a) Correct reef knot; (b) incorrect half-hitch.

- needle size and type
- length of material
- method of sterilisation
- date of manufacture
- batch number
- code number for re-ordering.

The expiry date is 5 years from manufacture. After this period, absorbable sutures will lose their strength and the time for absorption becomes unpredictable. The cost of the suture is actually very small when compared to the total cost of the experiment, and it is most unwise to use out of date sutures and risk wound breakdown.

## Suture patterns

The general aim when suturing is merely to appose the tissue margins is to allow healing – excessive tension on sutures should be avoided, as it will slow healing. There are many specialised suture techniques for particular tissues and specialised surgical texts should be consulted for these.

The basic *surgical knot* is common to all suture patterns. This can be hand or instrument tied and it is helpful to become familiar with both methods. Essentially, it is a square (reef) knot with an extra throw, that is right over left, left over right, right over left (see Figure 10.16).

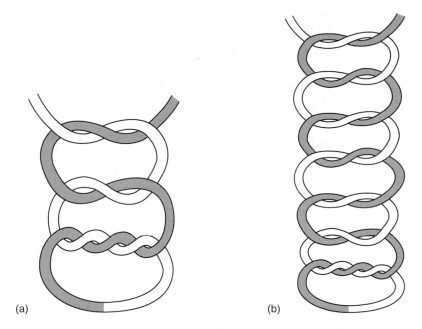

**Figure 10.17** The surgeon's knot. (a) Correct; (b) incorrect – excess bulk.

The method for tying the knot with instruments is to first place the stitch across the incision. Notice that there is a long end of suture material with the needle attached, and a short end. If the incision is parallel to the operator, place the needle holders parallel to the incision, between the long and the short end, and loop the long end around the needle holder in an inward direction. Grasp the short end and pull it through the loop. Movement of the surgeon's hands in opposite directions forms this first throw of the knot; note that the long end and the short end have changed places. The process is repeated to form the second throw, the needle holders being placed between the short end and the long end, parallel to the incision, the long end taken round the needle holders, going towards the centre. Grasp the short end in the needle holders. The surgeon now moves his hands, again in opposite directions, to form the second throw and lay the knot. A third throw formed in a similar manner will lock the knot securely and prevent it from becoming untied. Additional throws are unnecessary; they add no strength and will simply add bulk and more foreign material adding to the irritancy. Three throws are sufficient for most suture materials but for some slippery suture materials, or in wounds where there is some tension, it helps to use a surgeon's knot, that is the first throw is a double one (see Figure 10.17).

After tying the knot, the ends are trimmed. For buried sutures these need to be short, so that no excess foreign material is left on the wound, but they should not be cut so short that the knot becomes untied. For sutures that are to be removed, leaving a long end will facilitate the removal process, but they should not be left so long that the animal is encouraged to interfere with them. The exact length for trimming the sutures will be determined by experience. Knot security is obviously important and depends on the type of knot, the coefficient of friction of the suture material and the technique used for tying the knot. Some sutures are coated with wax or silicone to

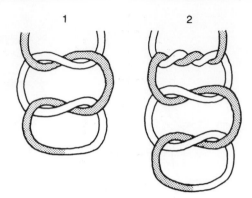

**Figure 10.18**   Knot used with coated Vicryl.

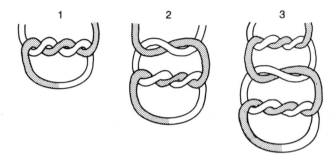

**Figure 10.19**   Knot used with PDS.

reduce tissue drag. This will reduce friction and decrease knot security. Thus for Vicryl and PDS, special knots are used (Figures 10.18 and 10.19).

The simplest knot that will provide security should be used, and the first throw should not be pulled so tight that the tissue becomes strangulated. Crushing clamps should not be applied to any part of the suture that remains in the tissue, as it will weaken the material.

*Suture patterns* can essentially be divided into *interrupted* and *continuous* patterns; in all interrupted patterns, a knot is tied after each suture is completed, whereas in a continuous pattern, the thread is repeatedly passed through the layers of tissue and only knotted at the beginning and end. Obviously, the former is slower but has the advantage of added security – if one suture breaks down, or one knot comes undone, the whole row is not lost. The latter is quicker but less secure.

To demonstrate the various patterns available, the closure of a midline abdominal incision can be considered. In closing such an incision, typically three layers of sutures would be used as follows: muscle, fat and either the subcuticular layer or the skin.

### Muscle layer

When suturing this layer, it is important to remember that the actual holding power of muscle is poor – the layers that surround it are much better (fascia and peritoneum

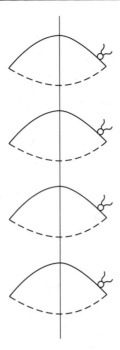

**Figure 10.20**   Simple interrupted suture pattern: good security, but slow to insert. Useful for skin and muscle.

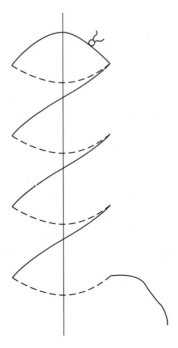

**Figure 10.21**   Simple continuous suture pattern: fast to insert, but poor security. Useful for fat tissues.

in this case), so when placing sutures in the abdominal body wall, it is vital to ensure the fascia and peritoneum (a silvery layer adherent to the under surface of the muscle) are both included in the suture.

A *simple interrupted pattern* is preferred here for added security (Figure 10.20).

## Fat

Simple interrupted sutures could also be used here, but in practice most people use a *simple continuous* pattern for speed (Figure 10.21). It is important that the suture is not pulled tight or fat necrosis will result.

## Subcuticular

This is essentially a *continuous horizontal* mattress suture in the subcutis, closing the wound with no suture material being left on the skin surface, thus reducing chances of interference from the animal (Figure 10.22).

## Skin

The *simple interrupted* suture will give the best security, but will take a long time to insert, increasing anaesthetic time. Better is the *cruciate* suture (Figure 10.23), which is quicker to insert, and still gives good security.

The *horizontal mattress* suture (Figure 10.24) has the disadvantage that it everts the wound edges which will predispose to infection and scarring along the wound line.

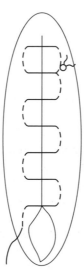

**Figure 10.22**    Subcuticular suture pattern: invisible on the surface; no interference from the animal.

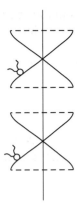

**Figure 10.23**   Cruciate mattress suture pattern: faster than simple interrupted; no eversion. Useful on skin.

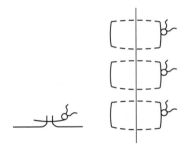

**Figure 10.24**   Horizontal mattress suture pattern: everting increases scarring.

## SUMMARY

When performing experimental procedures, you should aim to

- achieve asepsis and avoid post-operative infections
- minimise inflammation by using good techniques and appropriate instruments
- minimise haemorrhage by careful surgery and meticulous haemostasis
- produce good wound apposition by using suitable suture materials and patterns
- provide good post-operative care and minimise recovery time.

These can be achieved with a little preparation and practice. In many cases, there is considerable room for improvement in the techniques used for experimental surgery. Following the principles described above will result in improved science and better experimental data, as well as contributing to improved animal welfare. Your Named Veterinary Surgeon will be able to advise and guide you.

## FURTHER INFORMATION

Anderson, R.M. and Romfh, R.F. (1980). *Techniques in the Use of Surgical Tools*. Appleton-Century-Crofts, New York.

Bradfield, J.F., Schachtman, T.R., McLaughlin, R.M. and Steffan, E.K. (1992). Behavioural and physiologic effects of inapparent wound infection in rats. *Laboratory Animals* 42, 372–8.

Cunliffe-Beamer, T.L. (1990). Surgical techniques. In *Guidelines for the Wellbeing of Rodents in Research*. (ed. Guttman, H.). Proceedings of Conference Held at Scientist Centre for Animal Welfare, North Carolina.

Ethicon Publications and Catalogues: http://www.ethiconinc.com/

Kirk, R.W. and Bistner, S.I. (1981). *Handbook of Veterinary Procedures and Emergency Treatment*. W.B. Saunders Co., Philadelphia, London and Toronto.

Lang, C.M. (1982). *Animal Physiologic Surgery* (2nd edn). Springer-Verlag, New York.

Lumley, J.S.P. *et al.* (1990). *Essentials of Experimental Surgery*. Butterworths, London.

Marigold surgical gloves: http://www.stratfords.com/hand_protection/marigold_suretech_biogel_p.html

Slatter, D. (2003). *Textbook of Small Animal Surgery*. Saunders.

Strachan, C.J.L. and Wise, R. (eds.) (1979). *Surgical Sepsis*. Academic Press, London.

Swindle and Adams (eds.). Induced animal models of human disease. In *Experimental Surgery and Physiology*. Williams & Wilkins.

Van Dongen, J.J., Remie, R., Rensema, J.W. and van Wunnik, G.H.K. (1990). *Manual of Microsurgery on the Laboratory Rat*. Elsevier, Amsterdam.

Video. *Preparation and Draping of the Canine Surgical Patient*. Allan White Memorial Video Library, Unit for Veterinary Continuing Education, The Royal Veterinary College.

Video. *Minor Surgical Techniques*. Allan White Memorial Video Library, Unit for Veterinary Continuing Education, The Royal Veterinary College.

Wind, G.G. and Rich, N.M. (1983). *Principles of Surgical Technique*. Urban and Schwarzenberg, Baltimore.

# Chapter 11
# The project licence application

## INTRODUCTION

Section 5(1) of the Animals Scientific Procedures Act 1986 (ASPA) states 'A project licence (PPL) is a licence granted by the Secretary of State specifying a programme of work and authorising the application, as part of that programme, of specified regulated procedures to animals of specified descriptions at a specified place or specified places.'

Although this handbook is aimed primarily at the personal licensee, all work has to be authorised by a project licence. Project licences are issued to a person, who takes overall responsibility for the programme of work. The holder must be a UK resident, and is usually a senior researcher, who undertakes to direct and supervise the particular programme of work. This person must make sure that the work is done in such a way as to keep within the terms and conditions of the licence.

Project licences are only granted if the work falls into one or more particular categories, known as permissible purposes. These are:

(a) the prevention, diagnosis or treatment of disease in man, animals or plants
(b) the assessment, detection, regulation or modification of physiological conditions in man, animals or plants
(c) the protection of the natural environment in the interests of the health or welfare of man or animals
(d) the advancement of knowledge in biological or behavioural sciences
(e) education or training other than in primary or secondary schools
(f) forensic enquiries
(g) the breeding of animals for experimental or other scientific use.

Sometimes projects will fall into more than one category, in which case one purpose is given as the primary purpose, with others as secondary purposes. Education and training should not be combined with other permissible purposes (Box 11.1).

Sections 5.4 and 5.5 of the ASPA set out the main requirements of the Act with regard to project licences. Section 5.4 states that '... the Secretary of State shall

---

**Box 11.1** A project licence.

- Covers a research programme with a single theme or purpose.
- Issued to someone, who takes overall responsibility.
- Undertaken for a permissible purpose.

weight the likely adverse effects on the animals concerned against the benefit likely to accrue as a result of the programme to be specified in the licence.' Section 5.5 states that 'The Secretary of State shall not grant a project licence unless he is satisfied

(a) that the purpose of the programme to be specified in the licence cannot be achieved satisfactorily by any other reasonably practicable method not entailing the use of protected animals;
(b) that the regulated procedures to be used are those which use the minimum number of animals, involve animals with the lowest degree of neurophysiological sensitivity, cause the least pain, suffering, distress or lasting harm, and are most likely to produce satisfactory results.'

Thus, the requirement is that for each stated purpose (objective), the likely benefits should be weighed against the likely costs to the animals under a utilitarian framework (known as the 'cost–benefit analysis'), and also that the costs are minimised and the likely benefits are maximised. The project licence application, therefore, must contain sufficient information to allow an assessment to be made against these criteria for each objective stated. The likely benefit can be judged by considering the importance of the objectives, and the likelihood of achievement. The likely costs can be judged by considering the number and type of animals used, the severity of the procedures and the steps taken to control severity.

In addition, special justification is needed for the use of dogs, cats, equidae, primates or endangered species. Applications for projects proposing to use these species must demonstrate that no other species is suitable for the purpose, or that it is not practicable to obtain them.

Project licence standard condition 6 states, 'For any procedure, the degree of severity imposed shall be the minimum consistent with the attainment of the object-ives of the procedure, and this shall not exceed the severity limit attached to the procedure. The minimum number of animals of the lowest neurophysiological sensitivity shall be used in procedures causing the least pain, suffering, distress or lasting harm'. This places an ongoing requirement on the researcher to seek for refinement alternatives and to ensure that the conduct of the research minimises animal use throughout the lifetime of the project licence.

Schedule 2A to the Act requires that all procedures are carried out under general or local anaesthesia, unless the administration of the anaesthetic would be more traumatic than the experiment itself, or the use of anaesthesia is incompatible with the aims of the experiment. If anaesthesia is not possible, then analgesics or other appropriate methods must be used to minimise any pain, suffering, distress or lasting harm, and to prevent animals from experiencing severe pain, distress or suffering. Anaesthetised animals likely to suffer considerable pain once the anaesthesia has worn off must be treated with pain relieving means in good time, or immediately killed using a Schedule 1 method. If it is required that an animal will experience suffering as a necessary part of the experiment, this needs to be carefully justified. These requirements are reiterated in project licence standard conditions 6A, 6B and 6C.

A project licence remains in force for a maximum of 5 years, after which time it expires, and a new application must be submitted if the work is to continue. This provides the applicant and the Secretary of State with an opportunity to review the progress of the research programme, and implement any refinements that have been developed since the original application.

## THE PROJECT LICENCE APPLICATION

*'The carpenter's rule is "measure twice, cut once". You have to make sure that the blueprint, the first creation, is really what you want, that you've thought everything thorough. Then you put it into bricks and mortar. … You Begin with the End in Mind.'*

*Covey (1986).*

The key to a successful application is being very clear about what you want to achieve, that is defining clear objectives. The purpose of the application form is to obtain sufficient information about the proposed use of animals in regulated procedures to allow the Secretary of State to be able to make a judgement against the relevant criteria for project licences (see text and Box 11.2). He must be able to weigh the likely adverse effects on the animals concerned against the benefit likely to accrue, and be satisfied that there is full implementation of the three Rs. If sufficient information to make this judgement is not provided, the application will be rejected and will need to be revised. A project licence must stand alone: referring to techniques in papers or books is unlikely to be acceptable unless a copy of the relevant information is appended to the licence, so be sure to send copies of any such documents with the application. *Before completing an application form, read the notes for applicants thoroughly (see www.homeoffice.gov.uk/comrace/animals/index.html), and consult with the local Inspector.*

The application form is divided into a number of sections:

- *Sections 1–7* deal with personal information and are self-explanatory. The project title should describe the theme of the work in a way that is likely to remain valid for the whole of the project, for example 'Fetal and Neonatal Mineral Metabolism', 'The Biochemistry of Retinal Dystrophies', etc. The title should be less than 50 characters long.
- *Sections 8* and *9* deal with existing licence authorities and allow these to be tied up with new authorities.
- *Section 10* asks for experience relevant to the application (see below).
- *Section 11* lists the primary availability and gives the option of naming a deputy project licence holder.

---

**Box 11.2**   Criteria for project licences.

Section 5.4: Costs must be weighed against likely benefits.
Section 5.5(a): There must be no alternatives to the use of protected animals.
Section 5.5(b): The procedures must

- use the minimum number of animals,
- of lowest neurophysiological sensitivity,
- cause the least pain, suffering, distress or lasting harm,
- be most likely to succeed.

- *Section 12* is used to list any additional establishments, where work may be carried out. In this case, a nominated deputy should normally be based at each additional establishment and be in a position to direct work authorised under the project licence. Section 18 of the application should describe which parts of the programme of work will be carried out at each of the sites, and indicate whether animals undergoing regulated procedures will be moved between sites.
- *Section 13* should be completed if work is to be carried out at a place other than a designated establishment (PODE). Give details of the location(s) and the reference number(s) of the experimental protocols, which are intended to be carried out there. Show in Section 18 why it is necessary to conduct those experimental protocols at those locations.
- *Section 14* gives the permissible purpose. A 1 should be marked against the primary purpose, and 2 against any other purposes. Note that Education and Training should not be combined with any other purposes.
- *Section 15* relates to special categories of work, such as tobacco or alcohol research, which will require additional justification and assessment.
- *Section 16* asks for the duration of the project. A project licence is usually valid for a maximum of 5 years. They cannot be extended to last longer than 5 years and authority to continue work beyond this time will require a new licence, application for which must be made in sufficient time to allow due consideration.
- *Section 17* asks for the background, objectives and potential benefits relating to the proposed work.
- *Section 18* asks for a description of the plan of work.
- *Section 19* asks for a detailed description of the procedures to be carried out on the animals (see below).
- *Section 20* asks for an assessment of the overall severity of the project.
- *Section 21* asks for a declaration by the applicant that they have taken into consideration the three Rs, that they have sought advice from the NVS and NACWO, and have read the Home Office Guidance Notes.
- *Section 22* asks for a declaration by the certificate holder that facilities are available and that the application has successfully completed the local ethical review process.

The link between the structure of the project licence and the requirements of the Act may be illustrated simplistically as follows:

$$\text{Justification} = \frac{\text{Maximum benefit}}{\text{Minimum cost}}$$

$$= \frac{\text{Importance of objectives} \times \text{Probability of achievement}}{\text{Number of animals} \times \text{Degree of suffering}}$$

$$= \frac{\text{Section 17} \times \text{Sections 10, 11 and 18}}{\text{Section 19}} \quad \text{(of project licence)}$$

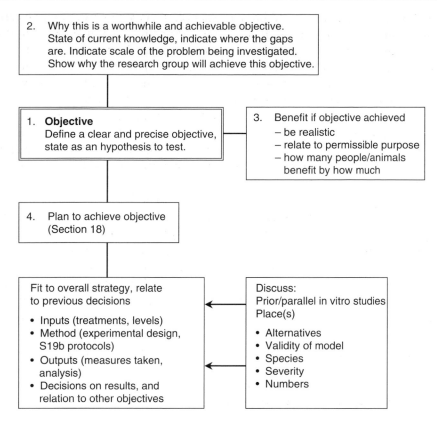

**Figure 11.1**   Steps in drawing up a project licence application.

## Maximising benefit

This can be judged by considering the importance of the studies to be undertaken and the likelihood of a successful outcome. The *importance of the objectives* will depend on such things as whether the work is a new approach in relation to existing knowledge, whether the project is realistic or over-ambitious, whether it has implications for other areas of research, whether it relates to areas of current concern and whether the potential benefits are to do with improved health, increasing scientific knowledge, educational, economic or forensic investigations.

The *probability of achievement* depends on the quality of the science, and this depends on the choice of model and experimental design, and takes into account the track record of the research group in that particular field.

The information is taken from *Section 10, Section 11, Section 17* and *Section 18* of the application form. Figure 11.1 shows the steps in constructing a project licence application.

*Section 10* shows that you are able to take overall responsibility for the programme of work, and for its proper design and conduct. This includes the scientific direction, management and control of the project, ensuring compliance with the terms and conditions of issue of the licence, the supervision of personal licence holders (PILs) working under the project and making annual returns. It shows how you are equipped by experience, training or qualifications to design and manage the programme of work. Completion of accredited training (see Chapter 1) is usually required although applicants who have recently held a project licence are not currently expected to undertake further mandatory training. However, it is necessary to keep up to date, and details of any other relevant training undertaken should be supplied. In addition to providing details of status, qualifications and experience, indicate your familiarity with

- the types of regulated procedures described in the application
- the ethical and legal considerations relevant to the use of animals
- the knowledge and skills required to design, conduct and analyse scientific experiments using living animals
- alternative and more refined methods, and how to find them.

*Section 11* lists the primary availability, which is usually the designated establishment where the work is to be carried out and where the licence holder is based. The nature of the facilities and staff are taken into consideration when judging the likelihood of success of a project. This section also allows a deputy to be named, who may assume responsibilities in the absence of the project licence holder, or assist with the day-to-day running of a programme of work. If no deputy is named, it should be clear how the project will be managed in the absence of the licence holder. The ultimate responsibility for the conduct of the programme of work remains with the project licence holder, but if a deputy has particular expertise in an area, this should be stated as it can have a bearing on the likelihood of success. The project licence applicant should provide details of the duties to be delegated to the deputy and explain how the deputy is equipped by qualification, training and experience to discharge those duties.

*Section 17* asks for the background, objectives and potential benefits for the proposed work. This provides the information to judge whether the objective is worth pursuing. *If the objectives are correctly specified, construction of the remainder of the application follows logically.* Begin by defining clear and precise objectives, which describe the information which is sought, rather than the methods which will be used to seek it. This can be achieved by breaking down the research project into a series of key questions to investigate. It can be useful to state the questions in the form of hypotheses to test, for example 'to test the hypothesis that cells of type A have function B', or 'does gene A have a role in the development of organ B', not 'to perform studies into the role of gene A'. Having identified the objectives, discuss the background that leads up to them. This should provide a full, balanced, up-to-date account of the current state of knowledge in the field of interest, indicating where the gaps are that the application intends to fill, and showing clearly how the objectives are derived. Include a list of references, and copy any key references to send in with the application.

The potential benefits should indicate how many humans, animals or plants may benefit by how much from the data arising from the work. Indicate the realistic likely outcomes following from the *specific objectives addressed in the programme of work*, as well as from study of the area of science as a whole, in the short and longer term. The benefits should link to the cited permissible purpose, for example if medical benefit has been described, there should be a likelihood of demonstrable medical benefit within the lifetime of the project licence. It is important to show what use will be made of the data, for example publication in journals, formulating guidelines and policies or treatment of patients, since the benefit from a programme of work will be nil if the data is not disseminated appropriately.

This section also asks for an overview of the research group's standing and previous contributions in the field. Summarise any progress made under existing or past project licence authorities, and the resources and skills of the research group. Also, show where the funding is to come from, and if the work has already been peer reviewed.

*Section 18* describes the plan, which will be used to achieve the objectives, and is used to determine the likelihood of success. Describe an overall strategy for achieving the objectives, which will include a discussion of previous or parallel *in vitro* studies and clinical work in human subjects, indicating how they fit together with the animal studies in a coherent programme of work. Identify criteria, which will be used at decision points, to determine whether the project proceeds further and in which direction. It should be made clear, how the individual protocols will be used in the achievement of the objectives. Flow charts can sometimes be helpful in showing how the protocols fit together to answer the questions.

Then, *for each objective*, consider the requirements of Section 5.5 (see above).

**Non-animal alternatives**   Justify the use of live animals in the achievement of each individual objective. Describe how the suitability and feasibility of any alternatives were assessed, and show why they were not suitable. Often, parts of an objective or programme of work can be achieved using *in vitro* methods, and this should be made clear.

**Least neurophysiological sensitivity, least severity, minimum numbers and most likely to achieve satisfactory results**   Show how these four elements are balanced to minimise animal suffering. Often, there is conflict between the elements (e.g. should more animals experience less suffering, or fewer animals experience more?), but in general, refinement should take precedence over reduction. Discuss the choice of species and (if relevant) strain of animal to be used, showing clearly why lower species will not suffice. Validate the animal model to be used, and show why it is the best one for the purpose, particularly if there are other models available of lower severity, for example they involve unclassified or mild work, or use a lower species. If the model is new, or there are many unknowns, pilot studies may be needed to determine unknowns (e.g. variability, time course) and determine end points appropriate to the objectives. In this case, the work will need to be carried out in stages, decisions being made following each stage as to the best way to proceed.

To minimise the numbers of animals, it is necessary to have very *clear objectives* of the experiment, understand and *control variation* through careful experimental designs, use an appropriate method of *statistical analysis* to extract the maximum data from the results, and then *interpret the results* carefully. Describe the experimental design to be used, including an explanation of the experimental unit, with consideration of how the design of the experiment and selection of the animal model minimise the number of animals needed to achieve the objective. Show how the number of animals per group is chosen (e.g. power analysis, resource allocation method), how the number of groups per experiment is selected and how this relates to the overall estimate of animals to be used in the project as a whole. Groups should be large enough to ensure the statistical validity of studies, but unnecessarily high levels of precision

**Table 11.1**   Features of different experimental designs (see Festing *et al.*, 2002).

| Design | Usage | Pros | Cons |
|---|---|---|---|
| Fully random | If uncontrollable variation sources unimportant | Simple, easy to understand (e.g. *t*-tests) | No control of nuisance effects |
| Block | To detect variability due to known sources | Improves precision | Can get too complex |
| Factorial | Tests effects of several factors (e.g. sex, age) simultaneously | Efficient information provision, can test for interaction | Factor interaction may be difficult to interpret |
| Repeat measure | Several measures on one individual (e.g. at different times) | Cuts out inter-individual variation | Sometimes not valid, for example if there is an order effect |
| Sequential | If data obtainable quickly, to minimise animal use | Results analysed along the way, can stop when significance reached | Expert advice needed |

are not acceptable as a basis for very large groups. Describe the treatments to be applied including control groups, and show how these are randomised across the experimental units: blocking may be required to account for known differences. Different designs of experiment may be useful depending on requirements (see Table 11.1 above): *it is wise to consult a statistician at the planning stage to determine the best way to approach the experiment.* Describe the measures to be taken, relating these outputs to the objective being pursued. Some consideration of how signal : noise ratio is to be maximised for each measure should be included, that is demonstrate how the model has been optimised. It should be clear how the results will be analysed to provide the answer to the question being asked, even if the analyses are carried out on blood, tissues or cells ex vivo. Show why each protocol is necessary, and why each step in each protocol is required, including an explanation of the time course of the experiment and how sampling points have been selected. Show that the procedures have been maximally refined, and at what point humane end points will be applied. It is expected that best practice will be employed.

Section 18b asks for any additional information regarding the three Rs of reduction, refinement and replacement, which has not been included elsewhere. However, ideally you should show how the three Rs are to be pursued as an integral part of the plan of work and in the relevant section 19b (vi), in which case it will not be necessary to repeat the information.

## *Special justifications*

The use of cats, dogs, equidae, non-human primates or endangered species requires particular justification in section 18; and for non-human primates, a supplement to section 18 (section 18c) must be completed. To justify the use of these species, show that no other species is suitable for the specified programme of work, or that it is impracticable to obtain them. History, custom and practice, size, cost or convenience are unlikely to provide sufficient justification. If Old World primates are to be used, show why New World species would not satisfy the needs of the work. It must be stated where the animals will be bred, and if it is likely that Old World primates will be exposed to procedures of more than mild severity for toxicological purposes. If animals are to come from a non-designated breeding centre (i.e imported), an application form must be completed by the project licence holder and submitted to the Home Office at least 2 weeks before their importation with full details of the transportation. A separate section 19b should be completed for procedures involving the use of non-human primates. Endangered species may only be used if the work is either research aimed at preservation of the species in question, or essential biomedical research, where the species in question exceptionally proves to be the only one suitable for those purposes.

The use of Schedule 2 species from non-designated suppliers or animals taken from the wild also require particular justification. The use of wild animals may require authority under other legislation (e.g. the Wildlife and Countryside Act). If wild animals are to be released in the course of regulated procedures, a separate section (18d) should be included, demonstrating that the maximum possible care will be taken to safeguard the animal's well-being, that the animal's state of health will allow it to be set free, and that the setting free of the animal will pose no danger to public health or the environment.

## Minimising costs

In order to determine the *cost to the animals*, there must be an assessment of the potential adverse effects on how many of which types of animal. The costs to the animals are determined from sections 18 and 19. Section 18 must justify fully the use of live animals, and describe how the number of animals is minimised, and this has been discussed above.

*Section 19* describes in detail the procedures which will be carried out, and the strategies to be employed to reduce suffering, such as anaesthesia, analgesia, supervision or early killing. It sets out exactly, what is to be done and what animals it may be performed on, and is in two parts. Section 19a is an index of the procedures described in section 19b. This provides an overview of the number of animals of which type are to be used in procedures of which severity. There should be a separate entry in section 19a for each section 19b protocol sheet. Each protocol sheet has a reference number, a short title and a severity limit (see Chapter 2). The kind of animal to be used and their stage of development must be specified, and an estimate given of the number to be used each year.

*Section 19b* consists of a series of individual protocol sheets. These ideally describe all the interventions to be carried out on a particular animal for the achievement of a particular purpose, covering the total use of the animal from the time of removal from stock to the time it is killed or otherwise discharged from control. The purpose of section 19b is to obtain sufficient detail of what is to happen to each animal to allow a realistic assessment of the likely severity of the procedures carried out on that animal.

---

**Box 11.3**   Examples of severity of common procedures.

*Mild*
- Small or infrequent blood sampling.
- Procedures in which the animal is killed before it shows more than minor changes from its normal behaviour (use of the *humane end point*).
- Minor surgical procedures under anaesthesia, for example, superficial biopsy, laparoscopy and vascular cannulation (non-surgical).

*Moderate*
- Surgical procedures where post-operative care and analgesia are reliably provided.
- Toxicity tests with defined *humane end points* (as opposed to lethality as the end point).

*Substantial*
- Major surgery causing post-operative suffering.
- Studies with significant morbidity or death as an end point.
- Procedures resulting in significant deviation from the normal state of health.

*Unclassified*
- Procedures performed under non-recovery general anaesthesia, or on decerebrate animals.

---

*Each protocol has a severity limit, which should be* either *mild, moderate, substantial* or, in the case of procedures carried out on decerebrate animals or wholly under terminal anaesthesia, *unclassified*. The severity limit should describe the *maximum* degree of severity likely to be seen in the animals and which is consistent with the objectives, regardless of the proportion of animals expected to reach that limit. It is not necessary to make allowance in the assessment for the unexpected. In procedures combining recovery and terminal techniques, the severity limit should relate to the recovery techniques.

Suggestions for the severity assessment of individual procedures are given in the Home Office Guidance Notes, and some examples are given in Box 11.3. The severity limit should take into account the possible immediate and long-term effects of the procedure, the nature of any likely adverse effects, the likely incidence of their occurrence and the action to be taken to minimise these effects. The administration of an anaesthetic is *not* taken into account. By limiting the occurrence of severe adverse effects, through careful monitoring and the implementation of a humane end point (see Chapter 4), it may be possible to place an otherwise moderate or substantial procedure into a lower severity limit. Adherence to the severity limit and observance of any other controls described in section 19b are required by the standard licence conditions. The three severity bands are not discrete entities, but form a spectrum across a wide range of adverse effects. If the severity limit of the procedure is exceeded, the Home Office Inspector must be informed.

Each protocol sheet should be in a form such that it can be handed to a personal licensee as a working document indicating how the procedure should be carried out, what adverse effects are likely, and what must be done to remain within the authorised severity limit. Section 19b (v) describes the interventions to be carried out. Begin with a brief statement of the purpose of the protocol, then list the interventions to be carried out in chronological order. For each intervention, an *anaesthetic code* should be given. These are

- AA – no anaesthesia throughout the procedure
- AB (L, G or R) – anaesthesia with recovery, which may be local, general or regional
- AC – anaesthesia without recovery
- AD – use of neuromuscular blockade.

Include any details which might be relevant to an assessment of severity, such as administration or sampling techniques, implantation of catheters or cannulae, creation of CNS lesions or nerve sections, surgical interventions, exposure to infectious agents and the fate of the animal at the end of the procedure. It may be necessary to include details of interventions, which are not themselves regulated. Any repetition or combination of techniques on individual animals must be clearly stated, and it should be clear if stages are optional. The duration of procedures should be stated where relevant. It is not necessary to describe here *why* the interventions are carried out: this should be clear from section 18.

While it is important to avoid ambiguity, try not to make the application over-specific since unnecessary inflexibility may cause difficulties in practice and lead to infringements over minor adjustments of technique. For example, it is unwise to specify exact volumes, frequencies, routes or agents, or compounds to be administered or sampled. It is better to avoid unnecessary technical detail and use appendices listing standard constraints, for example, dosing and sampling routes, limit volume/frequencies for dosing and sampling, which will allow flexibility without exceeding the stated severity limit. Limits may be described in section 18, or in section 19b (vi). Figure 11. 2 shows one way to approach the construction of a section 19b.

*Section 19b (vi)* should address the *potential* pain, suffering, distress or lasting harm, which may be done to the animals, even if the likely incidence of the effects is low. Show how the incidence, intensity and duration of potential adverse effects will be minimised. It should be possible from the information in this section for anyone who identifies abnormalities in an animal to determine whether this is a likely adverse effect of the procedures carried out, and if so the course of action to be taken to control the effects. Adverse effects relate to the immediate and long-term consequences of well-performed regulated procedures, not just of regulated procedures that went wrong. In this section, list all potential adverse effects together with the likely incidence and proposed methods of prevention or control. Severity can be reduced by *prevention*, involving continual refinement of the procedure; *alleviation*, involving the use of analgesics or special husbandry techniques; or *termination*, involving killing the animal at a defined humane end point to prevent potential distress. When drawing up section 19b (vi), it can be helpful to list the individual interventions, identify the range of possible adverse effects from each intervention, which covers both the physical intervention and any likely consequences from it, then discuss proposed control measures. An example is shown below in Figure 11.2. Define suitable end points for three eventualities:

1. when the research objectives have been achieved (scientific)
2. when they cannot be achieved (error)
3. when the severity exceeds the minimum necessary to achieve the objective (humane).

---

19b.   PROTOCOL SHEET                    Protocol reference number: **19b**  | 1 |

*Please give the following information, using separate sheets for each protocol listed in Section 19a. To insert an additional protocol sheet [double-click here]. This information is essential to determine the severity limit of the protocol, which must be observed as a condition of this project licence and of the licences of participating personal licensees.*

  (i)  Short title      | Antibody production |

  (ii)  Severity limit   | Mild |

  (iii)  Species, stage of development and estimated number to be used each year

> Rabbit, adult 50
> Rat, adult 100
> Mouse, adult 100

  (iv)  Details of previous licensed use

If the animals have been used, bred or surgically prepared under the authority of this or any other project licence, please indicate whether the use now proposed represents 'continued-use' or 're-use' – the *Notes to Applicants* and the Home Office *Guidance on the Operation of the Animals (Scientific Procedures) Act 1986* refer.

State whether continued-use or re-use

Sources: PPL numbers/protocol numbers/short titles or appropriate other details

  (v)  Description of the procedure. Read *Notes*

1. **AA** – A baseline test bleed may be taken from a superficial vein.
2. **AA** – Animals will be immunised subcutaneously/other route with antigen with or without adjuvant. Mice may also be immunised intraperitoneally.
3. **AA** – Booster immunisations will be given at intervals of typically 2–4 weeks on up to 4 occasions.
4. **AA** – Test bleeds will be taken from superficial veins 7–14 days after immunisation.
5. **AC** – Animals will be exsanguinated by cardiac puncture, or killed by a Schedule 1 method.

---

The end points should be clearly recognisable (see Chapter 4). The successful implementation of end points requires careful scheduling of experimental procedures, to ensure that there are staff available to perform the appropriate frequency and type of observations and interventions necessary to control severity. For further advice, see Chapters 4 and 8 and discuss the proposal with the NVS.

*Section 19b (vii)* covers the fate of the animals at the end of the procedure. When a series of regulated procedures for a particular purpose has finished, the animal must be humanely killed by a Schedule 1 method or other authorised method if it is likely

| | | |
|---|---|---|
| Test bleeds | Haemorrhage bruising | Good technique, apply pressure. If bleeding fails to stop within e.g. 5 minutes NVS advice may be sought and/or the animal killed by a Schedule 1 method. |
| | Infection | Aseptic technique will be used. If the animal develops systemic infection it will become distressed and the humane end point implemented as detailed below. |
| | Anaemia | Limit volumes for samples will be used.[1] The PCV may be monitored and if anaemia is detected the animal will not be bled or will be killed by a Schedule 1 method. |
| Immunisation | Pain | Limit volumes for injection will be used,[2] injections will be given by competent staff using best practice techniques. |
| | Infection | Aseptic techniques and sterile antigens will be used for administration. If abscesses develop, cleansing and treatment will be given as directed by NVS. Animals failing to respond to treatment will be killed using a Schedule 1 method. |
| | Granuloma formation | Care will be taken with adjuvant selection. Freund's complete adjuvant will not be used. |
| | Anaphylaxis | Care will be taken with species selection to avoid the likelihood of anaphylaxis. If animals exhibit signs of distress such as dyspnoea, cyanosis or collapse the NVS will be called and/or the animal will be killed by a Schedule 1 method. |
| Final bleed | Anaesthetic problems | Lightening of the anaesthetic could occur but will be avoided by regular monitoring and appropriate action. Animals showing signs of recovery such as muscle movements will be killed by a Schedule 1 method. |
| | Cardiac bleeding | Cardiac tamponade may develop. Animals developing this will become pale and may show a weak, irregular heartbeat. These animals will be killed by a Schedule 1 method immediately. |

[1] Limit volumes for sample: Not more than 10% of blood volume will be collected on any one occasion, and not more than 15% in a 28 day period. Blood volume is taken as 70 ml/kg

[2] Limit volumes for administration:

| Species | Intravenous (ml) | Intra-peritoneal (ml) | Intra-muscular (ml/site) | Sub-cutaneous (ml/site) | Intra-dermal (μl/site) |
|---|---|---|---|---|---|
| Mice | 0.2 | 1–2 | 0.05 | 0.5 | 100 |
| Rabbit | 1–10 | 10–15 | 0.25 | 3 | 100 |
| Rat | 1 | 2–4 | 0.1 | 2 | 100 |

A maximum of two sites will be used on any one occasion.

**Humane end point**: Animals will be monitored and a scoring sheet may be used to assess welfare. If an animal exceeds mild severity (as assessed using a selection of criteria including failure to groom, inappetance more than 48 h, weight loss more than 5–10% of age matched controls, increase or decrease in core temperature more than 1°C, increase or decrease in respiratory rate more than 30%, lethargy or mildly exaggerated responses), it will be humanely killed using a Schedule 1 method.

**Figure 11.2** Example of 19b protocol sheet. PPL form, from Home Office website, www.homeoffice.gov.uk/.

to suffer adverse effects. An animal may remain alive if it is not suffering or likely to suffer adverse effects, as determined by a veterinary surgeon or other suitably qualified person. Animals which are kept alive may be transferred to another protocol or project for continued use or re-use, be discharged from the controls of the Act, for example as a pet or to a farm, or be released to the wild. Note that any continued use, re-use or discharge of animals requires authority from the Secretary of State, and may require certification of fitness by a veterinary surgeon.

If after a series of regulated procedures for a particular purpose, the same animal is used again in the same or another protocol as a matter of scientific necessity, this constitutes continued use. This often applies to genetically modified animals, which are bred under one protocol, then transferred to other protocols for scientific use. If after a series of regulated procedures, the same animal is used again in the same or another protocol where a naïve animal would have sufficed, this constitutes re-use. Section 14 of the Act and paragraphs 5.60–5.66 of the Home Office Guidance Notes describe the constraints on the re-use of protected animals. There should be some justification in section 18 for the re-use of these animals, with a description given of the methods that will be used to limit the overall suffering to the animals. Animals which have been given a general anaesthetic for the first use may only be re-used if the procedure carried out under first anaesthetic was essential surgical preparation for the subsequent procedure, if the anaesthetic was given solely to immobilise the animal or if the second anaesthetic is terminal. It is unlikely that re-use will be authorised for animals that have experienced severe pain. Typically, re-use is requested for animals used for mild procedures such as blood sampling, where the cumulative effect of several uses is minimal. Any re-use or continued use must be authorised by the Secretary of State, and shown clearly in section 19b (vii) of the first protocol and section 19b (iv) of the second protocol.

Animals that are kept alive at the end of a series of regulated procedures remain at the designated establishment under the supervision of a veterinary surgeon. This applies to animals waiting to be re-used. Animals may be discharged from the controls of the Act with the consent of the Secretary of State if a veterinary surgeon certifies that they will not suffer if they are moved from the designated establishment. This typically applies to farm animals on epidemiological studies.

Animals may be released to the wild during the course of procedures provided they are fit, the procedures do not put the animals at a biological disadvantage, and they pose no danger to the public. Typically, this applies to field studies of wild animals, where, for example population dynamics are being studied.

## Section 20 – overall severity

Section 20 requires an assessment to be made of the overall severity of the project. If all the individual procedures are under terminal anaesthesia or on decerebrate animals, then the overall severity of the project is unclassified. Otherwise, the severity of the project should be assessed as *mild*, *moderate* or *substantial*. The assessment of overall severity reflects the overall level of cumulative suffering to be experienced, not just the single worst possible case. It takes into account the proportion of animals expected to experience pain, suffering, distress or lasting harm, the duration of the exposure to that harm, the nature and intensity of the adverse effects, and the actions to be taken to relieve suffering. Overall severity thus has qualitative and quantitative aspects and does not simply equate to the severity of the single most severe procedure. It is feasible for a project consisting of substantial severity procedures to have an overall severity limit of mild, if the incidence of substantial effects is limited to a small proportion of the animals for a short period of time. This assessment of overall severity is used to judge the 'cost' when making a cost–benefit analysis.

## THE APPLICATION PROCESS

A project licence application goes through a number of steps before being submitted to the Home Office (Box 11.4). If a programme of work is to continue beyond 5 years, it is wise to begin preparing a replacement application several months in advance of the expiry of the existing project. First, identify objectives to be pursued. If drafted correctly, the remainder of the application will follow logically from here. Objectives should describe the desired outcome, or the question to which the answer is sought, not the process that will be used. Having identified objectives, consider how they might be achieved using non-animal alternatives. If the objective is to obtain proof of concept or determine a mechanism, there may well be ways to achieve the objective using cell lines or lower species. Start looking for alternatives at this early stage, using organisations, such as FRAME, ECVAM, UFAW, HSUS, The Dr Hadwen Trust for Humane Research, The Humane Research Trust or databases, such as PREX, based at Utrecht University, to help. Once alternatives have been ruled out for all or part of the project, consider how the objectives might be achieved in the most refined manner. Refinements in technique can be identified by discussions with the NVS, NACWO, Home Office Inspector, and by consulting the organisations above. Reduction can be achieved by careful consideration of the experimental design and model to be used. Consult a statistician at an early stage to identify a suitable experimental design and method of analysis. Then draft the application making sure that the requirements of ASPA Section 5.5 have been addressed for each objective. Again, it can be helpful to consult the Inspector during this process to be sure that the relevant criteria are being addressed, and to read the notes to applicants thoroughly.

Once the application has been drafted, it will need to be submitted to the local ethical review process at the establishment, which requires that the application is reviewed by the NVS, NACWO, scientists and lay members. This process can take several days or weeks, and may require further revisions to the licence. The ethical

---

**Box 11.4**   Stages in making a project licence application.

- Start 9–12 months in advance.
- Identify clear objectives.
- Consider replacement – for example, use FRAME.
- Consider refinements – use NVS, NACWO, HOI, FRAME, etc.
- Consider reduction – consult a statistician.
- Draft application – consult HOI, read notes to applicants.
- Submit to ERP.
- Submit to Home Office.

review process will consider whether the work *should* be done, and whether the three Rs have been implemented fully. Following completion of the ethical review process, the application, duly signed by the certificate holder and applicant, may be sent to the Home Office for consideration. Remember to include any training certificates, and any key supporting references, which may help in understanding the application. The Home Office Inspector will review the application and aim to make contact within 20 working days. It may be necessary for more revisions to be made to the application, so be sure to leave enough time for this. It can take many months, and often several redrafts, for a project licence application to be granted.

## ASSESSMENT OF THE APPLICATION

Licence applications are assessed by Home Office Inspectors. The assessment process involves an estimation of the likely benefit and likely severity of the programme of work, and an ethical judgement of whether the balance of the likely benefit and the likely severity is acceptable. The decision whether or on what terms a licence or certificate (or an amendment) is granted is made by officials in a different branch of the Home Office (Animal Procedures and Coroners Unit, AP and CU), following advice from the Inspectorate.

Licences are assessed against the relevant legal criteria as described above, but there may also be additional policy or administrative criteria involved. For example, legally it is permissible to carry out regulated procedures on Great Apes; however, current policy prevents this. Current policy is described in the guidance notes.

The assessment is made on the basis of evidence contained in the application, which may include supporting material (e.g. training certificates or published scientific articles). Inspectors interpret the evidence with respect to the relevant criteria, and may also access further information in the public domain, before making a professional judgement whether the application meets the criteria. Also included are consideration of the training, experience and competence of staff and the husbandry and housing conditions of the animals. These are very important to the welfare of the animals, but are controlled not by the project licence but by other elements of the system, specifically the personal licence and the certificate of designation. Few of the elements of the assessment of project licences lend themselves to strict quantification. A balanced rational judgement is made based on the information provided.

In most cases, the assessment of an application involves one inspector. In some cases, the assessment involves more than one inspector, for example if an application requests availability at more than one establishment, or internal referral is needed. Where the application involves complex or unfamiliar scientific issues, or where there is scope for further replacement, reduction or refinement which the applicant is unwilling to accept, an external assessor may be asked to offer an expert opinion. Some types of application are automatically referred to the Animal Procedures Committee (e.g. applications for work of substantial severity on primates, work with wild caught primates and work on tobacco or cosmetics).

*You may not start any regulated procedure until a project licence covering the work has been granted by the Secretary of State.*

# PROJECT LICENCE MANAGEMENT

The project licence holder must take overall responsibility for the programme of work. This includes the scientific direction, ensuring that the work is done within the scope and conditions of the licence, and that only the species and number of animals listed on the licence are used in areas which are covered by a certificate of designation where the licence has availability. He must ensure that any personal licensees carrying out procedures within the project are appropriately licensed, trained and supervised (if this is stipulated) to do so, and are aware of the severity conditions of the licence. At all times, the project licence holder must seek reduction, refinement and replacement alternatives: implementation of the three Rs is an ongoing process, and if an alternative becomes available during the lifetime of a project licence, it should be used, regardless of the existing authorities. Project licence standard condition 6 requires the licence holder to implement refinements as they become available. Therefore, project licence holders must ensure that they remain up to date, by attending courses and reading journals as appropriate.

Full records should be kept of all regulated procedures carried out. Records should include:

- Project licence number, name of holder and deputy.
- Names of personal licensees involved.
- Details of procedure:
  - species
  - number of each species
  - sex and age at commencement of procedure
  - identification of animal (or batch)
  - date of start of procedure
  - any unexpected morbidity or mortality
  - re-use or continued use within the project
  - date of end of procedure.

Records should be kept of the fate of animals at end of procedures, which will be either released to the wild, released to private care, released for slaughter, killed within the establishment or re-used. In the latter case, the project licence to which it is to be transferred should be identified and a copy of the Home Office transfer form should be kept if applicable.

Project licence holders are required to make returns each year of the numbers and types of procedures that have been carried out and on what types of animals under the project licence during the previous 12 months. It is wise to keep records in such a format that makes the annual returns easy to compile.

Although PILs are responsible for checking that they have the appropriate authority on both personal and project licence, the project licence holder is responsible for ensuring that PILs, the NVS and the NACWO are familiar with the programme of work, which includes understanding sections 17–19, and the purpose of the procedures. The project licence holder is responsible for ensuring that PILs comply with the programme of work and are trained and supervised. There must be effective communication between the project licence holder, PILs, NVS and NACWO if the project is to be managed successfully. Project licence applicants must take responsibility for the day-to-day management of the project. Only sign an application form if you are prepared to accept these responsibilities.

## FURTHER INFORMATION

Covey, S.R. (1986). *The Seven Habits of Highly Effective People.* Simon & Schuster, New York.

Festing, M.F.W., Overend, P., Gaines Das, R., Cortina Borja, M. and Berdoy, M. (2002). The design of animal experiments. *Laboratory Animal Handbooks Number 14.* Royal Society of Medicine Press, London.

Festing, M.F.W. (1992). The scope for improving the design of laboratory animal experiments. *Laboratory Animals* 26, 256–67.

FRAME/UFAW (1998). *Selection and Use of Replacement Methods in Animal Experimentation.* UFAW, Wheathampstead.

Home Office (2001). *Notes to Applicants for Project Licences under the Animals (Scientific Procedures) Act 1986.*

HMSO (2000). *Guidance on the Operation of the Animals (Scientific Procedures) Act 1986.* The Stationery Office, London.

Mead, R. (1988). *The Design of Experiments.* Cambridge University Press, Cambridge.

## WEBSITES

Home Office website: www.homeoffice.gov.uk

Fund for the Replacement of Animals in Medical Experiments (FRAME): www.frame.org.uk

European Centre for the Validation of Alternative Methods: http://ecvam.jrc.it

Universities Federation for Animal Welfare: www.ufaw.org.uk

Humane Society of the United States: www.hsus.org

# Section 2
# Species

# Chapter 12
# Small laboratory animals

## RODENTS

Animals in the order Rodentia belong to a very successful order of placental mammals which can be found colonising almost all habitats. Despite their success, all members of the order are small, the largest member, the Capybara, being about the size of a small pig. Rodents have a number of distinguishing features, notably they have the typical open-rooted sharp teeth and hindgut microbial fermentation chambers of herbivores, and are coprophagic. Rodentia are divided into two suborders, the Sciurognathi and Hystricognathi (Figure 12.1).

## MOUSE

The mouse, *Mus musculus*, is the most commonly used laboratory animal. Many well-defined inbred strains and outbred stocks are available, for which the karyotypes are known. In fact, more is known about the genome of the mouse than any other species, which is one reason for its popularity as a research animal. There are many types of genetically modified mice available which are useful models for specific disease entities (see Chapter 13).

## Behaviour

Mice are social animals which can live in harmony, in groups with one male and several females, once their hierarchy is established. Pheromones act as mediators in

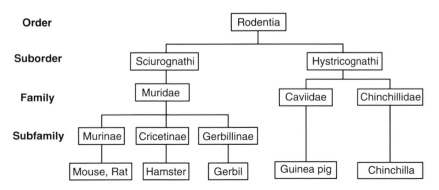

**Figure 12.1**   Rodent taxonomy (from Wilson & Reeder (1993) and Wilson & Cole (2000)).

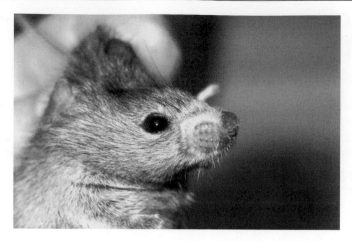

**Figure 12.2**    Barbering in the mouse.

communication between mice, and the influence of pheromones must be taken into account when managing a mouse colony. Pheromones are used to maintain stability in the colony and if they are removed each time the cage is cleaned, fighting will ensue and subordinate mice will be barbered, or possibly injured (Figure 12.2).

Providing environmental enrichment to provide places of refuge and the technique of leaving a little of the soiled bedding in the new cage to reduce the need to keep re-establishing the dominance hierarchy and territory marking will all help to reduce this. Some of the effects of pheromones are listed below:

- Stress in one mouse causes dispersal of other mice.
- Female mice attract male mice, and vice versa.
- Lactating females emit pheromones to attract the young.
- Foreign females will stimulate aggression by other female mice.
- Foreign males will provoke aggression from other male mice, and may cause recently mated females to abort (Bruce effect).
- Co-existing males emit pheromones to reduce aggression within the group, but which cause foreign males to avoid the territory.

There are also strain differences in behaviour. For example, male BALB/c mice are particularly aggressive, and fight wounds are common.

## Housing

Mice can be housed in conventional units where the pathogen status may be unknown, but more frequently are kept in barrier units with a defined and regularly monitored health status. Cages are usually of the shoebox type made of polycarbonate plastic. Bedding should be provided, such as wood chips or commercially prepared paper-based bedding (see Chapter 6). Adult males tend to fight, and are sometimes housed alone. Female mice are less aggressive, and can be kept in groups of familiar females. Females with litters will defend their young and are best separated while nursing. Keeping mice in compatible groups, and placing tubes and objects to climb on in the cage all enrich the environment and reduce stereotypic behaviour, such as barbering (see Figure 12.2).

## Feeding

Mice are usually fed ad lib with a complete pelleted mouse diet, from hoppers suspended above the floor to prevent faecal contamination. These should be cleaned weekly, but the cleaning routine will depend on factors, such as the housing system, stocking density, or presence of newborn litters. Generally, *mice will consume 3–5 g of pelleted diet daily*, but there are strain differences, and disease states and pregnancy affect the food requirements.

## Water

Water is required for lubrication of the food as well as hydration, so if insufficient fluid is available they have difficulty eating. It is supplied in automated systems or bottles. *The usual requirement is 6–7 ml water daily.* The disadvantage of automated systems when used with solid-bottomed cages is the risk of run out resulting in death of the animals either due to drowning or from chilling when they get wet. The water may need to be acidified or chlorinated to reduce contamination, particularly for immuno-compromised mice. When ill, mice drink very little and rapidly dehydrate. Medicines administered in the water are, therefore, unlikely to be effective, and care must be taken to ensure that adequate quantities of fluid are administered by other means (see Chapter 8).

## Environment

Mice have a large surface area to volume ratio and, therefore, lose heat rapidly and are sensitive to changes in ambient temperature. Much energy is expended in maintaining body temperature, and they cannot tolerate a reduction in room temperature. Mice are also susceptible to water loss. They cannot afford to sweat or pant to lose heat, as this would cause dehydration. In the wild they use behavioural mechanisms, such as burrowing to keep cool, which cannot be done in most laboratory housing. Therefore, maintenance of the correct environmental conditions is vital. To comply with the Home Office Code of Practice (CoP), mice require temperatures between 19°C and 23°C, humidity between 40% and 70%, 12–15 air changes per hour, and 12 h daylight daily. The light intensity should be 350–400 lux, except for albino mice. For these, it should be less than 60 lux to avoid damage to the retina. Mice are also very sensitive to ultrasound. Normal noise levels may sound quiet to the human ear, but they may be extremely loud for a mouse. Care should be taken to reduce ultrasound in rodent-keeping facilities.

## Breeding

Male mice reach puberty at 7 weeks, and females at 6 weeks. Females then cycle every 4–5 days. This is effected by photoperiod and the presence of others. Oestrus, mating

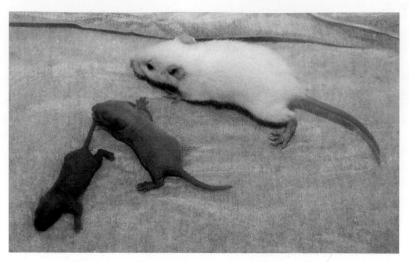

**Figure 12.3**    Ageing the rodent. (From left to right.) At 4 days old, the pup is blind and deaf with no hair. At 8 days old, the pup is still blind and deaf but is covered with fine hair. At 18 days old, the eyes and ears have opened, the hair coat is well developed and the animal is increasingly independent.

and ovulation tend to occur during the dark phase of the light cycle. Group-housed females will become anoestrus, but will resume cycling if a male is introduced. This is known as the Whitten effect, and can be used for synchronising oestrus or for timed matings. Mating results in the formation of a vaginal plug, which can be detected to confirm mating. Gestation lasts 19–21 days, and 4–15 pups may be born, depending on the strain. They are weaned at 3 weeks by which time they have fur and their eyes and ears are open (see Figure 12.3).

Mice may be bred using a harem system, with one male for two to six females, pregnant females being removed from the group to give birth, or may be kept together in a monogamous system. With the latter system, the young are removed before the next litter is born. Mice will breed until they are 12–18 months old, although the economic breeding life of most strains is around 6 months.

## Growth

Strains vary dramatically in rate of growth. In general, outbred stocks grow much faster than inbred strains (Figure 12.4).

## Handling

When handling small rodents, it may be advisable to remove the lid of the cage, rather than opening the flap in the lid, before catching the animal. Otherwise, they may hide beneath the food hopper, which makes them harder to catch and also increases the risk of being bitten. Mice move very fast, so you have to be quick and decisive to catch them:

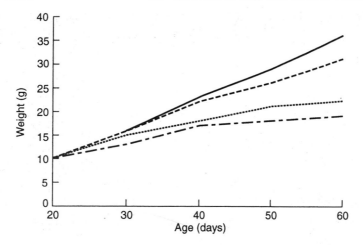

**Figure 12.4**    Growth curves for inbred (BALB/c) and outbred mice. (—) Outbred male;
(– – –) outbred female; (• • •) BALB/c male; (— · — ·) BALB/c female.

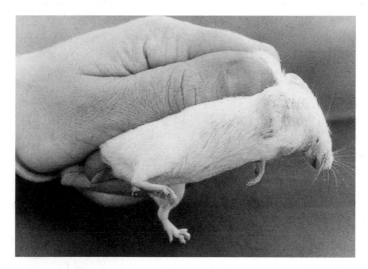

**Figure 12.5**    Handling the mouse.

- Grasp the base of the tail gently but firmly and lift the mouse. Mice may be carried short distances or transferred between boxes this way.
- Place the mouse down on a non-slip surface, such as the top of the cage, or your arm, without releasing the tail. The animal may then be sexed by lifting the tail to expose the perineum. The ano-genital distance in the male is approximately twice that seen in the female.
- Slide the thumb and index finger of the other hand up the animal's body and grasp the scruff of the neck to restrain the head.
- The animal is then secure and may be examined or injected safely. Extra restraint may be achieved by holding the tail with the fourth and fifth fingers (see Figure 12.5).

When handling newborn mice, it is important to transfer the mother to a separate cage first, to prevent any aggression from her. The pups can then be gently rolled into the palm of the hand. To avoid subsequent cannibalism by the mother, rub the hands in soiled bedding material to acquire pheromones before handling the pups, and rub the young with nest material after handling before replacing the mother. From 10 days of age, they can be handled as adults, but the mother should still be removed first.

## Pain and stress recognition

Different strains of mice may vary significantly in their responses to particular stimuli but, generally, an increase in sleeping time and weight loss will follow any procedure expected to cause pain. Affected animals show piloerection and hunched appearance and may be isolated from the rest of the group.

## Common diseases and health monitoring

Mice which are not kept under barrier conditions are likely to be carrying a number of commensal and potentially pathogenic organisms, and even barrier-reared animals can develop infections if there is a breakdown in the barrier. It is advisable to perform regular health screens on a representative number of animals from the colony in order to ascertain the health status, and to ensure that there are no potentially problematic organisms in the colony. There should be very few zoonoses in laboratory-bred mice in Britain. However, hantaan virus and lymphocytic choriomeningitis (LCM) virus can cause potentially fatal infections in man, and leptospirosis can cause undulating fevers and kidney damage. The researcher should be aware of these possibilities and take appropriate precautions.

Many viruses cause sub-clinical infections. Respiratory infections in particular must be avoided, since they increase the risks associated with anaesthesia and surgery. Sendai virus and pneumonia virus of mice can cause respiratory infections, which can be complicated by secondary infection with *Pasteurella pneumotropica* or other bacteria. Mouse hepatitis virus can cause a whole host of signs, from diarrhoea to neurological signs, interfering with many aspects of research. Minute virus of mice (MVM) and lactate dehydrogenase elevating virus (LDHV) are two viruses that commonly affect research data. MVM and many others can infect transplantable tumours and tissues, and LDHV causes increases in the levels of several enzymes, interfering with some projects. *Helicobacter* spp. have been found in mice and may be of particular significance in models of oncology and immunology. The researcher should be aware of any infections, which are likely to affect the research, and ensure that there is an appropriate screening programme in place to detect these infections before any problems are caused.

Recommendations for health monitoring of mouse colonies may be found in the Report of the FELASA Working Group on Health Monitoring of Rodent and Rabbit Colonies, *Laboratory Animals* (2002) 36, 20–42.

## Biological data and useful reference data

Biological data and useful reference data are given in Table 12.1.

**Table 12.1**    Useful data: mouse.

| Biological data | | Breeding data | |
|---|---|---|---|
| Adult weight (g) | Male   20–40 | Puberty (days) | 28–49 |
|  | Female 18–40 |  | average 42 |
| Diploid number | 40 | Age to breed male (days) | 70 |
| Food intake | 15 g/100 g | Age to breed female (days) | 60–84 |
|  | bodyweight | Gestation (days) | 19–21 |
| Water intake | 15 ml/100 g | Litter size | 4–15 |
|  | bodyweight | Birth weight (g) | 1–1.5 |
| Natural lifespan (years) | 1.5–3 | Weaning age (days) | 18–21* |
| Rectal temperature (°C) | 38–39 | Oestrous cycle (days) | 4–5 |
| Heart rate/min | 310–840 | Post-partum oestrus | Fertile |
| Blood pressure (mmHg) | | | |
| Systole | 133–160 | **Biochemical data** | |
| Diastole | 90–110 | Serum protein (g/dl) | 3.5–7.2 |
| Blood volume (ml/kg) | 60–75 | Albumin (g/dl) | 2.5–4.8 |
| Respiratory rate/min | 60–220 | Globulin (g/dl) | 0.6 |
| Tidal volume (ml) | 0.18 | Glucose (mg/dl) | 62–175 |
|  | | Blood urea nitrogen (mg/dl) | 12–28 |
| **Haematological data** | | Creatinine (mg/dl) | 0.3–1 |
| RBC ($\times 10^6$/mm$^3$) | 7–12.5 | Total bilirubin (mg/dl) | 0.1–0.9 |
| PCV (%) | 39–49 | Cholesterol (mg/dl) | 26–82 |
| Hb (g/dl) | 10.2–16.6 | | |
| WBC ($\times 10^3$/mm$^3$) | 6–15 | | |
| Neutrophils (%) | 10–40 | | |
| Lymphocytes (%) | 55–95 | | |
| Eosinophils (%) | 0–4 | | |
| Monocytes (%) | 0.1–3.5 | | |
| Basophils (%) | 0–0.3 | | |
| Platelets ($\times 10^3$/mm$^3$) | 160–410 | | |

*Date of weaning may need adjustment depending on weight of the animal.
(Note: There are strain variations especially in genetically modified mice.)

## Drug doses for anaesthesia in mice

Pre-anaesthetic fasting in mice is unnecessary, since vomiting on induction does not occur. Also fasting may result in depletion of glycogen reserves and the development of hypoglycaemia. It will, therefore, only be required if surgery on the gastrointestinal tract is to be undertaken and even then, since coprophagy is often not prevented, even removing the animal's food may not result in an empty stomach.

Drug doses are intended only as a guide and will have to be adjusted to take account of varying responses of different strains of mice to the drugs. Close monitoring of the animal is essential.

### Hypnorm (fentanyl/fluanisone) combinations

For surgical anaesthesia lasting 45–60 min, a mixture of one part Hypnorm: two parts sterile water for injection: one part midazolam can be given at the rate of 10 ml/kg intraperitonially (i.p.). To prolong the anaesthesia, additional doses of Hypnorm at 0.3 ml/kg every 30–40 min may be given. The fentanyl component can be reversed with naloxone (0.01–0.1 mg/kg intravenously (i.v.) or i.p.) to reduce the recovery time, or partially reversed with nalbuphine at 4 mg/kg i.p. or subcutaneously (s.c.) or butorphanol at 2.0 mg/kg i.p. or s.c. to provide continued analgesia.

Diazepam may be used instead of midazolam (0.4 ml/kg Hypnorm plus 5 mg/kg diazepam) but they may not be mixed in the same syringe since the diazepam, unlike midazolam, is not water soluble.

Fentanyl/medetomidine combinations in the mouse are not recommended, since there can be urinary retention leading to rupture of the bladder.

### Ketamine combinations

For surgical anaesthesia ketamine at 75 mg/kg i.p. with medetomidine at 0.5–1.0 mg/kg i.p. will produce 20–30 min of surgical anaesthesia, with rapid recovery if atipamezole (1 mg/kg s.c. or i.p.) is used as a reversal agent, or 2–4 h sleep time, if it is not. Ketamine (80–100 mg/kg) can also be given with xylazine (10 mg/kg) for similar results although the atipamezole is not so specific in its action to reverse the xylazine.

Ketamine at 150 mg/kg i.p. with diazepam at 5 mg/kg i.p., or acepromazine at 2.5 mg/kg i.p., produces light anaesthesia for 20 min with 2 h of sleep time.

### Saffan

Alphaxalone/alphadolone at 10–15 mg/kg will produce 5 min surgical anaesthesia, but only if given i.v. Recovery will take about 10 min.

### Propofol

Given i.v. at 26 mg/kg it may be useful for short-term anaesthesia or for induction prior to inhalation anaesthesia.

### Barbiturates

Pentobarbitone has a narrow safety margin and should only be used for terminal procedures and there will be marked respiratory depression. A dose of 45 mg/kg i.p. will have a variable effect in different strains with sleep time varying between 50 and 250 min, so over- or underdosage with this drug is a frequent occurrence, with all the unwanted sequelae.

### Inhaled agents

Isoflurane is the agent of choice. For induction, it can be used with an anaesthetic chamber and for maintenance given via a face mask.

### Other drugs

Doxapram may be administered at 5–10 mg/kg i.v. or i.p. to reverse respiratory depression and atropine at 0.05 mg/kg will reduce salivary and bronchial secretions.

## Drug doses for analgesia in mice

### Opioids

- *Buprenorphine*: 0.05–0.1 mg/kg s.c. or i.p. given 8 hourly. It is a partial μ-agonist; so reverses opioids, such as fentanyl, but maintains analgesia. It has a slow onset of about 40 min so must be given before the animal regains consciousness and feels pain, but it has a relatively long duration of action:
- *Butorphanol*: Give 1–5 mg/kg s.c. for 4 h of analgesia.
- *Codeine*: Give 60–90 mg/kg orally or 20 mg/kg s.c. for 4 h of analgesia.
- *Morphine*: Give 2–5 mg/kg s.c. for 2–4 h of analgesia.
- *Nalbuphine*: Give 4–8 mg/kg s.c. for 4 h of analgesia.
- *Pentazocine*: Give 10 mg/kg s.c. for 1 h of analgesia.
- *Pethidine*: Give 10–20 mg/kg s.c. for 2–3 h of analgesia.

### NSAIDs

- *Carprofen*: 2–4 mg/kg by s.c. injection gives 24 h of mild to moderate analgesia. For oral administration dissolve 50 mg (large animal solution) in 2500 ml water and give ad lib. For a 30 g mouse drinking 4.5 ml water a day, this will result in a daily intake of 4 mg/kg. The made-up solution is stable for at least 24 h.
- *Flunixin*: 2.5 mg/kg s.c. lasts 12 h.
- *Diclofenac*: 8 mg/kg orally.
- *Ibuprofen*: 30 mg/kg orally.

## RAT

Rats used in research are mainly derived from the brown or Norwegian rat, *Rattus norvegicus*. Outbred and inbred strains are available. Commonly used outbred strains include the Wistar and Sprague–Dawley varieties. Fewer inbred strains exist than for mice, but a commonly encountered one is the Lewis rat.

## Behaviour

Rats are usually friendly and amenable animals if handled gently, although there are some strain differences. They will become friendlier with more frequent handling. They are social animals and will live together in groups with little fighting provided they are not overcrowded. Rats have a tendency to be nocturnal. Feeding, drinking and mating all usually occur at night. Their eyesight is poor, and blind rats will behave as if perfectly normal. See www.ratlife.org for details of the normal behaviour of the laboratory rat.

## Housing

Rats may be kept in metal or plastic cages although there is debate about the use of mesh floors without bedding (see Chapter 6). If mesh floors are used, care must be taken to ensure that the mesh is small enough that young animals do not fall through it, but not so small that the rats catch their feet. Mesh floors are not suitable for breeding females, as nest building is not possible. In solid-bottomed cages paper-based commercial bedding, wood shavings or corn cobs may be used as bedding (see Chapter 6). Depending on the type of bedding used, the cage should be changed at least weekly; the cleaning regime will depend on the stocking density. Rats like to stand erect, and so cages with high lids are required.

## Feeding

Rats, like all rodents, are coprophagic. They can be fed ad lib on a complete pelleted rodent diet, from hoppers suspended above the floor of the cage. Food hoppers should be cleaned once or twice weekly. The diet should contain 20–27% protein. Higher protein levels than this may reduce reproduction efficiency. Rats are cautious eaters and will reject strange food. *Rats will eat 5–10 g feed per 100 g body weight daily.*

## Water

Water may be provided by sipper tubes or by automated watering systems. The system should be cleaned once or twice weekly. The water may need to be acidified or chlorinated to reduce contamination, particularly for immunocompromised rats. *Rats will drink 10 ml water per 100 g body weight daily.*

## Environment

Rats are less sensitive to temperature changes than mice, but should be kept between 19°C and 23°C. Young rats have much brown fat to assist in thermogenesis, the level of which reduces with age. The humidity should be 40–70%. Low humidity results in tail ring, in which an annular lesion appears around the tail, which may result in sloughing of the tail distal to the lesion. A 12-h light period is adequate for rats but, being nocturnal, bright light is deleterious, particularly for albino rats, and results in retinal degeneration. The level should be less than 400 lux, or 100 lux for albinos. Photoperiod affects the oestrus cycle, and 12–16 h light is best for optimal breeding. Ventilation is particularly important for rats, as many of their pathogens are aerosol borne. Twelve to fifteen air changes per hour is sufficient, provided the air is not recycled or an effective filter is present.

## Breeding

Puberty occurs at 50–60 days, and breeding begins at 3 months, when females weigh 250 g and males 300 g. They breed until they are 12–18 months old. Oestrus occurs every 4–5 days. The Whitten effect is less pronounced in rats than mice (synchronisation of oestrus in females by exposure to male pheromones), but does occur. Mating usually occurs at night, and a copulatory plug of gelatinous material is left in the vagina for 12–24 h, which then falls out and can be detected to confirm that mating has occurred. Gestation lasts 21–23 days. A litter of 6–12 pups is born in a shallow nest made by the female. Paper- or cotton-based bedding, wood shavings or specialised bedding materials (e.g. 'Vetbed' simulated fur bedding) can be supplied to aid in nest building. Ground corn cobs are not suitable for nest making. Weaning occurs at 21 days. If a female is disturbed in the immediate post-partum period, she may destroy her young, so extreme care must be taken when cleaning cages during this time.

Rats may be bred by monogamous or polygamous mating systems. With a monogamous system, the female will be mated at the post-partum oestrus, and the young are removed at weaning. This produces the maximum number of litters, but the male may interfere with the young. He can be removed at parturition, and returned to the female after the young are weaned. If the female is lactating during gestation, implantation can be delayed, leading to a 3–7-day increase in the length of gestation. A variation in the monogamous system exists in which a single male is moved between singly housed females, spending a week with each. One male is used for every seven females. Care must be taken to remove the male before parturition, or he may attack the litter. In polygamous systems, one male is housed with two to six females. Pregnant females are removed prior to parturition and returned after weaning. Females in this system produce more milk and have larger litters.

## Growth

Male rats exhibit prolonged growth, and bones do not become fully ossified until their 2nd year. Inbred and outbred rats differ slightly in their rates of growth (Figure 12.6).

## Handling

There are many ways of handling rats. In general, rats are amenable animals, which rarely bite if approached correctly, although there are strain differences.

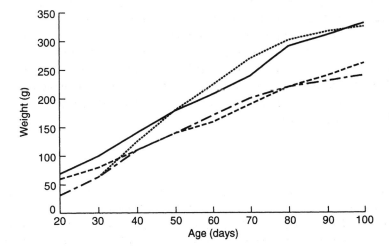

**Figure 12.6**   Growth curves for inbred and outbred rats. (—) Outbred male; (– – –) outbred female; (• • •) Lewis male; (— · — ·) BALB/c female.

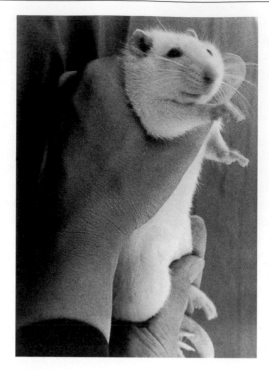

**Figure 12.7**    Handling the rat.

1.  Remove the lid of the cage, and grasp the rat by the base of the tail. Lift the animal from the cage and support it immediately on a non-slip surface, such as the arm or cage top. Rats should not be suspended by their tails for any length of time to avoid injury. Once supported on a surface, the animal may be sexed by lifting the tail to expose the perineum, as in mice.
2.  To restrain the animal for examination or procedures, once it has been transferred to a non-slip surface as above, slide the free hand up the animal's body to a position behind the shoulders. Position the thumb between the forelimbs so it rests under the chin to restrain the head, with the fingers behind the other forelimb. The animal may then be lifted, and the hindquarters held with the other hand (see Figure 12.7).
3.  Alternatively, for added restraint, complete Step 1 then slide the free hand up the animal's body, but press the elbows with the thumb and fingers to cause the forelegs to cross over under the chin. This method may be used if the animal is aggressive or unfriendly.

## Pain and stress recognition

Rats are naturally curious, and will explore in any new situations. Failure to stand erect and take an interest in their surroundings is an indicator of poor health. They are generally docile but become more aggressive and resist handling during repeated stressful procedures. Acute pain or distress is accompanied by vocalisation and struggling. They will lick or guard a painful area and will sit crouched. Sleep patterns will be disturbed and increased if pain and distress are present. The Harderian gland, a modified tear gland situated on the bulbar conjunctiva of the third eyelid, produces a porphyrin-rich secretion, which normally lubricates the eye. When the rat is stressed, this secretion tends to overflow onto the face, producing a red ring around the eye, which is characteristic of stress. This is known as chromodacryorrhoea. Red staining may also appear at the nose, as the secretion flows down the nasolacrimal duct. Video evidence shows that the three key signs of pain post-laparotomy in the rat are: back-arching, twitching and a cat-like stretch, in addition to showing reluctance to move.

## Common diseases and health monitoring

Rats are susceptible to a number of diseases which may be zoonotic, have effects on the animals when under stress, or affect research data. For example, Hantaan virus and Leptospirosis are zoonoses, Sendai virus, pneumonia virus of mice, SDAV/RCV and *Mycoplasma pulmonis* may all have effects on the respiratory system particularly in the stressed animal and Kilham rat virus may infect transplantable tissues and is teratogenic.

## Biological data and useful reference data

Biological data and useful reference data are shown in Table 12.2.

## Drug doses for anaesthesia in rats

### *Medetomidine + ketamine*

Inject i.p. at a dose rate of 0.5 mg/kg medetomidine + 60–75 mg/kg ketamine. For small rats medetomidine may be diluted 1:10 with sterile water and the ketamine added in the same syringe. Anaesthesia is achieved in a few minutes and lasts up to 30 min. For recovery in 5–10 min, reverse with atipamezole 1 mg/kg s.c.

### *Hypnorm (fentanyl/fluanisone) combinations*

If just sedation is required for minor procedures, use Hypnorm alone 0.3–0.6 ml/kg i.p. and then reverse with naloxone at 0.1 mg/kg.

Surgical anaesthesia with good muscle relaxation can be achieved for 30–40 min by giving 0.6 ml/kg Hypnorm with 2.5 mg/kg midazolam or diazepam i.p. If using midazolam, this may be mixed in the same syringe as the Hypnorm. Additional doses of Hypnorm at about 0.1 ml/kg intramuscularly (i.m.) every 30–40 min, may be used to prolong the anaesthesia if necessary.

The fentanyl component of Hypnorm may be reversed by naloxone 0.1 mg/kg i.p. or i.v. or buprenorphine 0.05 mg/kg s.c. or nalbuphine 0.1 mg/kg i.v., 1.0 mg/kg i.p. or s.c. or butorphanol 0.1 mg/kg i.v. or 2.0 mg/kg i.p. or s.c.

A dose rate of 300 µg/kg fentanyl with 300 µg/kg medetomidine i.p. will provide 45–60 min of surgical anaesthesia. Reverse with atipamezole 1 mg/kg s.c. plus either nalbuphine 1 mg/kg s.c. or butorphanol 0.1 mg/kg i.v. or 2.0 mg/kg i.p. or s.c. for recovery in about 8 min with post-operative analgesia.

**Table 12.2** Useful data: rat.

| *Biological data* | | | *Breeding data* | |
|---|---|---|---|---|
| Adult weight (g) | Male | 450–520 | Puberty (days) | 50–60 |
| | Female | 250–300 | Age to breed (days) | 65–110 |
| Diploid number | 42 | | Gestation (days) | 20–23 |
| Food intake | 5–10 g/100 g | | Litter size | 6–12 |
| | bodyweight | | Birth weight (g) | 5–6 |
| Water intake | 10 ml/100 g | | Weaning age (days) | 21 |
| | bodyweight | | Oestrous cycle (days) | 4–5 |
| Natural lifespan (years) | 3–4 | | Post-partum oestrus | Fertile |
| Rectal temperature (°C) | 36–40 | | | |
| Heart rate/min | 250–450 | | *Biochemical data* | |
| Blood pressure (mmHg) | | | Serum protein (g/dl) | 5.6–7.6 |
| Systole | 84–134 | | Albumin (g/dl) | 3.8–4.8 |
| Diastole | 60 | | Globulin (g/dl) | 1.8–3 |
| Blood volume (ml/kg) | 54–70 | | Glucose (mg/dl) | 50–135 |
| Respiratory rate/min | 70–115 | | Blood urea nitrogen (mg/dl) | 15–21 |
| Tidal volume (ml) | 0.6–2 | | Creatinine (mg/dl) | 0.2–0.8 |
| | | | Total bilirubin (mg/dl) | 0.2–0.55 |
| *Haematological data* | | | Cholesterol (mg/dl) | 40–130 |
| RBC ($\times\ 10^6$/mm$^3$) | 7–10 | | | |
| PCV (%) | 36–48 | | | |
| Hb (g/dl) | 11–18 | | | |
| WBC ($\times\ 10^3$/mm$^3$) | 6–17 | | | |
| Neutrophils (%) | 9–34 | | | |
| Lymphocytes (%) | 65–85 | | | |
| Eosinophils (%) | 0–6 | | | |
| Monocytes (%) | 0–5 | | | |
| Basophils (%) | 0–1.5 | | | |
| Platelets ($\times\ 10^3$/mm$^3$) | 500–1300 | | | |

## Ketamine combinations

A combination of 10 mg/kg xylazine + 90 mg/kg ketamine i.p. will achieve about 30 min of surgical anaesthesia. Ketamine (100 mg/kg i.p.) alone may be used just for sedation but does not produce surgical anaesthesia. Ketamine at 75 mg/kg i.p. may also be combined with acepromazine at 2.5 mg/kg i.p., or ketamine 75 mg/kg i.p. with diazepam at 5 mg/kg i.p. to produce a light level of anaesthesia lasting 20 min with a 2–3-h recovery time.

## Saffan

*Alphaxalone/alphadolone* (*Saffan*): 10–12 mg/kg i.v. (lateral tail vein) will produce surgical anaesthesia for about 5 min but incremental doses may easily be given to prolong the anaesthesia as necessary.

## *Propofol*

Given i.v. at 10 mg/kg propofol is useful for short-duration anaesthesia or for induction prior to inhalation anaesthesia.

## *Barbiturates*

Pentobarbitone has a narrow safety margin and should only be used for terminal procedures. If administered at 45 mg/kg i.p. it will produce anaesthesia lasting between 15 min and 1 h. However, there will be marked respiratory depression and high-mortality rate. Thiopentone can be used i.v. at 30 mg/kg.

## *Inhaled agents*

Isoflurane is the agent of choice. For induction it can be used with an anaesthetic chamber and for maintenance given via a face mask.

## *Other drugs*

Doxapram may be administered at 5–10 mg/kg s.c., i.v. or i.p. to reverse respiratory depression and atropine at 0.05 mg/kg will reduce salivary and bronchial secretions.

## Drug doses for analgesia in rats

### *Opioids*

- *Buprenorphine*: 0.1–0.25 mg/kg s.c. or orally given 8–12 hourly. It is a partial μ-agonist so reverses opioids, such as fentanyl but maintains analgesia. It has a slow onset of about 40 min so must be given before the animal regains consciousness and feels pain, but it has a relatively long duration of action.
- *Butorphanol*: Give 0.5–2.0 mg/kg s.c. for 4-h analgesia.
- *Codeine*: Give 60 mg/kg s.c. for 4-h analgesia.
- *Morphine*: Give 2–5 mg/kg s.c. for 2–4-h analgesia.
- *Nalbuphine*: Give 1–2 mg/kg s.c. for 3-h analgesia.
- *Pentazocine*: Give 10 mg/kg s.c. for 3–4-h analgesia.
- *Pethidine*: Give 10–20 mg/kg s.c. for 2–3-h analgesia.

### *NSAIDs*

- *Carprofen*: 2–5 mg/kg s.c. injection gives 24 h of mild to moderate analgesia. For oral administration dissolve 50 mg (large animal solution) in 1250 ml water and give ad lib. For a 600 g rat drinking 60 ml water a day this will result in a daily intake of 4 mg/kg. The made-up solution is stable for at least 24 h.
- *Diclofenac*: 10 mg/kg orally.
- *Flunixin*: 2.5 mg/kg s.c. lasts 12 h.
- *Phenylbutazone*: 20 mg/kg orally.

- *Aspirin*: 100 mg/kg orally lasts 4 h.
- *Ibuprofen*: 15 mg/kg orally lasts 4 h.

If the rat is eating, then continued analgesia may be provided by mixing the required amount of the drug in jelly so it is taken orally. The berry fruit flavours are preferred and the jelly also provides a source of fluids and glucose, which aids in post-operative recovery.

# HAMSTER

Hamsters are known widely for their cheek pouches, in which they gather food, to store in deep burrows, particularly when photoperiod is decreasing. The pouches are unusual in having no lymph drainage and, therefore, do not reject tissues transplanted to them. This is useful in immunological and other research. Several different varieties of hamster are used, the commonest one being the Golden or Syrian hamster, *Mesocricetus auratus*. Different strains are available.

## Behaviour

Hamsters are readily tamed, and rarely bite unless startled or handled roughly. Males are more docile than females. They are active at times during the day, but are mainly nocturnal, so most activity occurs at night. Hamsters are solitary animals, and will attack each other. Females will attack males except for a brief period during oestrus, and often attack other females. Groups of same sex animals may be maintained, if they are put together at weaning or before puberty. Territory marking is done using a secretion from the flank glands, which are visible, particularly in the male, as dark patches on each side.

## Housing

Hamsters, being solitary, prefer to be housed individually. They are adept at chewing through cages, so tough plastic cages with solid bottoms are used. If they do manage to escape, unlike rats and mice, they are unlikely to return to their cages. Deep-piled bedding is usually provided. Little waste is produced, and cages can be cleaned out one to two times weekly.

A breeding female must have deep bedding and soft nesting material, such as commercially produced paper-bedding material, or an inadequate nest will lead to her abandoning or killing her young. To avoid disturbing a nursing mother, cleaning out may be done every 2 weeks.

## Feeding

The nutritional requirements of hamsters have not been extensively studied. They are coprophagic, but may have different digestive systems to rats or mice. A diet with 16% protein, 5–7% fat and 60–65% carbohydrate would appear to be sufficient. *Hamsters eat 5–7g pelleted diet daily.*

As they have blunt noses, hamsters cannot feed from standard wire mesh suspended hoppers. They need hoppers with slots greater than 11 mm, so they can pull the food through onto the floor. Nursing females should be floor fed, or they become preoccupied with pulling food from the hopper and neglect their young. Food hoppers and drinking apparatus should be cleaned once or twice weekly.

## Water

*Hamsters need 10 ml water per 100 g body weight daily.*

Water bottles or automated systems can be used, but the sipper tubes must be stainless steel and not glass, as hamsters can bite through glass. For breeding animals, the sipper tubes should extend low into the cage so that neonates can reach them. Lactating females have a greater water requirement.

## Environment

Hamsters are originally from hot countries, and burrow to avoid heat. If unable to burrow, they tolerate heat poorly. Cold, however, may be tolerated quite well. If the temperature drops below 5°C, they can go into a state of pseudohibernation, from which they can be aroused by stimulation. If insufficient food is available, hibernation is delayed. Hamsters should be kept between 19°C and 23°C, and breeding animals need to be at the higher temperature. Relative humidity should be 40–60%. A 12–14-h period of light should be provided daily.

## Breeding

Puberty occurs at 32–42 days, and breeding usually starts at 6–10 weeks for females and 10–14 weeks for males, when they weigh 90–130 g. Fertility is lower in the winter. The female has oestrus every 4 days, and is receptive for a very short time. Gestation lasts 15.5–16 days. Between five and nine young are born. Due to the short gestation, they are small, weighing 2–3 g, and immature. An adequate nest is essential to provide warmth and security for the young, hence the need for nesting material. Weaning occurs at 20–25 days. Males and females are usually kept separately, and put together for a short period after dark for mating. If the female is not receptive and does not accept the male, he should be removed at once. Otherwise, he is removed at the end of the dark period, before the light part of the cycle begins. A system of monogamous pairs can be maintained if the male and female are put together before puberty and kept permanently together. Alternatively, females can be rotated through the male's cage at weekly intervals, one male being used for seven females, or a harem can be set up with several males and females together. The females are removed prior to parturition and returned after weaning. However, these systems can lead to fighting.

Hamsters commonly abandon or kill their young. This can be triggered by environmental disturbances, inadequate nesting material or early handling of mother and young. Sometimes when disturbed, females hide their young in their cheek pouches. While this affords the young some protection, it may also suffocate them. To avoid stressing a nursing mother, sufficient food and bedding for at least 1 week should be provided just prior to parturition, so that she does not have to be disturbed for 7 days post-partum. Fostering and hand rearing of young are usually unsuccessful, so it is difficult to rederive a colony by Caesarian section to control disease outbreaks.

## Handling

Hamsters have a tendency to bite if startled and should be picked up gently but firmly by cupping the animal in the hand. Hamsters have no tail, and large cheek pouches. They are restrained by grasping a *large* pinch of scruff and turning over into the hand as for mice. If insufficient scruff is grasped, the hamster will turn and bite. Additional restraint may be achieved by grasping skin along the back between the fingers and palm.

## Pain and stress recognition

Hamsters will show weight loss, extended sleep period and increased aggression or depression. Ocular discharge and diarrhoea may be associated with stress.

## Common diseases and health monitoring

Hamsters are relatively free from clinical diseases. They may get non-specific enteritis, known as 'wet tail', which is sometimes associated with *Salmonella* or *Campylobacter* infection, both of which are potentially zoonotic. They can also carry LCM and Sendai viruses, and these should be included in the regular health-screening programme.

## Biological data and useful reference data

Biological data and useful reference data are shown in Table 12.3.

## Drug doses for anaesthesia in the hamster

### Fentanyl/fluanisone combinations

For surgical procedures, combine Hypnorm at 0.5–1 ml/kg i.p. with midazolam at a dose of 5 mg/kg. Remember absorption from the peritoneal cavity may be variable, but the anaesthesia should last 20–40 min.

The Hypnorm may be reversed with naloxone 0.05 mg/kg, or for continued analgesia with nalbuphine 2.0 mg/kg s.c. or butorphanol 2.0 mg/kg s.c.

### Ketamine combinations

Ketamine 200 mg/kg plus xylazine 10 mg/kg i.p. will also produce surgical anaesthesia but with moderate respiratory depression. Ketamine 150 mg/kg i.m. can be given with acepromazine at 5 mg/kg i.m.

### Propofol

Propofol can be used at 10 mg/kg i.v.

**Table 12.3**  Useful data: hamster.

| Biological data | | Breeding data | |
|---|---|---|---|
| Adult weight (g) | Male 85–130 | Puberty (days) | 32–42 |
| | Female 95–150 | Age to breed male (weeks) | 10–14 |
| Diploid number | 44 | Age to breed female (weeks) | 6–10 |
| Food intake | 5 g/100 g | Gestation (days) | 15–16 |
| | bodyweight | Litter size | 5–9 |
| Water intake | 10 ml/100 g | Birth weight (g) | 2 |
| | bodyweight | Weaning age (days) | 20–25 |
| Natural lifespan (years) | 1–3 | Oestrous cycle (days) | 4 |
| Rectal temperature (°C) | 37–38 | Post-partum oestrus | Infertile |
| Heart rate/min | 250–500 | | |
| Blood pressure (mmHg) | | **Biochemical data** | |
| Systole | 150 | Serum protein (g/dl) | 4.5–7.5 |
| Diastole | 100 | Albumin (g/dl) | 2.6–4.1 |
| Blood volume (ml/kg) | 78 | Globulin (g/dl) | 2.7–4.2 |
| Respiratory rate/min | 35–135 | Glucose (mg/dl) | 60–150 |
| Tidal volume (ml) | 0.6–1.4 | Blood urea nitrogen (mg/dl) | 12–25 |
| | | Creatinine (mg/dl) | 0.91–0.99 |
| **Haematological data** | | Total bilirubin (mg/dl) | 0.25–0.6 |
| RBC ($\times 10^6$/mm$^3$) | 6–10 | Cholesterol (mg/dl) | 25–135 |
| PCV (%) | 36–55 | | |
| Hb (g/dl) | 10–16 | | |
| WBC ($\times 10^3$/mm$^3$) | 3–11 | | |
| Neutrophils (%) | 10–42 | | |
| Lymphocytes (%) | 50–95 | | |
| Eosinophils (%) | 0–4.5 | | |
| Monocytes (%) | 0–3 | | |
| Basophils (%) | 0–1 | | |
| Platelets ($\times 10^3$/mm$^3$) | 200–500 | | |

## Saffan

Alphaxalone/alphadolone (Saffan) may be given at 150 mg/kg i.p.

## Medetomidine

Medetomidine at 100 μg/kg s.c. produces sedation which will enable cheek pouch examination. Higher doses do not seem to produce more sedation, but medetomidine is useful as a premedicant to reduce stress when inducing gaseous anaesthesia. To reverse the medetomidine, use atipamezole at 1 mg/kg s.c.

## Barbiturates

A dose rate of 50–90 mg/kg pentobarbitone will produce anaesthesia but with a high-mortality rate as the safety margin is very low. Thiopentone can be given i.v. at 30 mg/kg.

## *Inhaled agents*

Isoflurane is the agent of choice. For induction it can be used with an anaesthetic chamber and for maintenance given via a face mask.

## *Other drugs*

Atropine 0.04 mg/kg s.c. when the animal is asleep to prevent secretions blocking the airway. For respiratory depression use doxapram 5–10 mg/kg.

## Analgesia

- *Buprenorphine* 0.5 mg/kg s.c.
- *Butorphanol* 0.4 mg/kg s.c.
- *Flunixin* 2.5 mg/kg s.c.
- *Pethidine* 20 mg/kg s.c.

## GERBIL

Over 100 species are included in this group, but the one used mainly for research is the Mongolian gerbil, *Meriones unguiculatus*. These are easy to keep, being hardy with few diseases. Most gerbils used are from outbred stocks, but an inbred strain is available (MON/Tum strain).

## Behaviour

Gerbils are generally docile creatures, which are easily handled and rarely bite. They are generally very active, and when approached, they will resist being caught. Normally, they exhibit exploratory behaviour in new surroundings, and if loose they do not hide but show curiosity and interest in the environment. In the wild they are crepuscular. Although friendly with people, unfamiliar adults caged together will be aggressive. Stable groups may be established by putting animals together before weaning. Normal social behaviour will then be seen, in which animals wrestle and groom each other.

Some young gerbils will display epileptiform seizures if stimulated, for example by handling or environmental disturbances. Should this occur, the best treatment is to leave the gerbil in a warm, dark, quiet place to recover. Drugs may be given following veterinary advice to control severe seizures. Frequent handling from an early age will reduce the frequency of seizures.

## Housing

Gerbils have similar husbandry needs to other rodents. They prefer solid floors to mesh, and need at least 2 cm depth of bedding for nest building, which occurs even if the female is not pregnant. Sawdust or shavings made from pine should not be used, as the fur tends to become matted with these materials. Gerbils need at least 15 cm space between the top of the bedding and the roof of the cage, as they like to sit erect. As gerbils tend to gnaw the cage, it should be of suitably strong material to resist attempts to escape. Very little urine is produced by gerbils, and their faecal pellets are small and hard. They are naturally clean animals, and cages usually need cleaning only at weekly intervals.

## Feeding

Like all rodents, gerbils are coprophagic. Eating is spread throughout the day and night. Standard rodent diets with 22% protein are adequate, but due to a unique lipid metabolism the dietary fat level must be below 4% to prevent the development of high blood cholesterol. Higher fat levels lead to obesity, and in females may cause infertility due to fat deposition around the genital tract. Standard food hoppers are normally used, but supplementary food may be put onto the floor for young gerbils until they become used to the hoppers. Pellets can also be soaked. *Gerbils consume 5–8 g of pelleted food daily.*

## Water

Gerbils, being desert animals, will cope with very little water, although older males tend to need more than younger animals. They produce very concentrated urine, and are resistant to water loss. Bottles or automated systems may be used, and care must be taken that the sipper tube is accessible to all individuals in the cage, including juveniles. *Gerbils do well with 4–7 ml water daily.*

## Environment

Due to their desert origin, gerbils can tolerate high temperatures and have a great ability to regulate their body temperature. They thrive between 19°C and 23°C. Humidity should be between 30% and 50%, and 12 h light should be provided daily at 350–400 lux. Ventilation should produce 12–15 air changes per hour.

## Breeding

Gerbils are less-efficient breeders than other rodents. Often, when mates are introduced fighting occurs, or if a long-time partner dies, the remaining partner will not breed again. Less aggression is seen if the introduction takes place on neutral territory. The best regime involves keeping gerbils in monogamous pairs and never separating them. If they are separated then reintroduced, they will probably fight. Puberty occurs from 6 weeks of age, and they are usually bred from 9 to 12 weeks. Oestrus occurs in the female every 4–6 days. Gestation lasts 24–26 days, unless the female is mated at the post-partum oestrus. In this case, lactation prolongs the gestation period to 27–48 days. To avoid post-partum mating, the male can be removed at parturition, but the separation should be for less than 2 weeks. Three to seven pups are born, and the male will assist in caring for them. Despite this, neonatal mortality is high. Weaning takes place at 21 days.

## Handling

Gerbils may be restrained using techniques as for mouse and rat. They may be picked up by grasping the base of the tail, then supporting the body with the other hand. Great care must be taken because if the shaft of the tail is held the skin may slip off.

## Pain and stress recognition

Gerbils will show weight loss, piloerection with a characteristic scruffy appearance and increased aggression or depression. Ocular discharge and diarrhoea may be associated with stress.

## Common diseases and health monitoring

Gerbils, like hamsters, are relatively free from clinical diseases. They can develop Tyzzers disease, a frequently fatal enteric infection which also affects the liver, can also carry LCM and Sendai viruses, and these should be included in the regular health-screening programme.

## Biological data and useful reference data

See Table 12.4.

**Table 12.4**   Useful data: gerbil.

| *Biological data* | | *Breeding data* | |
|---|---|---|---|
| Adult weight (g) | Male    65–100 | Puberty | Vaginal opening |
| | Female 55–85 | | 41 days (28 g) |
| Diploid number | 44 | Age to breed male (days) | 70–85 |
| Food intake | 5–8 g | Age to breed female | 65–85 |
| Water intake | 4–7 ml | (days) | |
| Natural lifespan (years) | 3–4 | Gestation (days) | 24–26 (27–48 |
| Rectal temperature (°C) | 37–38.5 | | if lactating) |
| Heart rate/min | 360 | Litter size | 3–7 |
| Blood volume (ml/kg) | 66–78 | Birth weight (g) | 2.5–3.5 depends |
| Respiratory rate/min | 90 | | on litter size |
| | | Weaning age (days) | 21 |
| *Haematological data* | | Oestrous cycle (days) | 4–5 |
| RBC ($\times 10^6$/mm$^3$) | 8–9* | Post-partum oestrus | Fertile |
| PCV (%) | 43–49 | | |
| Hb (g/dl) | 12.6–16.2 | *Biochemical data* | |
| WBC ($\times 10^3$/mm$^3$) | 7–15 | Serum protein (g/dl) | 4.3–12.5 |
| Neutrophils (%) | 5–34 | Albumin (g/dl) | 1.8–5.5 |
| Lymphocytes (%) | 60–95 | Globulin (g/dl) | 1.2–6 |
| Eosinophils (%) | 0–4 | Glucose (mg/dl) | 50–135 |
| Monocytes (%) | 0–3 | Blood urea nitrogen | 17–27 |
| Basophils (%) | 0–1 | (mg/dl) | |
| Platelets ($\times 10^3$/mm$^3$) | 400–600 | Creatinine (mg/dl) | 0.6–1.4 |
| | | Total bilirubin (mg/dl) | 0.2–0.6 |
| | | Cholesterol (mg/dl) | 90–150 |

*High levels of reticulocytes, stippled red blood cells, and polychromatic cells.

# Drug doses for anaesthesia in the gerbil

## Fentanyl/fluanisone combinations

For surgical procedures, use Hypnorm at 0.5–1 ml/kg i.p. combined with midazolam at a dose of 5 mg/kg i.p. The Hypnorm may be reversed with naloxone 0.05 mg/kg or for continued analgesia with nalbuphine 4.0 mg/kg i.p. or s.c., or butorphanol 2.0 mg/kg i.p. or buprenorphine 0.1 mg/kg s.c.

## Ketamine combinations

Ketamine 100 mg/kg plus xylazine 2 mg/kg i.p. may produce surgical anaesthesia in the gerbil but it is not reliable and causes moderate respiratory depression. Alternatively, ketamine at 50 mg/kg i.m. can be combined with diazepam at 5 mg/kg i.p.

## Saffan

Alphaxalone/alphadolone (Saffan) may be given at 150 mg/kg i.p.

## Medetomidine

Medetomidine at 100 μg/kg s.c. is useful as a premedicant to reduce stress when inducing gaseous anaesthesia. To reverse the medetomidine, use atipamezole at 1 mg/kg s.c.

## Barbiturates

A dose rate of 60–80 mg/kg pentobarbitone will produce anaesthesia but with a high-mortality rate as the safety margin is very low.

## Inhaled agents

Isoflurane is the agent of choice. For induction it can be used with an anaesthetic chamber and for maintenance given via a face mask.

## Other drugs

It is advisable to also use atropine 0.04 mg/kg s.c. when the animal is asleep to prevent secretions blocking the airway. For respiratory depression, use doxapram 5–10 mg/kg. Acepromazine may precipitate seizures.

## Analgesia

- *Buprenorphine*, 0.1–0.2 mg/kg s.c.
- *Butorphanol* 2.0 mg/kg i.p. or s.c.
- *Pethidine* 20 mg/kg s.c.

# GUINEA PIG

The guinea pig, *Cavia porcellus*, is a rodent that originated from South America. There are several different varieties of guinea pig available, including the short hair (English and American varieties), Abyssinian (which have hair in whorls), and Peruvian (which have long hair). Commonly used laboratory stocks are derived from the short-hair variety. The Dunkin–Hartley and Hartley guinea pigs are outbred stocks, and strains 2 and 13 are inbred strains.

## Behaviour

Guinea pigs are amenable animals which rarely bite. Naturally they are crepuscular, but in the laboratory they will be active for periods throughout the day and night. When startled, guinea pigs have a tendency either to become immobile or to stampede and vocalise, leading to the risk of trampling young and making capture difficult. Providing bolt-holes and barriers within the pen and frequent handling to habituate the animals will reduce the problem. The approach of a person will cause excitement, and the scatter reaction should be elicited as an attempt is made to capture a guinea pig. The normal behaviour is for the guinea pig to 'resist arrest' and vocalise strongly. If this does not occur it may indicate that there is a problem.

Group-housed familiar guinea pigs will soon establish a stable hierarchy, which is male dominated and maintained mainly by olfactory cues, but with some barbering and chewing of subordinate males. If unfamiliar males are placed together, fighting will ensue particularly in cramped conditions or if oestrous females are present. Guinea pigs are creatures of habit and become increasingly unable to cope with changes in routine as maturity approaches. If there are any changes in the type of food hopper or water bottle, or in the type of food or water, the guinea pig may be unable to adapt and cease eating and drinking. This is particularly disastrous with pregnant females. Similarly, if there are changes in the type of housing, problems may be encountered.

## Housing

As gregarious animals, guinea pigs like to be housed in groups. This may be in floor pens, or large plastic or steel cages. Although guinea pigs rarely jump, cages should have sides at least 23 cm high, and more height is required for open-topped floor pens (Figure 12.8). Guinea pigs thrive on solid floors, but are sometimes kept on slats or mesh if accustomed to these types of floor. Mesh floors may also predispose to footpad ulcers and increased stress levels, and are certainly contraindicated with experiments involving joints and feet.

Bedding materials provide comfort and a substrate for rooting behaviour. Materials such as wood shavings, paper-based bedding, ground corn cobs or sawdust may be used, together with hay. Fine shavings and sawdust alone may cling to moist areas, such as the perineum, and probably are best not given to breeding guinea pigs. Larger shavings are better for these animals. Guinea pigs are messy animals and will disperse opaque, creamy coloured urine and faecal pellets throughout the pen. All pens, cages, feeding receptacles and water bottles must be cleaned and disinfected at least weekly. Removal of urine scale may require the use of acidic-cleaning agents.

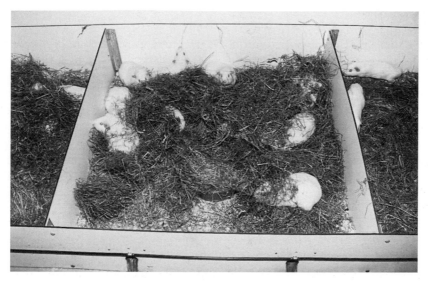

**Figure 12.8**   Guinea pigs housed in floor pens.

## Feeding and water

As guinea pigs are messy, food and water bowls placed on the floor will soon become soiled with bedding, urine and faeces, and should be suspended above the floor or cleaned frequently. There is a tendency to play with drinkers, which leads to messy floors, and bottles quickly become empty. Automated watering systems ensure a constant water supply, but in solid-floored systems, care must be taken to prevent flooding. All watering systems need to be checked and cleaned frequently. Any changes in watering system will upset the routine, and the guinea pig will need help to adapt. *The water requirement of a guinea pig is 10 ml/100 g body weight daily.*

Guinea pigs are fastidious eaters and will reject unfamiliar food. They require a pelleted, freshly milled complete guinea pig diet, not one designed for any other species. Supplements of hay may be given, but with care as digestive disturbances may result from an excessive amount, or from greens that have not been properly washed. *The food requirement is 6 g/100 g body weight daily.* However because much of the food is wasted more should be supplied. The food should contain 18–20% crude protein, and 10–16% fibre. Guinea pigs are unable to synthesise vitamin C, and require 5 mg/kg daily normally, and up to 30 mg/kg if pregnant. This can be supplied in the food or water, or by giving cabbage, kale or oranges. Food with added vitamin C must be used within 90 days of manufacture, or the vitamin C will degrade. Coprophagy does occur in the guinea pig, but may not be essential.

## Environment

Guinea pigs thrive at temperatures between 18°C and 26°C, with a humidity of 40% and 70%. They should have 12–15 air changes per hour, and 12–15 h light daily.

## Breeding

Female guinea pigs reach puberty from 5 to 6 weeks, and males from 8 weeks. The average is 9–10 weeks. Pairing should be done when the female is 400 g (at 2–3 months), and the male 650 g (3–4 months). One boar can be housed with one to ten females. The oestrous cycle of the female lasts 15–17 days, and she is receptive for 6–11 h. The vagina is covered by an epithelial membrane, which is intact except during oestrus and parturition, both of which are signalled by perforation of the membrane. Gestation lasts 59–72 days, depending on litter size. In the last week of gestation, the pubic symphysis separates under the influence of the hormone relaxin, and once the gap reaches 15 mm parturition will take place within 48 h. Females should have their first litter before reaching 7–8 months of age, or the symphysis will be unable to separate sufficiently and dystocia will result. In any case, there is often a high incidence of dystocia and fetal death. Abortions and stillbirths are common.

Female guinea pigs can breed until they are 20 months old. Thereafter, the litter size tends to drop and dystocia is more common. Neonatal guinea pigs are precocious, weighing 60–100 g, and they begin to eat solid food within a few days. Hand rearing is not difficult, making Caesarian rederivation of colonies quite easy. The young are not hungry until 12–24 h after birth, and can then be fed cows' milk or soaked guinea pig pellets. If the females are not kept in harem groups, the young may be removed at birth and hand reared, to allow the sow to be mated at the post-partum oestrus. Otherwise, weaning takes place at 180 g (15–28 days), or 21 days (165–240 g). Weaned males intended for breeding need to be weaned late or group housed to allow development of normal adult reproductive behaviour.

## Growth

The growth depends largely on the strain of guinea pig. Young guinea pigs should gain 2.5–3.5 g daily up to 60 days.

## Handling

Guinea pigs are easily startled, and they will vocalise and try to avoid capture when approached. They should be grasped quickly and smoothly, placing the thumb and fingers of one hand on either side of the shoulders, then lifted and the free hand placed beneath the hindquarters to support the weight. The guinea pig can then be turned over for i.p. injections or sexing. Positioning the thumb under the foreleg and beneath the chin as in the rat will provide additional restraint.

Alternatively, one hand may be placed under the thorax and the other under the rear feet. It is particularly important to support pregnant females with two hands (see Figure 12.9).

## Recognition of pain and stress

Guinea pigs are alert, apprehensive animals who will try to avoid capture and restraint. Any unusual sign of acceptance indicates the animal is unwell. Loud vocalisation

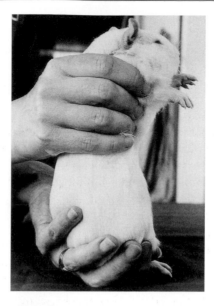

**Figure 12.9**    Handling the guinea pig.

accompanies even minor and transient pain. They often appear sleepy when in pain and rarely show aggression. They are stoical animals and it can be difficult to assess whether they are in pain from a single glance. A carefully used pain scoring assessment method should be employed (see Chapter 4).

## Common diseases and health monitoring

Relatively few infectious diseases are seen in guinea pigs. Guinea pigs are unique among non-primates in having a dietary need for vitamin C however, and will develop signs of deficiency, if fed diets that are not designed for guinea pigs, which have been stored incorrectly, or fed after the use by date, since vitamin C is labile and will degrade over a period of time. Most infectious diseases seen in guinea pigs are bacterial, with abscesses and non-specific infections most commonly encountered. However, guinea pigs can carry LCM virus (a zoonosis) and Sendai virus, and these two antigens should be included in regular screening programmes.

## Biological data and useful reference data

See Table 12.5.

## Drug doses for anaesthesia in the guinea pig

These are probably the most difficult rodents in which to achieve safe and effective general anaesthesia. The response to injectable agents is variable and post-anaesthetic complications, such as respiratory infection, generalised depression, inappetance and digestive disturbances, may frequently be seen. Many of these problems may be avoided

**Table 12.5**   Useful data: guinea pig.

| Biological data | | Breeding data | |
|---|---|---|---|
| Adult weight (g) | Male     850–1200 | Puberty (days) | Male 60 |
| | Female 700–900 | | Female 30 |
| Diploid number | 64 | Age to breed male | 3–4 months, |
| Food intake | 6 g/100 g | | 600–700 g |
| | bodyweight | Age to breed female | 2–3 months, |
| Water intake | 10 ml/100 g | | 300–450 g |
| | bodyweight | Gestation (days) | 59–72 |
| Natural lifespan (years) | 4–8 | Litter size | 2–5 |
| Rectal temperature (°C) | 37.2–40 | Birth weight (g) | 70–100 |
| Heart rate/min | 230–380 | Weaning age (weeks) | 3–4 |
| Blood pressure (mmHg) | | Oestrous cycle (days) | 15–17 |
|   Systole | 80–94 | Post-partum oestrus | Fertile |
|   Diastole | 55–58 | | |
| Blood volume (ml/kg) | 69–75 | **Biochemical data** | |
| Respiratory rate/min | 42–104 | Serum protein (g/dl) | 4.6–6.2 |
| Tidal volume (ml) | 2.3–5.3 | Albumin (g/dl) | 2.1–3.9 |
| | | Globulin (g/dl) | 1.7–2.6 |
| **Haematological data** | | Glucose (mg/dl) | 60–125 |
| RBC ($\times 10^6$/mm$^3$) | 4.5–7 | Blood urea nitrogen (mg/dl) | 9–31.5 |
| PCV (%) | 37–48 | Creatinine (mg/dl) | 0.6–2.2 |
| Hb (g/dl) | 11–15 | Total bilirubin (mg/dl) | 0.3–0.9 |
| WBC ($\times 10^3$/mm$^3$) | 7–18 | Cholesterol (mg/dl) | 20–43 |
| Neutrophils (%) | 28–44 | | |
| Lymphocytes (%) | 39–72 | | |
| Eosinophils (%) | 1–5 | | |
| Monocytes (%) | 3–12 | | |
| Basophils (%) | 0–3 | | |
| Platelets ($\times 10^3$/mm$^3$) | 250–850 | | |

by careful selection of anaesthetic agents and high standards of pre-, intra- and post-operative care.

Atropine (0.05 mg/kg s.c.) may be given to decrease airway obstruction. To counteract respiratory depression, use doxapram 5–15 mg/kg. The injection of both Hypnorm and ketamine in the guinea pig has been associated with tissue necrosis at the site leading to self-mutilation post-operatively.

## Sedation

For sedation alone Hypnorm (fentanyl/fluanisone) at 0.5 ml/kg i.m. can be used, but there will be poor muscle relaxation. Alternatively, use diazepam 2.5 mg/kg i.m. or acepromazine 2.5 mg/kg i.m.(hypotensive), or ketamine (100 mg/kg).

## Injectable general anaesthesia

### Fentanyl/fluanisone combinations

For surgical anaesthesia lasting about 45 min, combine Hypnorm 0.5–1.0 ml/kg with midazolam 2.5 mg/kg i.p. If continued anaesthesia is required, further doses of Hypnorm may be given at 0.5 ml/kg i.m. every 20–30 min. The fentanyl component can be reversed with naloxone (0.1 mg/kg) or, for continued analgesia with nalbuphine 1 mg/kg i.p. or s.c., or butorphanol 1 mg/kg i.p. or s.c., or buprenorphine 0.05 mg/kg i.p. or 0.01 mg/kg i.v.

If combining Hypnorm with diazepam, use 1 ml/kg Hypnorm plus 2.5 mg/kg diazepam.

Fentanyl 160 mg/kg and medetomidine 400 μg/kg i.p. will give about 20 min anaesthesia in the guinea pig, but it can be of rather variable depth. Nalbuphine (1 mg/kg) and atipamezole (1 mg/kg) can be used for reversal.

### Ketamine combinations

Xylazine and ketamine will give about 30 min of surgical anaesthesia (5 mg/kg xylazine s.c. plus 40 mg/kg ketamine i.m.). Ketamine may also be combined with diazepam (100 mg/kg ketamine plus 5 mg/kg diazepam i.m.), or with acepromazine (125 mg/kg ketamine plus 5 mg/kg acepromazine), or with medetomidine (40 mg/kg ketamine plus 250 μg/kg medetomidine). All these combinations give about 30 min anaesthesia with a 2–3 h recovery time. The response to the medetomidine component can be unpredictable in the guinea pig and is reversed with atipamezole (1 mg/kg).

### Saffan

A short period of surgical anaesthesia can be induced i.v. (ear vein) with alphaxalone/ alphadolone (Saffan) at the rate of 40 mg/kg. It may also be given i.p.

### Barbiturates

Pentobarbitone will induce anaesthesia lasting 15–60 min at 35 mg/kg i.p., but it has a very narrow safety margin and there will be a high-mortaility rate.

### Inhaled agents

Isoflurane is the agent of choice. For induction it can be used with an anaesthetic chamber and for maintenance given via a face mask.

## Dose of drugs for analgesia in the guinea pig

### Opioids

- *Buprenorphine*: 0.05 mg/kg s.c. lasts about 8 h.
- *Pethidine*: 10–20 mg/kg s.c. lasts 2–3 h.
- *Butorphanol*: 0.5 mg/kg s.c.

### NSAIDs

- *Flunixin*: 2.5 mg/kg i.m. or s.c.
- *Piroxicam*: 5.7 mg/kg orally.
- *Diclofenac*: 2 mg/kg orally.

- *Phenylbutazone*: 40 mg/kg orally.
- *Aspirin*: 85 mg/kg orally.

## RABBIT

The laboratory rabbit is derived from the domestic rabbit, *Oryctolagus cuniculus*, and belongs to the order Lagomorpha. Many stocks of rabbit are available, the commonest one seen in the laboratory being the New Zealand white, a large outbred stock. The smaller Dutch rabbit may also be encountered, and some inbred strains are available. Rabbits are listed in Schedule 2 to the Animals (Scientific Procedures) Act (ASPA), and must, therefore, be obtained only from accredited breeding or supplying establishments. Rabbits with coloured coats may be identified readily by their appearance. Other suitable methods of marking include microchip implants, wool dyes or marker pen. Tattoos or leg rings are less suitable, since tattooing may cause discomfort and leg rings applied when the animal is young may become too tight as the animal grows.

## Behaviour

Wild rabbits are crepuscular or nocturnal, becoming active and emerging from their burrows to feed at dusk or during the night. In the laboratory, periods of activity are seen throughout the day and night. Rabbits are social animals, which are able to utilise a complex, three-dimensional environment. If given sufficient space, domestic and laboratory rabbits will exhibit the full range of behaviours seen in their wild ancestors, including climbing up to a good vantage point, exploratory and tunnelling behaviour, social activity and aggression. Aggressive behaviour is seen most in breeding and pubertal animals, and adult males. Males are most aggressive when competing for food, territory or females. It is usual for them to be separated from 10 weeks of age to prevent fighting.

## Housing

In the laboratory, it is necessary to confine rabbits for practical reasons, but it is essential to provide sufficient room for the animals to perform the majority of their natural locomotory behaviours to prevent skeletal problems. Space is always limited, but careful design of housing will optimise the use of space. Cages designed to hold rabbits singly are unlikely to provide enough room to allow the rabbit to perform natural behaviour, resulting in prolonged periods of inactivity and increased stereotypic behaviour. This may also lead to hypoplasia of bone tissue and osteoporosis, with the increased risk of fractures and nerve damage leading to cage paralysis. Single caging should be used only where group housing is inappropriate, such as for adult males, or if an animal needs to be isolated for measurement of food and water intake. Pair housing in large cages may be an acceptable alternative in many circumstances.

Rabbits like to stretch out, and stand on their hind legs or climb onto ledges to gain a better view. Cages should allow the rabbit to stretch out in at least one direction and be tall enough for the animal to stand or even to house a box or shelf they can sit on. Environmental enrichment can be provided by giving hay, chew sticks or cardboard boxes to play with, and animals can be taken to exercise areas for short periods. Rabbits should always be housed where they can see other rabbits. Grid floors are generally provided if rabbits are kept in cages, and should be carefully designed to allow urine and faeces to drain without predisposing to sore hocks (pododermatitis). Trays beneath the grid should be lined with an absorbent pad to lock in the ammonia. Otherwise, high ammonia levels predispose the animal to the development of respiratory disease.

Rabbits will thrive particularly well if group housed in floor pens with high sides made from smooth impervious material. These can be constructed at low cost and will make good use of available space. Such pens can be used to house groups of compatible animals. The incidence of aggressive behaviour depends on many factors, including strain (Dutch rabbits are more aggressive than New Zealand Whites), sex, age and weight, pen size and construction, the relatedness of the individuals, and the proximity of other rabbits of the opposite sex. Animals to be group housed should be of similar weights, and it is important to provide ample dividers, cardboard boxes or large tubes within the pen so nervous or frightened animals have bolt-holes where they can hide from aggressive conspecifics. Continued monitoring of newly formed groups for excessive aggression is recommended. Groups of animals which can be successfully housed together include breeding females, if they are siblings or have been put together before or soon after weaning, a doe and litter, single sex groups of newly weaned animals, and stable groups of animals on procedure. Females group housed after puberty may develop pseudopregnancy, which can become a problem in breeding colonies. This will usually resolve once the animal leaves the group.

Rabbits communicate using olfactory cues, so this must be taken into consideration when designing rabbit housing. Rabbits will feel secure and confident if surrounded by their own smell, and are disturbed by excessive cleaning or the use of strong smelling disinfectants, etc. Floor pens should be deeply lined with bedding materials, such as straw, paper-based bedding materials or non-resinated sawdust, which do not have a strong smell. In these circumstances, rabbits will urinate and defaecate in latrine areas which can be cleaned frequently, but faecal matter will become spread throughout the pen and this should be cleaned out completely at least once every 2 weeks. Over-frequent cleaning, however, will simply result in increased territory marking and upset the animals' confidence.

Group housing in pens has many advantages over traditional single cages (see Figure 6.4). The improved welfare of group-housed animals manifests in improved physical and psychological well-being. Animals can exhibit natural behaviour and interact socially which reduces stereotypy, they tend to be calmer and more docile, the increased opportunity for locomotory behaviour reduces osteoporosis and cage paralysis, and improved ventilation leads to fewer respiratory problems. In addition, floor pens are more economic to purchase and maintain than conventional cages. On the other hand, there may be increased aggressive behaviour and stress particularly in unstable and incompatible groups, identification and treatment of individuals is more difficult, and exposure of staff to soiled bedding may increase the risks of laboratory animal allergy.

Overall, the standard laboratory cage provides an environment that is unlikely to satisfy the psychological, behavioural and physiological needs of rabbits. Group housing has inherent problems that can be overcome with careful husbandry and environmental enrichment, but it overcomes many of the disadvantages of housing rabbits in cages.

Rabbit cages should be cleaned at least weekly. They produce copious, turbid urine, which may be yellow to dark red, due to the presence of a varying quantity of porphyrins. The urine tends to leave scale on the litter trays due to the calcium content, and so they may need to be cleaned with acidic agents. Absorbent tray liners help to lock in ammonia and to reduce the scale problem.

## Feeding

Rabbits are coprophagic, and this is an important part of their digestion. They require a diet with a high-fibre content, and although much fibre remains undigested, it is required for bulk and reduces the incidence of hairballs and diarrhoea. A diet with 12–22% fibre, and 12% protein for maintenance or 15–17% protein for growth is recommended. Ad lib feeding for rabbits in cages may sometimes result in obesity. Overeating may be a stereotypic behaviour, and is seldom seen in floor-housed rabbits. Providing environmental enrichment and a variety of foodstuffs can reduce this problem. Hay may be given as a supplement to provide fibre and as a plaything. High-energy diets are required for rabbits which are reproducing and for the dwarf breeds, with 10,500 kJ/kg feed. For maintenance, 8800 kJ/kg is sufficient. *Rabbits need 5 g of high-energy food per 100 g body weight daily.*

As gut flora play an important part in digestion, changes in diet should be done gradually, over a 4–5-day period, to allow the flora to adapt. Failure to do this will result in diarrhoea or anorexia.

## Water

Water should be supplied ad lib, and be fresh and clean. Automatic systems are often used. *Rabbits normally consume 10 ml water/100 g body weight. Lactating does may drink up to 90 ml/100 g body weight.* Rabbits have a tendency to play with water bottles, so they should be checked frequently to ensure they are not empty, and that the floor has not become wet.

## Environment

Rabbits require temperatures between 16°C and 20°C. Neonates cannot maintain their body temperatures until they are 7 days old, so they must be kept in a warm environment. Humidity should be kept between 40% and 60%. Females require 14–16 h of light daily, and males eight to ten, with or without periods of twilight. Shorter light cycles may result in reduced sexual activity in the autumn. Low-intensity light should be provided for albino animals. Rabbits can hear in the ultrasound range, from 2 to 16 kHz and possibly up to 42 kHz, so care should be taken not to expose them to excessive ultrasound. Background noise can help to prevent the animals from being startled by sudden noises. Ventilation is particularly important for rabbits. They are susceptible to respiratory diseases, and poor ventilation allows a build-up of ammonia, which predisposes to these. Draughtless ventilation and efficient tray liners for caged animals, reduce the ammonia level. At least 12–15 air changes per hour should be provided.

# Breeding

Females begin breeding at 4–9 months, males at 6–10 months. Rabbits are induced ovulators, and have no oestrus cycle as such. They are receptive for 7–10 days, then inactive for 1–2 days. Does are also receptive at intervals during pregnancy and lactation. There is some seasonal effect, but if day length is maintained and particularly if the temperature is high, breeding will take place all year. Breeding efficiency falls after 7–11 litters, or 3–4 years. Docile animals should be selected for breeding. Various mating systems exist. Group-housed does can be taken individually to the buck, or a buck may be taken to a group of two to five does, and removed after mating or after a few minutes if mating does not occur. Coitus induces ovulation and results in pregnancy lasting 31–32 days in 75% of does. Care should be taken in handling the doe during gestation, as the pregnancy is easily aborted. The doe must have a clean nest box in the last week of gestation. The cage may have a solid floor together with a raised wire floor on which there is plenty of bedding. This construction keeps the nest dry and clean. A doe will scatter its young if the nest is dirty, or if it smells of disinfectant. The doe will line her nest with hair. A cardboard box placed on its side makes a cheap and disposable nest box. Does usually kitten in the morning, and between four and six kits are born, although this varies with the breed. It is rare for them to be eaten by the doe unless there is a deformity or they are dead, but it may also happen if the doe is inexperienced or if there is some environmental disturbance. Does will rarely retrieve their young if they crawl out of the nest, hence the need for a good nest box. Young are only suckled for 5–10 min once daily, in the morning, and lactation lasts 6–8 weeks. Hand rearing of rabbits is relatively easy. Does may be rebred shortly after parturition, but more usually are mated after weaning.

# Growth

Growth varies with the breed of rabbit.

# Handling

Rabbits are generally docile and amenable, can be readily trained, and rarely bite if handled correctly. The animal will become accustomed to handling, which will facilitate the performance of procedures. There are a number of particular considerations when handling rabbits. The animal should *never* be lifted by the ears, and the back must be supported at all times, otherwise contractions of the strong spinal muscles during struggling can result in injuries to the spine. Rabbits have powerful hind legs, and the handler must be careful to avoid being kicked or scratched. Before removing a rabbit from a cage or floor pen, orientate the rabbit so it is facing you. Grasp the animal by the scruff, avoiding the ears, and lift the front end. Then you can either slide the free hand beneath the rabbit, placing the thumb and little finger in front of the hind legs to extend them, and then lift the animal, or the free hand can be placed behind the animal's hindquarters and the animal scooped towards you. Once the animal has been lifted clear of the cage or pen, it should be carried held against the chest

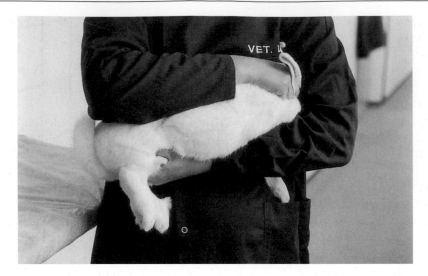

**Figure 12.10**    Handling the rabbit.

or resting on the arm with its head tucked under the armpit, with the scruff securely held and the back and hindquarters supported at all times (see Figure 12.10).

To sex adult rabbits, place the animal on a non-slip surface or support it on your knee. Hold the animal by the scruff and lift the head, scooping the hindquarters under the animal so it sits on its haunches. While still holding the scruff, the free hand can be used to expose the genitalia. Alternatively, the head can be controlled by placing the thumb and third finger each side of the head and the index finger between the ears. The other hand can then be placed under the abdomen, and the rabbit turned over onto the knee for sexing, its back being supported by the forearm.

## Pain and stress recognition

A rabbit will often react to painful procedures with stoic acceptance. This may relate to feral behaviour where concealment is important for survival. A rabbit in pain is usually characterised by reduced food and water intake and limited movement. There may be apparent photosensitivity and ocular discharge with protrusion of the third eyelid. Faecal staining of the coat, digestive disturbances and dehydration may also be seen.

## Common diseases and health monitoring

Rabbits suffer from very few viral diseases, but myxomatosis and viral haemorrhagic disease of rabbits are both potentially fatal. Vaccines are now available for both of these diseases. Myxomatosis is commonly encountered in wild and pet rabbits, and can be brought unwittingly into the laboratory by personnel who have contacted the virus outside or by insect vectors. Protective clothing and a good standard of hygiene are essential to prevent this. Viral haemorrhagic disease of rabbits is often characterised by sudden death, and it is currently rare in laboratory-reared stock. Rabbits suffer from a number of bacterial infections, the most important of which is

*Pasteurella multocida*. *Pasteurella* is mainly a respiratory pathogen, which can be carried sub-clinically in the upper respiratory tract, causing problems when the animal is stressed. Signs may vary from sudden death, pneumonia, meningitis, generalised septicaemia or subcutaneous abscesses to snuffles. A common manifestation is recurrent conjunctivitis caused by persistent infection of the tear ducts. Treatment may reduce the symptoms of *Pasteurella*, but it will not eradicate it. If this organism is present in a colony, it is essential to maintain adequate environmental conditions particularly humidity, ensure meticulous hygiene, keep the stocking density low and avoid stress. The stress of scientific procedures often precipitates an outbreak of clinical disease, and if this occurs ideally the colony should be culled and clean animals bought in after fumigation of the room. Use of specific pathogen-free animals, reared and kept in a clean environment has controlled this problem in many research units.

Diarrhoea is another common disease problem in rabbits. There are many causes including sudden diet changes, coccidial (intestinal parasite) infestation and infectious causes. Mucoid enteropathy is a common, often fatal, finding in growing rabbits. It is multifactorial, and seems to be associated with an inadequate level of fibre in the diet (less than 15%) and stress. There may or may not be an infectious component. Inappetence is another commonly encountered problem, associated with environment or diet changes, hairballs or sub-clinical diseases. This can cause a rapid loss of condition and should be treated promptly. In general, many of the commonest diseases of rabbits are husbandry related, so it is very important that the diet, housing, environment and general management of rabbits are kept up to a high standard.

## Biological data and useful reference data

See Table 12.6.

## Drug doses for anaesthesia in the rabbit

In this species the combination of stress and general anaesthesia can lead to cardiac and respiratory arrest. It is, therefore, very important to keep both the pre- and postoperative stresses to the absolute minimum.

If there is respiratory depression or cyanosis, doxapram may be given at 2–5 mg/kg i.v.

## Sedation/premedication

*For sedation use*
- *Medetomidine* 250 μg/kg s.c. This can rapidly be reversed with *atipamezole* 0.2 mg/kg into the ear vein.
- *Acepromazine* 1 mg/kg will produce moderate sedation but is hypotensive.
- *Diazepam* or *midazolam* 0.5–2 mg/kg i.v. or i.m. produces quite good sedation.
- *Hypnorm* 0.2 ml/kg i.m. produces sedation and analgesia but poor muscle relaxation which lasts for about 20 min with full recovery taking more than an hour unless specific reversal with *naloxone* (0.1 mg/kg i.m.) is used.
- *Ketamine* alone at 50 mg/kg i.m. produces sedation and immobilisation lasting about 30 min.
- *Xylazine* alone at 3 mg/kg i.m. will produce heavy sedation with some analgesia.

**Table 12.6**    Useful data: rabbit.

| *Biological data* | | *Breeding data* | |
|---|---|---|---|
| Adult weight (g) | 900–6000 | Puberty (days) | 90–120 |
| Diploid number | 44 | Age to breed male (months) | 6–10 |
| Food intake | 5 g/100 g | Age to breed female (months) | 4–9 |
| | bodyweight | Gestation (days) | 30–32 |
| Water intake | 10 ml/100 g | Litter size | 4–10 |
| | bodyweight | Birth weight (g) | 30–70 |
| Natural lifespan (years) | 6–12 | Weaning age (weeks) | 4–8 |
| Rectal temperature (°C) | 38.5–40 | Oestrous cycle | Induced |
| Heart rate/min | 130–325 | | ovulator |
| Blood pressure (mmHg) | | Post-partum oestrus | None |
|   Systole | 90–130 | | (not used) |
|   Diastole | 60–90 | | |
| Blood volume (ml/kg) | 57–65 | *Biochemical data* | |
| Respiratory rate/min | 30–60 | Serum protein (g/dl) | 5.4–7.5 |
| Tidal volume (ml/kg) | 4–6 | Albumin (g/dl) | 2.7–4.6 |
| | | Globulin (g/dl) | 1.5–2.8 |
| *Haematological data* | | Glucose (mg/dl) | 75–150 |
| RBC ($\times 10^6/mm^3$) | 4–7 | Blood urea nitrogen | 17–23.5 |
| PCV (%) | 36–48 |   (mg/dl) | |
| Hb (g/dl) | 10–15.5 | Creatinine (mg/dl) | 0.8–1.8 |
| WBC ($\times 10^3/mm^3$) | 9–11 | Total bilirubin (mg/dl) | 0.25–0.74 |
| Neutrophils (%) | 20–75* | Cholesterol (mg/dl) | 35–53 |
| Lymphocytes (%) | 30–85 | | |
| Eosinophils (%) | 0–4 | | |
| Monocytes (%) | 1–4 | | |
| Basophils (%) | 2–7 | | |
| Platelets ($\times 10^3/mm^3$) | 250–270 | | |

*Neutrophils often resemble eosinophils due to cytoplasmic granules.

## Injectable anaesthesia

An i.v. induction can be carried out very easily in the rabbit using the marginal ear vein. Before giving the injection, apply local anaesthetic cream (EMLA cream, Astra).

### Hypnorm

*Hypnorm* 0.3 ml/kg i.m. as a premedicant, followed after about 10–15 min by *midazolam* or *diazepam* at 2 mg/kg i.v. for induction will give about 40 min of surgical anaesthesia with good muscle relaxation. Longer periods of anaesthesia can be produced by giving additional doses of Hypnorm at about 0.1 ml/kg i.v. every 30–40 min. It may be reversed with *naloxone* 0.1 mg/kg, or for continued analgesia with *buprenorphine* 0.01 mg/kg or *nalbuphine* 0.1 mg/kg i.v.

### Saffan

*Alphaxalone/alphadolone* (Saffan) 6–9 mg/kg i.v. will produce a light plane of anaesthesia but higher doses may be needed for surgery which can lead to sudden apnoea and cardiac arrest. It is good for long-term light anaesthesia or for a smooth induction followed by gaseous anaesthesia with isoflurane for maintenance.

### Medetomidine

*Medetomidine* can be combined with *fentanyl* for full anaesthesia. 330 μg/kg medetomidine plus 8 μg/kg fentanyl i.v. will give about 40 min anaesthesia and can be reversed with 1 mg/kg *atipamezole* plus 1 mg/kg *nalbuphine* both given i.v.

### Ketamine combinations

*Ketamine* (10–25 mg/kg i.m.) can be combined with *medetomidine* (500 μg/kg i.m.), or at 25–35 mg/kg i.m. with xylazine (3–5 mg/kg i.m.) to produce surgical anaesthesia lasting about 30 min. Combined with *acepromazine* (75 mg/kg kctaminc and 5 mg/kg acepromazine i.m.) or with *diazepam or midazolam* (25 mg/kg ketamine and 5 mg/kg of the benzodiazepine i.m.) a light plane of anaesthesia is produced.

### Propofol

*Propofol* given i.v. at 10 mg/kg will produce short-term anaesthesia lasting 5 min and is a useful induction agent prior to using gaseous anaesthesia. Similarly, *thiopentone* 30 mg/kg i.v. will produce short-term anaesthesia. With *propofol* total i.v. anaesthesia can be given by infusion at a rate of 0.2–0.6 mg/kg/min.

## Non-recovery anaesthesia

*Pentobarbitone* at 30 mg/kg i.v. will induce surgical anaesthesia but has a very narrow safety margin. Respiratory arrest often occurs before a plane of surgical anaesthesia has been reached so there is a high rate of mortality.

### Inhaled agents

Isoflurane is the agent of choice. Inhaled agents should not be used for induction of anaesthesia since the rabbit will find this stressful and will hold its breath and show prolonged periods of apnoea. It is better to induce anaesthesia with an injectable agent and then use inhalational agents for maintenance via a face mask or endotracheal tube with a T-piece or Bain co-axial circuit. The larynx should be sprayed with lignocaine before intubation is attempted to reduce the risk of laryngospasm. Visualisation of the larynx in the rabbit requires the use of a Wisconsin laryngoscope blade (size 0 or 1), however, the rabbit can also be easily intubated without seeing the larynx. The rabbit is placed in sternal recumbency, its head gripped and extended upward. The tongue is pulled gently forwards taking care to bring it out to the side of the teeth so that it is not damaged. The endotracheal tube, lubricated with local anaesthetic gel, is advanced over the tongue towards the larynx. Careful observation of the chest wall will indicate when the rabbit breathes in. The tube is advanced through the larynx when it opens on inspiration.

## Doses of drugs for analgesia in the rabbit

### *Opioids*

- *Buprenorphine*: 0.01–0.05 mg/kg s.c. or i.v. will last for 8–12 h.
- *Butorphanol*: 0.1–0.5 mg/kg i.v. will last for 4 h.
- *Morphine*: 2–5 mg/kg s.c. or i.m. will last 2–4 h.
- *Nalbuphine*: 1–2 mg/kg i.v. will last 4–5 h.
- *Pentazocine*: 5 mg/kg i.v. will last 2–4 h.
- *Pethidine*: 10 mg/kg s.c. or i.m. will last 2–3 h.

### *NSAIDs*

- *Carprofen*: 1.5 mg/kg orally twice daily.
- *Flunixin*: 1.1 mg/kg s.c. or i.m. given twice daily.
- *Ketoprofen*: 1.0 mg/kg i.m.
- *Aspirin*: 100 mg/kg orally will give about 4 h relief from mild pain.
- *Ibuprofen*: 10 mg/kg i.v.

## FURTHER INFORMATION

Alexander, D.J. and Clark, G.C. (1980). A simple method of oral endotracheal intubation in rabbits. *Laboratory Animal Science* 30, 871–73.

Blouin, A. and Cormier, Y. (1987). Endotracheal intubation in guinea pigs by direct laryngoscopy. *Laboratory Animal Science* 37, 244–45.

Conlon, K.C., Corbally, M.T., Bading, J.R. and Brennan, M.F. (1990). Atraumatic endotracheal intubation in small rabbits. *Laboratory Animal Science* 40(2), 221–22.

Davies, A., Dallak, M. and Moores, C. (1996). Oral endotracheal intubation of rabbits (Oryctolagus cuniculus). *Laboratory Animals* 30, 182–83.

Field, K. and Sibold, A.L. (1999). *The Laboratory Hamster and Gerbil*. CRC Press.

Flecknell, P.A. and Liles, J.H. (1990). Assessment of the analgesic action of opioid agonist–antagonists in the rabbit. *Journal of the Association of Veterinary Anaesthetists* 17, 24–29.

Foster, H.L., Small, J.D. and Fox, J.G. (eds.) (1983). *The Mouse in Biomedical Research*, vol. 3. Academic Press, New York.

Greenman, D.L., Bryant, P., Kodell, R.L. and Sheldon, W. (1982). Influence of cage shelf level on retinal atrophy in mice. *Laboratory Animal Science* 32, 440–50.

Harkness, J.E. and Wagner, J.E. (1989). *The Biology and Medicine of Rabbit and Rodents*. Lea and Febiger.

Hillyer, E.V. and Quesenberry, K.E. (1997). *Ferrets, Rabbits and Rodents*. W.B. Saunders.

*ILAR Nutrient Requirements of Laboratory Animals* (4th edn). 1995.

Liles, J.H. and Flecknell, P.A. (1992). The use of non-steroidal anti-inflammatory drugs for the relief of pain in laboratory rodents and rabbits: a review. *Laboratory Animals* 26, 241–55.

McKellar, Q.A. (1989). Drug dosages for small mammals. *In Practice* 11, 57–61.

National Research Council (1989). *Immunodeficient Rodents: A Guide to their Immunology, Husbandry and Use*. National Academy Press.

National Research Council (1991). *Companion Guide to Infectious Diseases of Rats and Mice*. National Academy Press.

National Research Council (1991). *Infectious Diseases of Rats and Mice*. National Academy Press.

National Research Council (1996). *Laboratory Animal Management: Rodents*. National Academy Press.

Nau, R. and Schunck, O. (1993). Cannulation of the lateral saphenous vein – a rapid method to gain access to the venous circulation in anaesthetized guinea-pigs. *Laboratory Animals* 27, 23–25.

Popesko, P., Rajtova, V. and Horak, J. (1993). *A Colour Atlas of Anatomy of Small Laboratory Animals Volume 1: Rabbit, Guinea Pig. Volume 2: Rat, Mouse, Hamster*. Wolfe Publishing Ltd.

Refinements in rabbit husbandry. (1993). Second report of the BVAAWF/FRAME/RSPCA/ UFAW Joint Working Group on refinement. *Laboratory Animals*, 27, 301–29.

Report of the Rodent Refinement Working Party. (1998) Refining rodent husbandry: the mouse. *Laboratory Animals* 32, 233–59.

Report of the FELASA Working Group on Health Monitoring of Rodent and Rabbit Colonies. (2002). Recommendations for the health monitoring of rodent and rabbit colonies in breeding and experimental units. *Laboratory Animals* 36, 20–42.

Sharp, P. and LaRegina, M. (1998). *The Laboratory Rat*. CRC Press.

Smith, B.L., Flåøyen and Embling, P.P. (1993). A simple gag for the intragastric dosing of guineapigs (*Cavia porcellus*). *Laboratory Animals* 27, 286–88.

Suckow, M.A., Danneman, P. and Brayton, C. (2001). *The Laboratory Mouse*. CRC Press.

Suckow, M.A. and Douglas, F.A. (1997). *The Laboratory Rabbit*. CRC Press.

Terril-Robb, L. and Clemons, D. (1998). *The Laboratory Guinea Pig*. CRC Press.

Video: *Practical Animal Handling 1. Small Mammals*. BVA Animal Welfare Foundation.

Waynforth, H.B. and Flecknell, P.A. (1992). *Experimental and Surgical Technique in the Rat* (2nd edn). Academic Press, London.

Whary, M., Peper, R., Borkowski, G., Lawrence, W. and Ferguson, F. (1993). The effect of group housing on the research use of the laboratory rabbit. *Laboratory Animals* 27, 330–41.

Wilson, D.E. and Reeder, D.M. (1993). *Mammal Species of the World: A Taxonomic and Geographic Reference*. Smithsonian Institution.

Wilson, D.E. and Cole, F.R. (2000). *Common Names of Mammals of the World*. Smithsonian Institution.

# Chapter 13
# Genetically modified animals and harmful mutants

## INTRODUCTION

As our knowledge of genetics increases, more and more medical conditions are seen to result from the genotype. In order to understand the workings of genes and identify the causes of disease, increasing use is being made in biomedical research of genetically modified (GM) and harmful mutant (HM) animals. In 2001, 2.6 million scientific procedures were carried out, of which 24% were on GM animals, and 9.4% on HMs. More than 99% of GM and HM animals used were rodents or fish. These were used in many areas of biomedical research, including:

- studies of human diseases, such as cystic fibrosis, often using mice;
- projects to understand gene function, often using *Drosophila*, *Xenopus* or zebra fish;
- production of therapeutic proteins, for example collecting enzymes from the milk of GM sheep;
- projects to investigate the feasibility of xenotransplantation (organ transplants between different species);
- projects to enhance the health of farm animals, for example by increasing disease resistance or promoting growth.

## Definitions

The *genotype* of an animal describes the genetic makeup of the animal. This is determined by the genes inherited from the animal's parents.

The *phenotype* of an animal describes its overall physical characteristics, which depend on the genetic makeup of the animal, and the interaction of the genotype with the environment.

A *GM animal* is one in which the genotype has been altered deliberately by the insertion or deletion of DNA, in a way that does not occur naturally through mating or recombination of genes. Methods used for genetic modification include transgenesis (insertion of additional genes from the same or another species), or targeting of specific changes in genes or chromosomes, either by deletion of genes (knockouts), or addition of genes (knockins).

An *HM animal* is one in which the genome has been altered by the point mutation or chromosomal changes which do not involve insertion or deletion of DNA. HMs may arise spontaneously (e.g. the nude mouse, which is athymic and cannot mount a specific immune response), or be induced deliberately by mutagenesis, where viruses, chemicals or radiation are used to cause random changes in the genes.

A *cloned animal* is one that has been derived by inserting nuclear material from one cell into another, often an oocyte. This may also be called *nuclear transfer* or *cell nuclear replacement*.

A *genetically altered animal* is one in which the heritable DNA has been manipulated deliberately, using any of the methods described above.

# CREATION OF GENETICALLY ALTERED ANIMALS

## Selective inbreeding

In any population, there is a considerable amount of genetic variation. This is caused by spontaneous mutations in the genome, which occur due to mistakes in copying of genetic material during cell division, or natural exposure to radiation or oxidative damage. Natural mutations occur at a low rate of about one in 10,000–100,000 individuals. The variations in genotype result in variations in the phenotype of animals, and this sometimes confers advantages on some animals over others in particular environments. This is the basis of natural selection, in which particular characteristics give an animal an advantage over its peers, so that it is more likely to survive and reproduce. Selective inbreeding of animals to produce a particular favoured characteristic is a form of natural selection, and has been in progress ever since animals became domesticated. The various recognised breeds of dogs, cats and farm animals are a result of this selective inbreeding, as are the genetically stable lines of inbred rats and mice commonly used in research. The method is very simple: animals that bear the desired characteristics are chosen to breed, those that do not are discarded. However, many characteristics are poorly heritable, being controlled by many genes, so selective inbreeding is a very slow and inefficient way to increase the frequency of a particular gene in a population. Also, there can be undesirable side effects. Selecting for some genes often results in the perpetuation of other, deleterious or recessive genes, leading to genetic diseases. Many inbred strains of mice and rats carry recessive genes, and are susceptible to particular diseases or exhibit poor growth or fertility.

## Mutagenesis

The rate of spontaneous mutation can be increased by exposing animals to chemical mutagens, viruses or radiation. Animals exposed to these show an increased level of genetic mutation, which is seen in their offspring. These offspring show random genetic changes and chromosomal rearrangements with resulting phenotypic changes. The study of phenotypic changes brought about by mutagenesis in conjunction with analysis of the genetic changes sheds light on the function of particular genes. The alkylating agent ethylnitrosurea (ENU) is a powerful mutagen in male mice, causing mainly point mutations in premeiotic stem cells. Many of the mutants produced by ENU result in some loss of function, although gain of function may also occur. Large-scale mutagenesis screens have been carried out in *Drosophila*, *C. elegans* and zebra fish, and more recently in mice. Mutagenesis can be very efficient in mice. The frequency of mutation is about 1/1000 for a specific locus, depending on the strain, dosage and treatment regimen. A large number of F1 founder animals may be produced from a single-treated male. These F1 mice can either be analysed directly for dominant mutations, or bred further to study recessive phenotypes. With dominant mutations, a clinical phenotype may only be observed in the homozygous state, but changes of specific parameters, that is, a reduction in the activity of enzymes, can often be detected in heterozygotes. Recessive mutations can only be diagnosed in homozygotes.

## Transgenesis

This technique involves the microinjection of DNA containing the genes of interest into a fertilised egg, and implanting the resulting embryo into a recipient female. The eggs are usually collected from a female who has been injected with hormones to make her superovulate: this maximises the yield of eggs from a single animal. The female is killed at a certain time after mating, and fertilised eggs collected. Eggs are held still with a pipette and injected with DNA using very fine syringes under a microscope. Following injection, the eggs are implanted into the fallopian tubes of female mice rendered pseudopregnant by mating with a sterile or vasectomised male. The additional genes integrate into the genome of the embryo, and lead to changes in the phenotype of the individual produced. The genes introduced may be from the same or another species, so for example animals may be 'humanised' by microinjecting human genes. Transgenesis has been used very successfully in mice and also in rats, poultry, fish and farm animals. However, there is little control over the site of integration of the foreign DNA, multiple copies may integrate, integration may result in the disruption of other genes, and there may be no effect if the gene of interest is recessive and only one of a homologous pair of chromosomes carries the gene. Also, the effect of the transgene may depend on the background strain of the animal, effects being seen in one strain but not others, depending on the other genes present.

## Embryonic stem cell manipulation

This technique was developed to overcome some of the problems encountered with microinjection into fertilised eggs. Embryonic stem (ES) cells can be grown in culture, and targeted changes made to particular genes. These modified cells are then injected into an early embryo to produce a chimaera, containing both modified and unmodified cells. These are then implanted into a recipient female. If the modified cells become egg or sperm cells, the changes in DNA can be perpetuated. Manipulation of ES cells can also be used to stop the function of a particular gene, producing a 'knockout' animal, or to add in a piece of DNA to change the way a particular protein is produced or regulated, producing a 'knock-in' animal. It is also possible to delete or add in large regions of a chromosome with many genes, modelling such conditions as Down's syndrome. However, success with ES cells has been limited to a few mouse strains.

## Cell nuclear replacement or cloning

Nuclear material from one cell is inserted into another, enucleated cell, often an oocyte; thus the resulting animal is essentially derived from a single parent by asexual means. The mitochondrial DNA of the resulting offspring is derived from the recipient cell, and the nuclear DNA from the donor. There may or may not have been genetic modification of the donor DNA prior to transfer, that is, the techniques of cloning and genetic modification may be combined.

## LEGISLATIVE REQUIREMENTS

The generation and use of GM and HM animals are strictly controlled, both by the Animals (Scientific Procedures) Act 1986 (ASPA), and by health and safety legislation. A regulated procedure under ASPA is one that may cause pain, suffering, distress or lasting harm, and is carried out on a protected animal for a scientific purpose. There is an ongoing requirement for regulated procedures to be refined, and as technology advances, the techniques involved in generating HM and GM animals will, therefore, need to be refined. Several techniques used to generate and maintain GM and HM animals are regulated procedures, and, therefore, require authority on both project and personal licences. Standard protocols for techniques typically used in the generation and maintenance of transgenic animals can be found on the Home Office Website.

**Superovulation**  Injecting the donor female with hormones is regulated, since it involves an injection, and there may be the potential for harm caused by the hormones.

**Microinjection or embryonic stem cell manipulation**  The injection of DNA into a fertilised egg or manipulation of the genes in an ES cell are regulated procedures, since they may result in harm to the embryo and the consequences of the procedure last beyond the mid-point of gestation, when the embryo becomes a protected animal (see Chapter 2).

**Implantation**  Reimplanting modified embryos in the recipient female involves surgery, which is regulated.

**Vasectomy**  The preparation of sterile male animals for mating with recipient females to induce pseudopregnancy is regulated; however, the actual mating is not!

**Exposure to mutagens**  Injection of chemical mutagens or exposure to radiation are regulated, since they involve potential harm to the animal involved, and also have consequences for the next generation.

**Breeding and maintenance**  For both GM and HM animals, conception is a regulated procedure, since this is deliberately done, albeit indirectly, to produce an individual embryo whose genetic makeup *may* result in harm, and the potential for harm persists beyond the mid-point of gestation. Therefore, the maintenance of colonies of GM or HM animals is regulated, the number of regulated procedures equating to the number of embryos carrying the potentially harmful gene, which develop beyond the mid-point of gestation. As the potential adverse effects of genetic modification persist throughout the animal's life, project licence authority is required to hold these animals. When a project licence expires, the animals must be transferred to another suitable project licence, or killed: cryopreserved embryos may be held, but cannot be allowed to develop in culture beyond mid-gestation (or inserted into a protected animal) without appropriate project licence authority. If no adverse effects are seen after a new GM line has been bred to homozygosity for two generations, it may be possible to apply to the Home Office for discharge from the controls of the Act.

There is considerable public concern about the safety of genetic modification; therefore, the Health and Safety Executive (HSE) monitors and regulates all experiments involving genetic modification from a human and environmental safety point of view. The human health risks from work with genetically modified organisms (GMOs) are assessed under the GMO (Contained Use) Regulations 2000, and the environmental risk assessment is undertaken under the GMO (Risk Assessment) (Records and Exemptions) Regulations 1996. These regulations apply to work with both genetically modified micro-organisms (GMMs, or biological agents), and to GM animals. Premises where such work is done have to be registered with the HSE under the GMO (Contained Use) Regulations 2000, and have a GM safety committee. Laboratories proposing to begin work involving genetic modification must notify the HSE and describe the work to be carried out, the HSE then review the proposal and may consult with other government departments or the Advisory Committee on Genetic Modification. In certain circumstances, individual activities may need to be notified to the HSE prior to commencement. It is likely that all work with GMMs and work with GM animals, where the animal is more hazardous than its unmodified parent, will fall into this category. The HSE may inspect laboratories periodically to ensure compliance with the regulations, which require that the GMOs are suitably contained, that the risks to health and safety are assessed and controlled, and that carcases are properly disposed of.

The GMO (Risk Assessment) (Records and Exemptions) Regulations 1996 (made under the Environmental Protection Act 1990) require that anyone keeping GM animals (or plants) must carry out an assessment of the risks to the environment, including an assessment of the hazards arising from the escape of animals, and the risk of animals escaping.

The release of any GMO or GMM is covered by the GMOs (Deliberate Release) Regulations 1992 and 1995, and the Environmental Protection Act 1990. Such a release may only be authorised by the Secretary of State for the Environment, Food and Rural Affairs.

## MONITORING GENETICALLY MODIFIED AND HARMFUL MUTANT ANIMALS

GM and HM animals need to be monitored for the purity of the genetic line, the health status of the animals and the welfare consequences of the genetic modification.

## Genetic analysis

Following genetic modification of fertilised eggs of embryos, it is usual to test the off-spring produced to make sure that the desired genes have integrated or been affected as required. It may be possible to determine this from the phenotype: sometimes the modified genes produce obvious effects such as coat colour changes, otherwise tissue samples may need to be analysed for the genes of interest. The least invasive method possible should be used for this. Methods such as saliva sampling or blood sampling may be possible if the gene can be amplified from tiny amounts of DNA using techniques such as polymerase chain reaction (PCR) prior to analysis. If not and the amount of DNA needed is greater, it may be necessary to take a biopsy from the ear or tail. The smallest amount of tissue should be taken, and anaesthesia should be given first (this can be local). It is not normally necessary to take more than 5 mm from the tail tip for tissue analysis. Larger samples than this need to be adequately justified.

## Health monitoring

The Code of Practice for the Housing and Care of Animals in Designated Breeding and Supplying Establishments requires that a suitable microbiological health screening programme should be implemented. The breeding of GM and HM animals is no different. Indeed, it is expected that only animals of a high health status will be produced, since these animals are likely to be sent to other units and it is desirable that no rederivation programme is required before introduction into other animal units. Health monitoring should be done as for any strain of animals (see Chapter 6). Sentinel animals of a normal strain can be used in most circumstances to monitor the health of a GM or HM colony; however, sometimes GM or HM strains show particular susceptibility to certain diseases and sentinels will not suffice. If GM or HM animals are likely to be moved away from the designated establishment for screening, this should be indicated in the project licence, and authority from the Home Office may be needed in advance of such movements. It should be noted that some GM or HM strains are particularly unsuitable for health screening: immunocompromised animals, for example, may not be able to make antibodies, and will produce false negatives in serological tests for pathogens.

## Welfare considerations

There are considerable concerns about the effects of the genetic modification on the welfare of animals. The integration of a transgene within an endogenous gene may affect gene function (insertional mutations), inappropriate transgene expression may expose the animal to biologically active transgene-derived proteins, and the technologies employed in generating transgenic and cloned animals may result in an increased incidence of fetal and neonatal losses. This is particularly noted in farm animals, where the development of unusually large or otherwise abnormal offspring (large offspring syndrome) may lead to difficult parturition. New gene constructs may have unexpected adverse effects on the animal, producing obvious or subtle changes in the phenotype. It is expected that GM and HM animals will be monitored carefully for adverse effects, using scoring systems, such as those described in Chapter 4 (see also van der Meer *et al.*, 2001 and van Reenen *et al.*, 2001). Detailed assessment of every new transgenic animal may be impractical: it can have considerable implications in terms of staff time and resources, and interference with neonatal animals may cause the mother to reject her young. It may be preferable to develop a two-tiered system, with simple screening of parameters, such as litter size, birth weight and activity used to identify those animals which are more likely to be affected. These may then be subjected to more detailed scrutiny, either as neonates or after weaning. The welfare of affected animals may then be improved by revising husbandry methods, for example fostering if the GM animals are poor mothers, floor feeding if locomotion is affected, barrier rearing if they are immune compromised.

Many normal animals are used in the generation of GM or HM animals, and if the techniques used are inefficient, many of these animals are wasted. Researchers should strive to maximise the efficiency of the techniques used to generate new lines, obtaining training in novel techniques where appropriate. Many offspring produced in the initial stages may not be transgenic, and for lines maintained in a heterozygous state there will be a proportion of animals in every litter which are not carrying the gene of interest. In order to fully implement the three Rs, efforts should be made to utilise these normal animals as much as possible.

## MANAGEMENT OF GENETICALLY MODIFIED AND HARMFUL MUTANT ANIMALS

### Records

It is essential to keep careful records of GM and HM animals. Project licence holders should keep records of the efficiency of the generation programme (e.g. number of animals used per construct, pregnancy rates, percentage success in generating viable new modifications), the genotypes/phenotypes produced, the results of health screening, any deaths or welfare problems identified, the breeding performance of each GM or HM line and the fate of the animals produced. It is essential to be able to identify GM and HM animals accurately if the breeding programme is to be successful and if records are to be accurate. GM and HM animals often look just like other animals, and it can be difficult to keep track of which animals carry which genes, and animals which escape from cages may have to be killed if it cannot be determined where they came from. Identification can be done in many ways, including microchips and tattoos, which are preferred methods. Ear notching can be done, but the marks can be difficult to interpret. The use of toe clipping as a means of identification is not considered to be best practice and very clear justification for its use would be required. Methods of identification that cause no more than momentary or transient discomfort and no lasting harm are not regulated procedures; however, it is likely that toe clipping would require project and personal licence authority.

### Fate of animals

Often, GM or HM animals will be killed by a Schedule 1 method at various stages of pregnancy or after birth for *in vitro* analysis, in which case no further licence authority is needed. Alternatively, they may be used in other protocols within the project, or other projects with authority to use animals of that type. This constitutes continued use, and requires authority in the relevant project licences. Authority can also be obtained by using a Home Office transfer form.

If embryos are sent for cryopreservation, this should be stated in the project licence. The production of the GM or HM embryo is regulated if the animal goes on beyond the mid-point of gestation. Therefore, the production of GM or HM embryos for cryopreservation with the intention that they should be revived in the future requires project and personal licence authority, as does reimplantation into a recipient female, although the techniques involved in cryopreservation itself do not.

If genetically altered animals are sent out of the UK to scientific establishments abroad, it is necessary to obtain the permission of the Secretary of State for them to be discharged from the controls of the Act. This can be obtained by using a Home Office transfer form.

## Annual returns

Each GM or HM embryo which survives beyond the mid-point of gestation has undergone a regulated procedure during microinjection of DNA or conception following conventional breeding, and, therefore, requires project and personal licence authority. However, fetal, larval and embryonic forms are not counted for the purposes of the annual returns, so it is not necessary to make an estimate of the number of embryos produced. The number of GM or HM animals actually born should be counted; some of these may subsequently be found not to carry the mutation, in which case the method of sampling used for genetic analysis may be the only regulated procedure they have had.

## SUMMARY

The use of GM and HM animals has contributed greatly to the advancement of science in recent years, and this use is increasing. However, there is concern over their use in terms of human health and safety and animal welfare, and, therefore, the generation and use of such animals is strictly controlled. Before beginning any work which involves the generation of GM or HM animals, it is essential to obtain authority from the Home Office for the work, and to discuss the proposal with the HSE to ensure compliance with health and safety legislation.

## FURTHER INFORMATION

BVA AWF/FRAME/RSPCA/UFAW Joint Working Group on Retirement (2003). Retirement and reduction in production of genetically modified mice. *Laboratory Animals* 37 (Suppl. 1), July.

Home Office (1995). *Code of Practice for the Housing and Care of Animals in Designated Breeding and Supplying Establishments*. The Stationery Office, London.

Home Office (2001). *Supplementary Guidance on Projects to Produce and Maintain Genetically Modified Animals*. Available from Home Office Website.

Home Office (2002). *Statistics of Scientific Procedures on Living Animals, Great Britain 2001.* The Stationery Office, London.

Letourneau, D.K. and Burrows, B.E. (2002). *Genetically Engineered Organisms: Assessing Environmental and Human Health Effects.* CRC Press.

The Royal Society (2001). *The Use of Genetically Modified Animals.* The Royal Society, London.

van der Meer, M., Rolls, A., Baumans, V., Olivier, B. and van Zutphen, L.F. (2001). Use of score sheets for welfare assessment of transgenic mice. *Laboratory Animals* 35(4), 379 –89.

van Reenen, C.G., Meuwissen, T.H., Hopster, H., Oldenbroek, K., Kruip, T.H. and Blokhuis H.J. (2001). Transgenesis may affect farm animal welfare: a case for systematic risk assessment. *Journal of Animal Science* 79(7), 1763–79.

# Chapter 14
# Carnivores

Although the majority of animals used in research are rodents, some studies require the use of higher species, including carnivores. In 2001, approximately 11,600 carnivores were used in research in the UK, mainly for applied studies such as safety testing of drugs. This represents less than 0.5% of the total number of animals used in research. Approximately 8000 of these animals were dogs, with cats and ferrets accounting for most of the remainder.

Cats and dogs in particular are familiar as household pets to most people, and are afforded particular protection under the Animals (Scientific Procedures) Act 1986 (ASPA). Particular justification is required before project licences using cats or dogs will be granted by the Home Office, and in general they may only be obtained from accredited breeding establishments, although in particular circumstances animals from the general population may be used. For example, clinical cases may be used with the permission of the owners for research into the efficacy of treatments or control of pain after surgery.

## DOG

The dog, *Canis familiaris*, has been domesticated for thousands of years. Dogs can be useful models for many human diseases, such as muscular dystrophy and cardiovascular diseases, and they are particularly suited to studies requiring close monitoring and frequent sampling. Many breeds are recognised, varying in size and temperament, and purpose bred laboratory dogs are usually beagles, which are of medium size and generally have a good temperament. Dogs kept in the laboratory in the UK must be permanently marked for identification purposes, for example, with a tattoo in the ear flap, or with a microchip implanted between the shoulders.

### Behaviour

Dogs are gregarious animals, and in the wild they live together in packs, with males and females having dominance hierarchies, and demonstrate a complex range of social behaviour. Members of the pack co-operate in hunting, etc. Dogs should be kept in groups in the laboratory if possible, with care being taken to ensure that subordinate members of the group are not deprived, and can get sufficient food and water. Single housing should only occur in exceptional circumstances, and such dogs should be able to see and hear other dogs. The social status of the animal in the group can be important, since it can affect their behaviour and biochemical parameters such as cortisol levels. Dogs can also form social relationships with human beings, and well socialised dogs are much easier to handle and make better experimental subjects than

**Table 14.1**    Useful data: dog (beagle).

| *Biological data* | | *Breeding data* | |
|---|---|---|---|
| Adult weight (kg) | 10–15 | Puberty (months) | 7–8 (male) |
| Diploid number | 78 | | 8–14 (female) |
| Daily food intake | 18 g/kg of complete dry diet | Age to breed (years) | |
| | | Male | 1–2 |
| Daily water intake | 1200 ml* | Female | 1–2 |
| Natural lifespan (years) | 10–15 (larger breeds have shorter lifespans) | Gestation (days) (average 63) | 59–67 |
| | | Litter size | 1–12 (usually 4–6) |
| Rectal temperature (°C) | 37.9–39.9 | | |
| Heart rate/min | 70–160 | Birth weight (g) | 250 |
| Blood pressure (mmHg) | | Weaning age (weeks) | 4–6 |
| Systole | 95–136 | Oestrous cycle | Monoestrous. |
| Diastole | 43–66 | | Oestrus |
| Blood volume (ml/kg) | 76–107 | | interval of |
| Respiratory rate/min | 22 | | 7–8 months |
| Tidal volume (ml) | 251–432 | Post-partum oestrus | No |
| *Haematological data* | | *Biochemical data* | |
| RBC ($\times 10^6$/mm$^3$) | 5.5–8.5 | Serum protein (g/dl) | 6–7.5 |
| PCV (%) | 37–55 | Albumin (g/dl) | 3–4 |
| Hb (g/dl) | 12–18 | Globulin (g/dl) | 2.4–3.7 |
| WBC ($\times 10^3$/mm$^3$) | 6–17 | Glucose (mg/dl) | 54–99 |
| Neutrophils (%) | 60–70 | Blood urea nitrogen (mmol/l) | 3.5–7.5 |
| Lymphocytes (%) | 12–30 | | |
| Eosinophils (%) | 2–10 | Creatinine (μmol/l) | <120 |
| Monocytes (%) | 3–10 | Total bilirubin (μmol/l) | <5.0 |
| Basophils (%) | Rare | Cholesterol (mmol/l) | 4–7 |
| Platelets ($\times 10^3$/mm$^3$) | 200–900 | | |

*Variation with size and diet composition.

unsocialised dogs, as the former are much less stressed by handling and procedures. Dogs are intelligent and learn readily, which can be useful in the laboratory. They should be trained to accept being in a subordinate role, with the handler dominant. They can easily be trained to accept the presence of a handler, and to co-operate during procedures. Purpose bred laboratory dogs will in general have been raised in a pack environment with the opportunity to experience natural social behaviour and are, therefore, more likely to be temperamentally suited to the laboratory than pet or stray dogs of unknown background.

Dogs need to be socialised to man and other dogs as puppies, between 3 and 8 weeks of age, or they may be unapproachable by 14 weeks. Social contact at an early age is, therefore, vital and must be maintained if the dog is to remain friendly. Puppies should be allowed to mix and play together from a young age, so they may interact with peers and take part in complex social behaviour.

Male dogs are generally more aggressive than females, but this varies with the breed. Beagles tend to be placid, amenable dogs, which adds to their usefulness in the laboratory. Unfamiliar adults, however, may be hostile or nervous of one another, and should only be mixed with extreme care.

Dogs have many methods of communication, with other dogs and people, using behaviour, vocalisation and olfactory signals. It is possible for the handler to learn the signals associated with greeting, nervousness, submission and aggression, making interaction with the animals easier. Males mark territory by cocking their legs, and frequent cleaning of the pen often results in frequent urination to re-mark the territory. A balance has to be struck between the requirements of the people and those of the dogs. Dogs can be encouraged to urinate in particular places by the selective use of odour eliminators. These will inhibit territory marking if used in areas which are required to be clean, such as the bed area and feeding area.

## Housing

Dogs are active animals, which need a lot of exercise and a complex environment. They can be kept in indoor pens, with or without outside runs. Flexible pen designs allow partitions to be put in or removed as necessary, linking adjacent pens together so the dogs can interact as a group or be separated for procedures. Pens need to provide stimulation for the dogs, and may include platforms to allow the dogs to look out of the pens, closed in areas for privacy, and toys such as chew sticks or balls. There must be facilities for adequate exercise, either in the individual runs or in a communal exercise yard where dogs can go in pairs or groups and interact with each other and with the handler. Cages are unsuitable for dogs long term as there is little room for exercise or human contact. Environments that are inadequate will lead to stereotypic behaviour and poor welfare.

The floors and walls of the accommodation area need to be of smooth, impervious material, which can withstand frequent cleaning. Partitions should be paw and nose proof to prevent aggressive encounters between neighbouring dogs and to reduce disease transmission, and flooring should be non-slip to prevent injuries to the dogs or handlers. Noise can be a significant problem in dog accommodation, and thought should be given to constructing pens of materials which are less noisy than traditional stainless steel. There must be a warm dry area for the dog to sleep in, containing a suitable bed and comfortable bedding material, with underfloor or overbed heating.

If the runs are large enough, there will be no soiling of the bedding area, but faecal material should be removed from all areas daily, and the pen thoroughly washed once or twice weekly. The exercise run should be cleaned more frequently. Puppies are not as clean as adults, and pens for nursing bitches may need to be cleaned two to three times daily. Scattering bedding material such as sawdust on the floors can help absorb waste and keep the pen and the dogs clean.

## Feeding

Dogs are monogastric carnivores, which can eat a variety of foodstuffs. Many commercial tinned and dry diets are available. Tinned foods are usually given with a cereal-based biscuit. Dry or semi-moist diets are complete, and just need to be fed with water. These can be fed ad lib, so the dog adopts a little-and-often pattern of feeding. If there is a tendency to obesity, the quantity may be restricted. Feeding infrequent, large meals of dry food predisposes to acute gastric dilatation and should be avoided. Sudden changes in diet are not accepted well and may lead to digestive disturbances. Cold food is less well tolerated than warm food. Attention should be given to the provision of a suitable diet post-operatively, which should be appetising but not so rich as to predispose to diarrhoea. Diets usually contain 22% protein and 5% fat. Dogs are very adaptable and deficiencies are rare. *A 13 kg beagle needs 0.8 kg canned food or 0.25 kg dry food daily for maintenance.*

The ration should be increased by 30% for the last 3 weeks of gestation, and raised to 3 or 4 times maintenance during lactation. For peak lactation, a high-energy food with a high calcium level should be fed, to prevent metabolic problems such as hypocalcaemia.

## Water

Water should be provided ad libitum. *The total water requirement is 70–80 ml/kg/day.* An adult beagle needs approximately 1 l daily, which will be provided by food and water. Dogs fed on dry diets will need more water than those on moist diets.

## Environment

Dogs are very adaptable. They can cope with temperatures between 15 and 24°C, and lower temperatures are tolerated if there are no draughts and the dogs are in groups. Extremes should be avoided. Neonatal dogs require 30–32°C: some of this is provided by the bitch but the air should be at least 26–28°C for the first 5 days. By 4 weeks, 24°C is adequate. Ventilation providing 8–12 air changes per hour is sufficient, and natural daylight is preferred. If this is not possible, a 12:12 light:dark cycle is acceptable.

## Breeding

Puberty is reached at 7–8 months in the male and 8–14 months in the female. Bitches are monoestrous: each cycle is followed by a period of anoestrus lasting 4–14 months. The cycle starts with pro-oestrus, in which there is a sanguinous discharge. The discharge reduces as the bitch enters oestrus, after 6–10 days. The bitch is receptive for 6–12 days, then enters metoestrus, when activity declines. The bitch only permits mounting during oestrus, and the male and female will 'tie' for 20–30 min during copulation. Ovulation is spontaneous and pseudopregnancy is common in the bitch. Oestrus can occur at any months of the year, but is most common in the spring.

Gestation lasts 59–67 days. An average of six puppies is born, at intervals of up to 1 h. Puppies will begin feeding immediately after birth. Puppies must get colostrum during the first 24 h, and are fed initially every 2–4 h. The bitch licks the puppies to stimulate respiration at first, then regularly licks the perineal area of each puppy to stimulate urination and defaecation for the first 3 weeks.

Puppies can start to eat solids from about 3 weeks, and may be weaned at 6 weeks. Growing puppies need to eat twice the maintenance level of an adult of similar size.

To breed dogs in packs, one male is put with up to 12 bitches, and bitches are removed from the pack for whelping. Alternatively, bitches can be kept in pairs and moved in with the male 10 days after the onset of pro-oestrus for 5 days.

## Growth and development

Puppies are born with their eyes and ears closed and unable to stand. They will normally stand at about 10 days, and can walk by day 21. The eyes and ears open by day 10–14. Puppies should multiply their birth weight by a factor of 40 or 50 in their first year. Adult weight is reached at 9 months. Before this, they must be fed sufficient for maintenance and growth.

## Handling

When approaching dogs, first offer the back of a hand for the animal to sniff, since an open hand may be interpreted as a threat and be bitten. The lead and collar, or the scruff of the neck if there is no lead, can be grasped in the other hand once the dog has accepted the person.

To lift a dog, approach the dog from the left hand side. Restrain the head with the left hand by holding its collar or scruff (gently), and lift the dog by placing the right arm over the body of the dog and taking its weight on its sternum. Alternatively, the dog may be lifted by placing one arm around the chest in front of the forelegs and the other behind the hindlegs, holding on to the outer legs. If a dog is nervous or aggressive, it may be muzzled, using a ready made plastic or fabric muzzle, or with a tape (see Figure 14.1).

For cephalic venepuncture, it is helpful to hold the dog on a table. An assistant places their left arm under the dog's neck and holds its head firmly against their chest. The right arm is then placed over the thorax, and the right elbow is used to hold the dog's chest against the person's chest. The first two fingers of the right hand are placed behind the dog's elbow to hold the foreleg out, and the thumb is placed firmly over the top of the leg to raise the vein (see Figure 14.2). Good results are obtained if the thumb is first placed towards the inside of the leg then rotated outwards slightly, as this brings the vein on to the top of the leg. The quick release tourniquet can also be used (see Figure 9.7).

These methods may be modified for facilitating the administration of medicines.

## Pain and stress recognition

It is important to be familiar with the individual dog's normal temperament to be able to notice the changes brought about by the presence of pain. A dog in pain is generally quieter and less alert than usual, with a 'hangdog' look. There may be stiffness or an unwillingness to move, with inappetance, shivering or panting. With less severe pain, dogs are often restless, but if in severe pain they tend to lie still and crouch. They

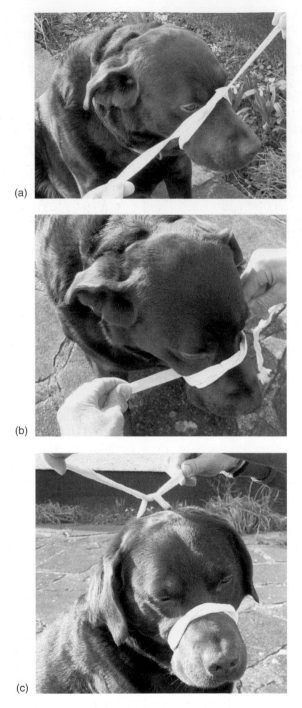

(a)

(b)

(c)

**Figure 14.1**    How to put a tape muzzle on a dog.

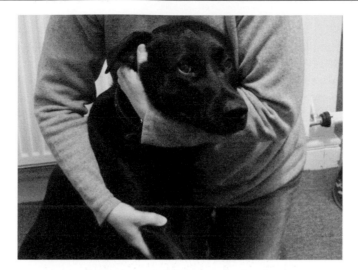

**Figure 14.2**   Holding a dog for cephalic venepuncture.

may whimper or howl, and growl without provocation. They may bite and scratch at painful areas and may become more vicious or aggressive. Observe closely to see if the animal is guarding a painful area, by altering its normal pattern of behaviour to avoid moving a painful part.

## Common diseases and health monitoring

Breeding colonies tend to consist of relatively stable populations of dogs, with major risks for disease entry being personnel or new arrivals. Disease entry can be minimised by providing quarantine facilities and serological screening for new arrivals, and by personnel adhering to strict entry requirements. For research facilities, where animals are introduced on a more frequent basis, new arrivals should be acquired from known sources with clean health records, effectively quarantined on arrival, and given a veterinary health check as soon as possible.

Colonies of dogs should have a regular health monitoring programme, including regular veterinary health checks, routine screening and investigation of any unusual occurrences and illnesses. Routine laboratory screening of approximately 10 dogs of different ages every 3 months is recommended (FELASA, 1998). Samples of blood, tonsillar tissue, skin/hair and faeces should be analysed for a range of diseases. The results of the most recent health screen should be considered when interpreting experimental data: anomalous data may be recorded if there has been an outbreak of disease in the colony. Fortunately, most of the major diseases of dogs are preventable by regular vaccination: screening for such diseases in vaccinated dogs is not necessary. Other diseases can be prevented by good hygiene and by regular preventive treatments, for example, for ecto- and endoparasites.

Diseases to be included in the health monitoring programme include zoonoses (which can be passed to humans), diseases which may cause clinical disease in the animals, and diseases which although subclinical may interfere with research data.

## *Zoonoses*

*Rabies* is a fatal zoonosis, against which dogs may need to be vaccinated unless there is rabies free status in the country. *Leptospira* spp. cause an unpleasant flu-like illness in man called Weil's disease, which can be fatal. *Salmonella* spp. or *Campylobacter jejuni* can cause enteric disease. *Toxocara canis* is a roundworm, which can be passed to people in dog faeces, causing a variety of lesions and possibly blindness. Dogs can contract and transmit ringworm, a fungal infection.

## *Subclinical and clinical diseases*

The major diseases of dogs which should be included in a screening programme or routine vaccinations are canine distemper, parvovirus, canine adenovirus type 1, and canine parainfluenza virus. Other diseases usually included in vaccines are *Bordetella bronchiseptica* (one cause of kennel cough) and *Leptospira* spp. Other pathogens that may need to be monitored include coronavirus and rotavirus, and internal and external parasites.

## *Diseases affecting research*

Depending on the research, many diseases can confound results. Respiratory or cardiovascular research may by affected by diseases such as kennel cough. *Toxocara* infections interfere with toxicology studies because migration of larvae through the viscera causes histological lesions, which may be misinterpreted.

In any case, a healthy dog that is well socialised and used to people will be the best experimental subject, as well as being fun to work with.

## Biological data and useful reference data

See Table 14.1.

## Anaesthesia

### *Pre-anaesthetic preparation*

A period of at least 12 h starvation should precede anaesthesia in the dog. It is not necessary to withold water. Premedication is essential to alleviate any anxiety and ensure a smooth induction and recovery from anaesthesia. *After premedication, the doses of induction agents required to produce general anaesthesia may be markedly reduced*.

### *Sedation/premedication*

*Drying agents: Atropine* (0.05 mg/kg) s.c. is used in routine premedication prior to general anaesthesia and prior to Hypnorm, alfentanil or xylazine sedation. Alternatively, *glycopyrollate* can be used at 2–8 μg/kg i.v. or i.m. These reduce salivary secretions.

*Acepromazine* 0.03–0.1 mg/kg i.m. produces sedation and hypotension but no analgesia. It can be used at 0.05 mg/kg in combination with opioids:

- pethidine 2 mg/kg i.m.
- morphine 0.1 mg/kg i.m. or s.c.

- buprenorphine 0.01 mg/kg i.v., i.m., s.c.
- butorphanol 0.2 mg/kg i.v., i.m.

*Fentanyl-fluanisone* (Hypnorm) (0.5 ml/kg i.m.) or fentanyl 2–5 µg/kg i.v. followed by diazepam or midazolam at 0.25 mg/kg i.v. 30 min later will also give sedation.

$\alpha_2$-Agonists: *xylazine* (2.0 mg/kg) i.m. produces good sedation with mild analgesia. It often produces vomiting, bradycardia, heart block and hyperglycaemia. Heart effects are abolished by atropine. *Medetomidine* produces sedation and analgesia, which are dose related. It can be given s.c., i.m. or i.v., the dose range being 10–80 µg/kg. Maximum effect is reached in 10–15 min. Blood pressure falls and breathing may become irregular, with cyanosis, but $pO_2$ is maintained. *Atipamezole* reverses the effects of medetomidine and xylazine. To reverse medetomidine, give an equal volume of atipamezole (if using the trade names Domitor and Antisedan which contain the drugs at 1 mg/ml and 5 mg/ml, respectively), and to reverse xylazine, atipamezole at 200 mg/kg reverses the effects of 3 mg/kg xylazine.

## General anaesthesia: injectable agents

Intravenous (i.v.) injection is easy using the cephalic vein on the anterior surface of the forelimb (see Figure 14.2).

- *Propofol* (Rapinovet or Diprivan): 5–7.5 mg/kg i.v. This is suitable for induction or maintenance by continuous infusion.
- *Thiopentone* (Intraval): 10–20 mg/kg of 1.25–2.5% solution. Care must be taken to ensure none of the drug goes perivascularly, since it is highly alkaline and causes tissue to slough. There may be a period of apnoea on induction.
- *Ketamine* combinations: ketamine 0.2–0.4 mg/kg i.v. with diazepam 0.2 mg/kg i.v. or ketamine 2.5 mg/kg i.m. with medetomidine 0.05 mg/kg i.m. or ketamine 5 mg/kg i.v. with xylazine 1–2 mg/kg i.v. or i.m.

## General anaesthesia: inhalation agents

These should not be used for induction as dogs resent this procedure. They are usually used for maintenance after induction with injectable agents and endotracheal intubation. *Isoflurane* and *halothane* both produce stable anaesthesia with good analgesia and muscle relaxation.

## Analgesia

### Opioids

If combined with barbiturates, these can cause respiratory depression.

- *Buprenorphine* 0.01–0.02 mg/kg s.c., i.m. or i.v. may be used pre-, intra- or post-operatively and will produce the longest relief from pain lasting 6–8 h.
- *Pethidine* 5 mg/kg i.m. post-operatively, lasts 2–3 h.
- *Fentanyl* 0.001–0.007 mg/kg can be given i.v. during surgery to increase analgesia.
- *Butorphanol* 0.4 mg/kg s.c. or i.m. 3–4 hourly.
- *Nalbuphine* 0.5–2.0 mg/kg s.c. or i.m. 3–8 hourly.

- *Pentazocine* 2 mg/kg i.m. 4 hourly.
- *Morphine* 0.5–5.0 mg/kg s.c. or i.m. 4 hourly. For epidural analgesia, 0.1 mg/kg epidurally over 30–60 s, latent period 30–60 min, duration 10–23 h.

## *Non-steroidal anti-inflammatory drugs*

- *Carprofen* 4 mg/kg pre-operatively or intra-operatively i.v. or s.c. lasts 18 h.
- *Ketoprofen* 2 mg/kg s.c., i.m. or i.v. for the first dose then 1 mg/kg orally daily for up to 5 days.
- *Meloxicam* 0.2 mg/kg orally daily for up to 21 days, then 0.1 mg/kg daily.
- *Flunixin* 1 mg/kg, give by *slow* i.v. injection or s.c., but not i.m. Do not give more than three doses. Not suitable for pre- or intra-operative use, but useful in acute pain, and endotoxic or septic shock.
- *Mefenamic acid* 5–20 mg/kg orally every 12 h initially, reducing to 48–72 hourly.
- *Piroxicam* 0.3 mg/kg every 48 h orally.
- *Ibuprofen* 5–10 mg/kg orally, 24–48 hourly.
- *Paracetamol* 10 mg/kg orally given 6 hourly for mild pain only, poor anti-inflammatory action.
- *Phenylbutazone* 2–20 mg/kg per day orally in divided doses.
- *Aspirin* 10–25 mg/kg orally, lasts 4–6 h, for relief from milder pain.

## CAT

The domestic cat, *Felis catus*, may be derived from the wildcat, *Felis sylvestris libyca*. Cats are true carnivores and hunters, using their good sight, smell and hearing to find prey. The reflective tapetum lucidum in the eye allows for particularly good night vision.

Several breeds of cat are available, but purpose bred non-pedigree cats are usually used in the laboratory. Cats kept in the laboratory in the UK must also be permanently marked for identification purposes, for example, with a tattoo or a microchip.

## Behaviour

Cats are intelligent, highly specialised hunters. They are solitary animals, but have the capacity to be sociable. Cats spend 60% of their time asleep, and the remainder of the time is spent exploring and marking their territory. Feral cats are nocturnal, and mark territories with urine and secretions from their anal glands. Males (toms) defend large territories covering the smaller territories of several females (queens), and are polygamous. The social organisation of feral cats depends on the availability of resources: where food is obtained only by hunting, they tend to be solitary since the supply of food may not support a social group. If prey is more plentiful, their territories may overlap. If food is supplied in abundance but in one location, such as occurs where humans are involved, cats will live together in colonies, consisting of matrilineal groups of related females and their offspring. Young males move away from the group

**Table 14.2**  Useful data: cat.

| Biological data | | Breeding data | |
|---|---|---|---|
| Adult weight (kg) | 2.5–3.5 | Puberty (months) | Male 8–9 female |
| Diploid number | 38 | | 5–12 |
| Daily food intake (g) | 200 | Age to breed (years) | |
| Daily water intake (ml) | 200–300* | Male | 1 |
| Natural lifespan (years) | 12–18 | Female | 1 |
| Rectal temperature (°C) | 38.1–39.2 | Gestation (days) | 58–72 (average |
| Heart rate/min | 110–140 | | 63) |
| Blood pressure (mmHg) | | Litter size | 3–5 |
| Systole | 120 | Birth weight (g) | 110–120 |
| Diastole | 75 | Weaning age (weeks) | 4–6 |
| Blood volume (ml/kg) | 47–65 | Oestrous cycle | Seasonal |
| Respiratory rate/min | 26 | | polyoestrus. |
| Tidal volume (ml) | 34 | | Cycles 2–3 weeks |
| | | | long January to |
| Haematological data | | | September. |
| RBC ($\times 10^6/mm^3$) | 5–10 | | Induced |
| PCV (%) | 30–45 | | ovulator |
| Hb (g/dl) | 8–15 | Post-partum oestrus | No |
| WBC ($\times 10^3/mm^3$) | 5.5–19.5 | | |
| Neutrophils (%) | 35–75 | Biochemical data | |
| Lymphocytes (%) | 20–55 | Serum protein (g/dl) | 6–7.5 |
| Eosinophils (%) | 2–12 | Albumin (g/dl) | 2.5–4.0 |
| Monocytes (%) | 1–4 | Globulin (g/dl) | 2.5–3.8 |
| Basophils (%) | Rare | Glucose (mg/dl) | 81–108 |
| Platelets ($\times 10^3/mm^3$) | 300–700 | Blood urea nitrogen | 3.5–8.0 |
| | | (mmol/l) | |
| | | Creatinine ($\mu$mol/l) | <180 |
| | | Total bilirubin ($\mu$mol/l) | < 4 |
| | | Cholesterol (mmol/l) | 2–4 |

*Depends on composition of diet.

when they are 2–3 years old, challenging older established males for access to groups of females as they mature.

Cats communicate by vocalisation, facial expression, postural changes and scent. They will demonstrate affection and aggression towards other cats and people, but if unused to people will be nervous if approached. They are sensitive to the attitudes of staff, and a gentle caring approach will soon result in friendly cats.

Young cats are playful and agile, and need to be kept in groups in large cages with many playthings. Adult females can be put together and will be amicable after the first few days. Adult males, however, will fight over females, so only the dominant males mate. Males that are not littermates are usually separated at 4–6 months.

## Housing

Housing for cats needs to allow them to exhibit a wide range of complex behaviours. Even in an enriched environment, cats may exhibit stereotypic behaviour due to lack of space. Cats may be kept indoors or outdoors. Group housing is best, with single caging for adult males, pregnant females, and queens with litters for the first 4–6 weeks. Singly housed cats should be allowed to exercise daily, and should be able to see other cats. In a breeding group, a large area is needed with lots of toys, perches, shelves and refuges, where kittens can play and where the cats can escape to. Perches and shelves should be sterilised regularly. Keeping the stocking density low and maintaining stable groups reduces stress on the cats.

All cats require scratching posts and sleeping boxes, which may be hung from the wall to facilitate cleaning. Solid floors are best. A dirt tray must be provided away from the sleeping area for urination and defaecation. These must be cleaned out at least once daily, and the rest of the room once or twice weekly.

## Feeding

Cats are hunters that tend to take small prey, having small meals spread throughout a 24 h period. However, they can readily adapt to the feeding patterns used in laboratories. Cats have a very high protein requirement, and specific requirements for particular amino acids (taurine and arginine). Protein must constitute at least 30% of the diet on a dry matter basis. Cats also become bored easily, and variety is preferred. Many commercial diets are available, tinned, dry and semi-moist. Food must be fed fresh, with no rancid fat, or it will be rejected. Twice daily feeding of tinned food with ad lib dry food overnight allows little-and-often feeding with no deterioration of the food. Food bowls may be placed directly on the floor or suspended from the wall, but must be able to be cleaned daily to remove stale food.

## Water

On a dry diet, cats will drink 200–300 ml daily, and much less on tinned diets. Cats dislike drinking from nozzles, so automatically filling bowls are best. Although many adult cats like milk, they do not need it and it can cause dietary disturbances due to lactose intolerance.

## Environment

In outdoor units, the environment is not controlled. Cats cope well but have litters mainly in spring and summer. In closed units the photoperiod can be controlled, and with a 12-h light cycle litters are spread throughout the year. The temperature needs to be between 21 and 25°C, with humidity between 45 and 65%. Providing heated beds or cooler areas allows cats to have some choice over the environment. Ventilation must be draught-free, and 10–15 air changes per hour is sufficient. Filters must be placed over the vents to prevent them from becoming blocked with hair. Background noise helps keep cats calm. In very quiet environments cats will startle easily.

## Breeding

Puberty is reached at 5–12 months, but breeding does not usually take place until 1 year. Outdoor cats breed seasonally, with females receptive from winter to summer.

Indoor cats breed all year under 12 : 12 light cycles. Females are polyoestrous, with cycles lasting 14–24 days. Oestrus is signalled by vocalisation (calling), and postural changes (lordosis). Anoestrous females will reject the male. Coitus induces ovulation, and it is normal for several matings to be required before ovulation occurs. In a harem, one or two males may be kept with a group of females. The dominant male mates with the majority of the females, however, the date of mating and paternity of the kittens may be unknown. Alternatively, males can be kept separately and females taken to the tom for mating. Oestrus lasts about 4 days if mating occurs, and up to 10 days in the absence of mating.

Pregnant females should be removed from the colony from 10 days before birth, but should be allowed to mix with the other females for short periods in the morning and afternoon so as not to lose their places in the hierarchy. Queens like to give birth in seclusion, and a box or bed should be provided in the nesting area. Gestation lasts about 63 days. There may be between 1 and 10 kittens in the litter (average 4). Once kittens are 6 weeks old, they and their mother can return to the group.

## Growth

Kittens are born weighing 90–140 g, and should gain 80–100 g weekly. Kittens need to feed very soon after birth, and need highly concentrated protein-rich milk for up to seven weeks, but can be weaned as early as 4 weeks, although 6–8 weeks is preferred. They start eating solids from around 3–4 weeks. They are born blind and virtually deaf. The eyes open at around 6 days, vision being fully developed by 16 weeks, and hearing is fully developed by 4 weeks. Newborn kittens have poor motor ability. They can stand by 3 weeks, but motor control is not fully developed until 11 weeks. The female stimulates the kittens to urinate and defaecate by licking their perineal areas: this may continue until the kittens are 6–7 weeks old. Kittens gain experience of hunting behaviour by interacting with prey brought to the nest by their mothers in the feral situation, and in the domestic situation by playing with toys. It is important that kittens gain experience with people between 2 and 7 weeks of age. Cats show more rapid development and are more likely to be friendly if handled regularly from birth.

## Handling

Cats are dignified creatures which respond to gentle handling and a quiet approach. A cat should first be allowed to familiarise itself with the smell of the handler by sniffing the back of the hand, as for dogs. Generally, cats are amenable and can be held for minor procedures and examinations by holding them gently but firmly around the shoulders (see Figure 14.3). Most cats can be picked up by placing one hand under the thorax and the other behind the rear end. Difficult cats can be restrained by grasping the scruff. Care must be taken though as the cat will still be able to reach the handler with its claws. Particularly vicious cats may be wrapped in a towel or blanket, or placed in a crush cage and given a sedative.

For venepuncture, the method described for the dog can be used (see Figure 9.10).

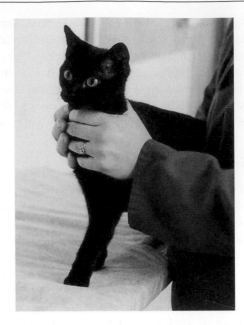

**Figure 14.3**    Restraining a cat.

## Pain and stress recognition

Healthy cats are alert, inquisitive, and exhibit frequent grooming behaviour. Cats in pain tend to be quiet and subdued and stop eating and grooming. Some react more violently, especially to acute and/or severe pain with frenzied activity or even dementia. Previously friendly cats may become aggressive when handled or approached if they are in pain. Vocalisation is variable as cats in pain will generally remain silent until attempts are made to move them, when they may howl and growl. Purring is not always a sign of health and contentment, as very sick cats frequently purr.

## Common diseases and health monitoring

Cats are available from barrier units which are free from disease. However, there are many common diseases that may be contracted in the laboratory and there should be a screening programme in place to monitor for these. As for dogs FELASA (1998) recommends screening at least 10 individuals from the colony every 3 months. All cats should have regular health checks, including twice yearly dental examinations.

### *Zoonotic diseases*

*Toxoplasma gondii* can cause an unpleasant flu-like illness in people, and it may be carried by cats. Routine screening should include serological testing for this organism. It can cause abortion in women if contracted during the first third of pregnancy, so advice should be sought from the Occupational Health Physician if you are pregnant and intend to work with cats.

Ringworm is a fungal skin infection which can cause sore or itchy lesions in people, and some mite infestations can be transmitted to people. If skin lesions are found on an experimental cat, contact the named veterinary surgeon or the named animal care and welfare officer. Remember that ringworm can also pass from people to cats, and it can be difficult to eradicate in cats, so take care not to introduce disease into the animal house, by wearing appropriate protective clothing.

Cat scratch disease is rare, but can cause chronic disease in elderly or immuno-compromised people bitten or scratched by a cat. The organisms responsible may be carried asymptomatically by up to 40% of cats. Care must be taken to use good hand-ling techniques and chemical restraint if necessary to avoid personal injury.

## Subclinical and clinical diseases

The main diseases of concern are cat flu (feline rhinotracheitis and calicivirus), infec-tious enteritis (feline panleucopaenia), feline leukaemia (FELV), feline infectious peritonitis (FIP) and feline immunodeficiency virus (FIV).

Cat flu is a common disease characterised by sneezing, ocular and nasal discharges, mouth ulcers and conjunctivitis. It is very common in grouped cats, and can be brought in by personnel who have contacted the disease in cats at home. Most forms of cat flu are preventable by vaccination, and this must be done every year to prevent any problems. In adults, the disease is usually mild and self-limiting, but it can prove fatal to kittens.

Infectious enteritis is a highly infectious, frequently fatal disease, which can be dev-astating to the colony. Vaccination is very effective and again this must be done yearly.

FELV and FIV can be carried asymptomatically for many years without causing any signs. The infectivity is relatively low, but both viruses spread most readily in the multi-cat environment found in the laboratory. These viruses can be detected by sero-logical screening, which should be done regularly. There is now a vaccine against leukaemia virus, but not yet against immunodeficiency virus, so any incoming animals must be screened for this virus before entering the colony.

The bacterial diseases to be monitored include *Bordetella bronchiseptica* and *Sal-monella*, and the cats should be checked regularly for evidence of parasitic infestation.

## Diseases affecting research

Any or all of the diseases mentioned may affect research. Cats are often used in neuro-logical studies: dietary deficiencies may affect vision, early infection with infectious enteritis virus can affect cerebellar development, and non-specific middle ear infections are common in kittens. If you suspect any problems with your research, contact the Named Veterinary Surgeon or the Named Animal Care and Welfare Officer for advice.

## Biological data and useful reference data

See Table 14.2.

## Anaesthesia

### Pre-anaesthetic preparation

The main consideration when anaesthetising a cat is the need to avoid stress on induc-tion, which can provoke laryngospasm. Premedication is essential to alleviate anxiety and ensure a smooth induction and recovery from anaesthesia. A period of 12 h starvation should precede anaesthesia. Water restriction is not necessary. *After premedication, the doses of induction agents required to produce general anaesthesia may be markedly reduced.*

## Sedation/premedication

- *Atropine* 0.05 mg/kg i.m. is advisable as a pre-medicant, especially if it is intended to intubate or to use ketamine.
- *Medetomidine* 50–100 μg/kg i.m. produces sedation in 10–15 min and lasts 30–180 min depending on the dose used. It may provoke vomiting shortly after injection. It can be rapidly reversed with *atipamezole* at 2½ times the previous dose of medetomidine, that is, if using Domitor and Antisedan, use half the volume of Antisedan to the volume of Domitor that was given.
- *Xylazine* 1–2 mg/kg i.m. or s.c. gives good sedation for 30–40 min but provokes vomiting. It is useful in combination with ketamine for full anaesthesia (see below).
- *Ketamine* 10–20 mg/kg i.m. gives moderate sedation with analgesia for 30–45 min but can be painful on injection. The increased muscle tone and lack of palpebral reflexes can be a problem, so the use of a bland ophthalmic ointment is important. It is better combined with midazolam (5 mg/kg ketamine with 0.25 mg/kg midazolam).
- *Acepromazine* 0.05–0.1 mg/kg i.m. or s.c. (or 1–3 mg/kg orally 1 h before sedation is required) is less reliable as a sedative but tranquilises adequately prior to induction and reduces post operative excitement due to barbiturates or alphaxolone/ alphadolone. Note that it causes hypotension.
- *Diazepam* can be used alone for sedation at 0.1–0.4 mg/kg i.v. or i.m.

## General anaesthesia: injectable agents

- *Alphaxalone/alphadolone*: 9 mg/kg i.v. produces 10 min surgical anaesthesia with good relaxation. Thereafter, incremental doses of 3 mg/kg can be given or a continuous infusion at 0.2 mg/kg/min. Swelling of the paws and ears may be noticed on recovery.
- *Ketamine* at 15–30 mg/kg in combination with *xylazine* 1 mg/kg i.m. or s.c. produces anaesthesia with good muscle relaxation. It is necessary to monitor the respiration and heart rates carefully.
- *Ketamine* 2.5–7.5 mg/kg i.m. can also be combined with *medetomidine* 80 μg/kg i.m. The onset of anaesthesia takes 3–4 min and lasts 30–60 min depending on the dose of ketamine used. Atipamezole can be used to reverse the medetomidine (see above for dose).
- *Barbiturates*: *thiopentone* 10 mg/kg of a 1.25% solution given i.v. with care to ensure that it does not go perivascularly, will give 5 min of light general anaesthesia. It is best given following premedication with, for example, acepromazine and used for induction prior to inhalation anaesthesia.
- *Propofol* at 7.5 mg/kg i.v. gives a few minutes anaesthesia with smooth rapid recovery. It is also useful for induction and can be used for continuous i.v. infusion.

## *General anaesthesia: inhalation*

This is not a suitable method for induction of anaesthesia in the cat as modern injectable agents are much better, but it is a very satisfactory method of maintaining anaesthesia. To avoid laryngospasm on intubation, first spray the larynx with 2% lignocaine then intubate with care using a 3–4 mm tube (for adults). T-piece or Bain circuits are ideal and suitable inhalation agents include isoflurane and halothane.

## Long-term anaesthesia

A well-maintained inhalational technique with the animal intubated has much to commend it but if the experimental design does not permit this, injectable alternatives exist. Rapidly metabolised agents whose effects are non-cumulative are the best choice.

*Alphaxalone/alphadolone (Saffan)* 9 mg/kg i.v. for induction followed by either incremental injections at 3 mg/kg or as a continuous infusion at 0.2 mg/kg/min, or *propofol* 7.5 mg/kg i.v. followed by incremental doses at 2 mg/kg thereafter.

## Analgesia

Opioids can be used in cats but care must be taken not to overdose. NSAIDs are generally poorly metabolised in cats and must also be used with caution. The potential difficulties in providing safe analgesia for cats should not be used as an excuse to preclude the use of analgesics completely.

## *Opioids*

- *Buprenorphine* 0.01 mg/kg s.c. or i.m. lasts at least 8 h
- *Nalbuphine* 1.5–3.0 mg/kg i.v. lasts 3 h
- *Pethidine* 2.5–10 mg/kg s.c. or i.m. lasts up to 2 h
- *Pentazocine* 2 mg/kg s.c. or i.m. lasts at least 4 h
- *Butorphanol* 0.4 mg/kg s.c. lasts 6 h
- *Morphine* 0.1 mg/kg s.c. or i.m. lasts at least 4 h

## *NSAIDs*

- *Carprofen* 4 mg/kg i.v. or i.m. may be given pre-operatively followed by 2 mg/kg p.o. 12 hourly post-operatively. After seven days this should be reduced to once every 24 h.
- *Meloxicam* 0.3 mg/kg i.v. or s.c. once, or 0.1 mg/kg p.o. 24 hourly for a maximum of 4 days.
- *Ketoprofen* 2 mg/kg s.c. daily for up to 3 days or 1 mg/kg orally daily for up to 5 days.
- *Flunixin* 1 mg/kg i.m, i.v. or p.o. preferably a single dose, but a maximum of 3 days.
- *Aspirin* 10–20 mg/kg orally is best used only as a single dose as it shows some toxicity in the cat. It can be repeated if necessary but dose only every 72 h maximum.
- *Phenylbutazone* 6–8 mg/kg orally daily.
- *Paracetamol* is toxic in the cat.

# FERRET

The ferret, *Mustela putorius furo*, is important as a laboratory animal as a carnivore which is small enough to be kept easily in the laboratory. There are two main varieties, the fitch ferret, which is buff with a black mask and points, and the albino. Domestic ferrets do not seem to exist in the wild, and are believed to be a domesticated form of the wild European Polecat. They appear to have been used by humans for at least 2000 years. References to ferret-like animals used for hunting have been found in ancient Greek and Roman records.

## Behaviour

Ferrets have a reputation for being aggressive, which is ill deserved. They are usually friendly, particularly if handled frequently from an early age. In strange surroundings, they can be nervous and may bite, particularly if roughly handled. Females with litters are protective and may also bite. Ferrets are curious, agile animals, which like to explore and burrow, and they will make good use of three-dimensional environments containing playthings and multilevel perches between which the animals can move.

Generally, unless breeding, ferrets like to be group housed, and young ferrets will readily play together. Ferrets communicate by using musk glands, which are situated lateral to the anus. The secretion may also be expressed when excited or frightened, or during the breeding season.

**Table 14.3**    Useful data: ferret.

| Biological data | | Breeding data | |
|---|---|---|---|
| Adult weight (g)[a] | 600–2000 | Puberty (months) | 9–12 |
| Food intake (g)[b] | 50–75 | Age to breed (days) | |
| Water intake (ml) | 75–100 | Male | 365 |
| Natural lifespan (years) | 5–9 | Female | 275 |
| Rectal temperature (°C) | 39 | Gestation (days) | 38–44 |
| Heart rate/min | 250 | | average 42 |
| Blood pressure (mmHg) | | Litter size | 8 |
| Systole | 110–140 | Birth weight (g) | 6–12 |
| Diastole | 31–35 | Weaning age (weeks) | 6–7 |
| Respiratory rate/min | 33–36 | Oestrous cycle | Induced |
| Diploid number | 40 | | ovulator |
| **Haematological data** | | **Biochemical data** | |
| RBC ($\times 10^6$/mm$^3$) | 6.8–12.2 | Serum protein (g/dl) | 5.1–7.4 |
| PCV (%) | 42–61 | Albumin (g/dl) | 2.6–3.8 |
| Hb (g/dl) | 15–18 | Globulin (g/dl) | 2.5–4.8 |
| WBC ($\times 10^3$/mm$^3$) | 4–19 | Glucose (mg/dl) | 94–207 |
| Neutrophils (%) | 11–84 | Blood urea nitrogen (mg/dl) | 10–45 |
| Lymphocytes (%) | 12–54 | Creatinine (mg/dl) | 0.4–0.9 |
| Eosinophils (%) | 0–7 | Total bilirubin (mg/dl) | <1 |
| Monocytes (%) | 0–9 | Cholesterol (mg/dl) | 64–296 |
| Basophils (%) | 0–2 | | |
| Platelets ($\times 10^3$/mm$^3$) | 297–910 | | |

[a] Both sexes show a periodic weight fluctuation of 30–40%. Fat is laid down in autumn and lost in winter.
[b] Dry carnivore pelleted diet. This should be fed soaked in hot water to form a paste for ferrets.

# Housing

Housing for ferrets needs to be particularly secure. Their slender bodies and extreme flexibility allow them to exploit the smallest gaps, and they are notorious escapers. Ferrets are gregarious animals, which should be housed together, except for females with kits, and males during the breeding season. Ferrets prefer solid floors with bedding such as sawdust or shavings rather than grid floors. They tend to urinate and defaecate in one latrine area, keeping the rest of the cage clean, so cleaning out is only necessary once or twice weekly. Ferrets can be trained to use a litter box. Plastic tubes, boxes and paper bags will add to the richness of the environment, and the animals will readily explore and play with them. However, ferrets are also prone to chewing and eating such objects, so they should be chosen with care to avoid intestinal foreign bodies. Nest boxes provide security and warmth for females with litters, and a solid partition at the bottom of the cage door will reduce bedding loss and prevent the young from falling out.

# Feeding

The nutritional requirements of ferrets have not been extensively studied. They have little ability to digest fibre, and they eat to energy requirements, so on moist cat food they can become protein deficient, leading to infertility. They cope well on mink diet, or on dry cat food supplemented with liver. They can also be fed a complete high protein dry carnivore diet (32% protein), which is usually soaked for ferrets and fed as a stiff paste. Food is usually provided in open bowls once daily, and the bowls should be cleaned after each meal. *Ferrets eat 50–75 g dry diet or 150 g soaked pellets daily.*

# Water

Water is given ad lib from bottles or cups. Galvanised water and food bowls should not be used for ferrets as they are susceptible to zinc toxicity.

# Environment

Ferrets are intelligent creatures, and enjoy a varied environment with places to hide and explore. They are agile and like to climb, and branches within the cage are well used. The temperature should be between 15 and 24°C, and the humidity 45–65%. Ferrets can tolerate low temperatures, but are susceptible to heat exhaustion above 30°C. Good ventilation is required. A 12-hour light cycle is usual, but changes in the light cycle can be used to manipulate the breeding cycle.

# Breeding

Puberty occurs at 9–12 months, in the spring following birth. Breeding is seasonal. In the northern hemisphere, females (jills) are active March to August, and males (hobs) December to July. This season is light dependent, oestrus being triggered by increasing day length, and artificial lighting can induce oestrus early and prolong the season. Testicular development in the male increases during the breeding season and decreases after July. Females are induced ovulators, with no obvious breeding cycle. The vulva of the female enlarges to signal oestrus at the beginning of the breeding season, and if not mated ovulation does not occur. In this event, persistent oestrus may develop, in which the prolonged high levels of oestrogen can lead to bone marrow depression. To prevent persistent oestrus, it is advisable to spay female ferrets that are not to be bred.

Oestrous females should be taken to the male for mating about 14 days after the onset of vulval swelling. The male will grasp the female by the scruff of the neck and drag her around the cage. Mating can take several hours and may be rough and noisy. Coitus results in ovulation after 30–35 h. If unfertilised, pseudopregnancy may develop. Otherwise, gestation lasts around 42 days, and 7–8 kits are born. Dystocia (difficult birth) is fairly common in ferrets, and if a jill has been straining to give birth for more than 2 or 3 h, veterinary advice should be sought. Weaning occurs at 6–7 weeks. If bred early in the year, a female may have two litters in a year.

## Growth

Kits weigh 6–12 g at birth. They have voracious appetites, attaching to the nipples immediately after birth if possible, and staying there. They begin eating solid food by 2–3 weeks, and can be weaned at 6–8 weeks. Adult weight is reached by four months of age, and males are twice the size of females. They are born blind and deaf: the eyes open at 28–34 days, and they hear from 32 days. They begin moving around before the eyes open.

## Handling

Although friendly, ferrets will bite if startled. They have relatively poor eyesight, and will bite a tentatively proffered finger, thinking it is a prey object. All movements towards ferrets should be smooth and deliberate. Talking to the animal will alert him to the presence of the handler. Approach the ferret by distracting him with a cloth or sleeve held in one hand, then grasp him with the other hand using an over the shoulder grip, or with the thumb and forefinger encircling the neck with the other fingers under the forelimbs (see Figure 14.4). Lift the animal up and support the hind quarters with the other hand. Ferrets will normally wriggle when first picked up, but should soon calm down. See also Figure 9.8 for jugular venepuncture in the ferret.

## Pain and stress recognition

Ferrets are alert, inquisitive creatures which should be active and explore vigorously once they are awake. A ferret in distress will not explore its environment and will show little interest in what is going on around it. If approached it may react with aggression and try to bite. The eyes may become puffy and half closed, and the coat will be ungroomed and take on a scruffy appearance.

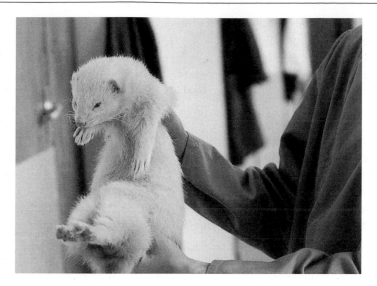

**Figure 14.4**   Handling a ferret.

## Common diseases and health monitoring

### Zoonotic diseases

Ferrets may carry a number of enteric pathogens, such as *Salmonella* and *Campylobacter*, so good hygiene is essential.

### Subclinical and clinical diseases

Ferrets are susceptible to human influenza, which can be severe in the ferret. Care should be taken to wear a mask when dealing with ferrets if you have a respiratory infection.

Canine distemper virus can cause an acute fatal disease in ferrets. Animals entering the colony should be of known health status and should be tested serologically to avoid bringing the disease in, or a vaccination policy should be employed.

Aleutian disease virus can cause many symptoms, including neurological signs and hypergammaglobulinaemia, and often affects breeding performance. It can be detected by serology on a small blood sample, and positive animals should be removed from the colony. There is no treatment or vaccine available.

Persistent oestrus can lead to bone marrow suppression and associated problems including severe anaemia. This is very difficult to reverse, so it must be prevented by either spaying non-breeding females, changing the lighting to the winter cycle, hormone treatment as directed by the veterinary surgeon, or housing with a vasectomised male to induce ovulation.

### Diseases affecting research

Many diseases can potentially affect research. Ferrets are often used in auditory research, and may suffer from ear mite infestation. Aleutian disease virus can interfere with neurological research, and any respiratory infection will increase the chances of anaesthetic deaths.

## Biological data and useful reference data

See Table 14.3.

## Anaesthesia

Ferrets should be fasted for 3–4 h prior to induction to minimise the risk of vomiting. Longer periods of fasting are not necessary, since the gut transit time is short, and may lead to hypoglycaemia.

### *Sedation and premedication*

- *Atropine sulphate* at 0.05 mg/kg s.c. reduces salivary secretions prior to general anaesthesia.
- *Medetomidine* at 100 μg/kg i.v., i.m. or s.c. produces good sedation and loss of the righting reflex in 5–10 min. It can be reversed rapidly with 1 mg/kg *atipamezole*.
- *Midazolam* (0.2 mg/kg) with *ketamine* (10 mg/kg) given together i.m. produce good short term sedation with relaxation, suitable for minor procedures.
- *Ketamine* 20–30 mg/kg i.m. produces sedation but poor relaxation. *Diazepam* or *midazolam* at 2 mg/kg i.m. both reduce anxiety prior to induction of general anaesthesia.
- *Hypnorm* may be used at 0.3–0.5 ml/kg i.m. but muscle relaxation is poor.

### *Injectable anaesthesia*

- *Medetomidine and ketamine*: 100–120 μg/kg medetomidine and 4–8 mg/kg ketamine given together i.m. produces surgical anaesthesia lasting 60 min or more, but with some respiratory depression. This is reversed by an equal volume of atipamezole i.m., for example, for 0.5–1 kg ferret, use 0.12 ml. Domitor and 0.08 ml ketamine together, and reverse with 0.12 ml Antisedan.
- *Ketamine and xylazine*: 25 mg/kg ketamine i.m. and 1–4 mg/kg xylazine i.m. will give 30–60 min of good surgical anaesthesia.
- *Ketamine and benzodiazepines*: 25 mg/kg ketamine with 2 mg/kg diazepam or midazolam i.m. produces 30 min surgical anaesthesia.
- *Alphaxolone/alphadolone (Saffan)* at 12 mg/kg i.v. may be given into the cephalic vein if there is a competent person available to restrain the animal; or into the jugular vein after sedation. Incremental doses of 6–8 mg/kg may be used for maintenance.
- *Propofol* at 10 mg/kg can also be used for total i.v. anaesthesia.

### *Other drugs*

- *Doxapram* at 1–2 mg/kg i.v. can be used to reverse respiratory depression. Repeat after 20 min if necessary.
- *Naloxone* 0.05 mg/kg i.v. or i.m. reverses the effects of opioids.

# Analgesia

## *Opioids*

- *Buprenorphine* 0.05 mg/kg s.c. or i.m. lasts up to 12 h
- *Butorphanol* 0.25 mg/kg s.c.
- *Morphine* 0.25 mg/kg

## *NSAIDs*

- *Flunixin* 0.5–2.0 mg/kg s.c.
- *Ketoprofen* 2 mg/kg s.c. given once daily
- *Aspirin* 200 mg/kg p.o.

## FURTHER INFORMATION

FELASA (1998). FELASA recommendations for the health monitoring of breeding colonies and experimental units of cats, dogs and pigs. *Laboratory Animals* 32, 1–17.

Lloyd, M. (1999). *Ferrets: Health, Husbandry and Diseases*. Blackwell Science, Oxford.

Martin, B. (1998). *The Laboratory Cat*. CRC Press.

National Research Council (1994). *Laboratory Animal Management: Dogs*. National Academy Press.

Otto, G., Rosenblad, W.D. and Fox, J.G. (1993). Practical venepuncture techniques in the ferret. *Laboratory Animals* 27, 26–29.

Poole, T. (ed.) (1999). *The UFAW Handbook on the Care and Management of Laboratory Animals. Vol.1: Terrestrial Vertebrates*, 7th edition. Blackwell Science, Oxford.

Taylor, P.M. (1985). Analgesia in the dog and the cat. *In Practice* 7, 5–13.

# Chapter 15
# **Primates**

The order primates includes a wide variety of mammals ranging from the pygmy mouse lemur, which weighs just 25–38 g, to the gorilla which can weigh up to 170 kg. See Figure 15.1 for a simplified classification of primates. Two suborders are recognised:

- Strepsirhine primates, which includes lemurs, lorises and bushbabies.
- Haplorhine primates, which includes tarsiers, monkeys, apes and man.

The most commonly used primates in the laboratory are monkeys, principally marmosets and macaques. Monkeys are included in Schedule 2 to the Animals (Scientific Procedures) Act (ASPA), and must, therefore, be acquired only from an accredited breeding or supplying establishment. In addition, primates are covered by CITES, most laboratory species appearing in Appendix II ('threatened' species), and international trade in monkeys, and tissues from monkeys, is thus strictly controlled.

The Haplorhini divide into Old World monkeys, the Cercopithecoidea, from Africa and Asia; the New World monkeys, the Ceboidea, from South America; and the Tarsioidea from South-east Asia. The main anatomical differences between the two principal infraorders are summarised in Table 15.1. These groups also differ in biological needs, and will be dealt with separately.

## SUPPLY OF NON-HUMAN PRIMATES

Any project licence applicant wishing to use non-human primates must complete Section 18c, detailing why it is essential to use them and giving justification for the use of Old World rather than New World monkeys, if applicable. The use of wild-caught primates in laboratories has been banned in the European Union (EU), unless there is exceptional and specific justification for their use. Project licence applications

**Table 15.1** Differences between New World and Old World monkeys.

| New World monkeys (Platyrrhini) | Old World monkeys (Catarrhini) |
| --- | --- |
| Broad nosed | Narrow nosed |
| Need vitamin $D_3$ if not exposed to UV light | No need for dietary vitamin $D_3$ |
| May have prehensile tail | No prehensile tail |
| No callus over ischial tuberosities | May have ischial calluses |
| No opposable thumbs | Opposable thumbs |
| Three premolar teeth each side | Two premolar teeth each side |

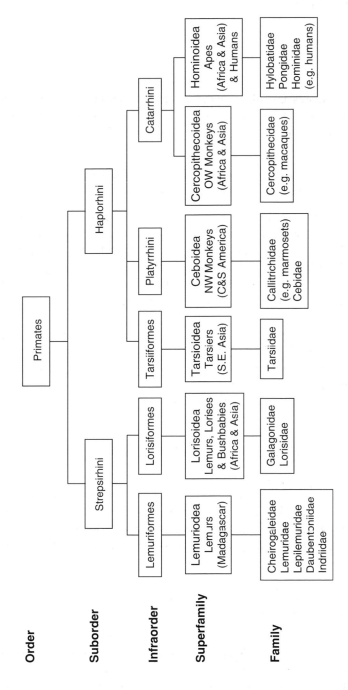

**TAXONOMIC LEVEL**

**Order**

Primates

**Suborder**

Strepsirhini

Haplorhini

**Infraorder**

Lemuriformes

Lorisiformes

Tarsiiformes

Platyrrhini

Catarrhini

**Superfamily**

Lemuriodea
Lemurs
(Madagascar)

Lorisoidea
Lemurs, Lorises
& Bushbabies
(Africa & Asia)

Tarsioidea
Tarsiers
(S.E. Asia)

Ceboidea
NW Monkeys
(C&S America)

Cercopithecoidea
OW Monkeys
(Africa & Asia)

Hominoidea
Apes
(Africa & Asia)
& Humans

**Family**

Cheirogaleidae
Lemuridae
Lepilemuridae
Daubentoniidae
Indriidae

Galagonidae
Lorisidae

Tarsiidae

Callitrichidae
(e.g. marmosets)
Cebidae

Cercopithecidae
(e.g. macaques)

Hylobatidae
Pongidae
Hominidae
(e.g. humans)

**Figure 15.1**  A simplified classification of primates.

requesting the use of such animals will automatically be referred to the Animal Procedures Committee. However, the import of purpose-bred monkeys from colonies outside the EU is permitted. Primates are Schedule 2 animals, so non-designated sources must be approved by the Home Office. Prior to approval, the Home Office will require details of the establishment, including staff numbers and training, involvement of attending veterinarians, demographics of the primate colonies, housing conditions and health surveillance, as well as details of the proposed transport arrangements. The aim is to ensure that only $F_2$ animals and beyond are supplied for use in research (i.e. those animals which are second-generation captive bred).

A designated establishment which intends to import non-human primates will have the intended source identified on the Certificate of Designation and on the relevant project licences. In addition, the project licence holder wishing to use imported monkeys will need to obtain separate authorisation for the acquisition and transport of each consignment of animals. Lifetime records must be kept for such animals. Primates must be permanently identified in some way. The alternatives being: numbered discs on collars for marmosets, tattoos, or microchip transponders implanted under the skin.

## PSYCHOLOGICAL WELL-BEING

The United States Animal Welfare Act 1985 requires researchers 'to provide a physical environment adequate to promote the psychological well-being of primates'. There are individual differences seen in primates (e.g. relaxed versus anxious individuals), both in nature and in the laboratory. Due to the differences, housing animals in social groups creates a more socially relevant context in which to study behavioural and physiological processes in the laboratory, but this also brings some potential problems that have to be overcome by good management programmes.

There is no specific measurement of psychological well-being, but four components can be considered together to build up a picture of the psychological condition of the animal. These are:

1. The physical health of the animal.
2. The behavioural repertoire of the animal.
3. An assessment of the stress the animal is under to determine whether or not it is chronically distressed.
4. An assessment of the animal's coping skills when presented with novelty. This will evaluate if it is inquisitive and explorative or if it reverts to an abnormal response and if so, how long it takes to return to baseline level. This will give an indication of the animal's resilience.

It can be seen that none of these parameters alone will give a clear picture of the animal's psychological well-being. A singly housed animal may well be in excellent physical health because it is not exposed to the risk of infections from other animals, there is no competition for food, and no chance of wounding by companions. Although it will suffer the stress of social deprivation, it will not be trying to maintain its position in a social hierarchy. However, such animals frequently show a poor behavioural repertoire with abnormal and even self-harming behaviours and do not have well-developed coping skills. Conversely, the benefit of social housing is that the environment is dynamic, variable and unpredictable; so, there is little habituation, but there are increased risks of infection, wounding and competition for food. With good management strategies these risks can be minimised but not altogether removed.

Companionship will promote psychological well-being but social living must be viewed as a component of psychological well-being, not synonymous with it. It depends to some extent whether the monkey is a high- or low-ranking individual. Even long-term cage-mates may have periods of social instability, but primates have mechanisms for conflict resolution and in a compatible pair one member will be subordinate. This does not mean it is picked on or harassed and does not mean deprivation; it is simply a means to resolve and reduce conflict that is mutually beneficial to both animals. Once the animals are in social groups, the problems of disease transmission diminish since they are unlikely to be sources of new pathogens for each other. Although social contact is desirable, and having two reasonably compatible animals confined in a cage together may be better than each animal being alone, there need to be other forms of enrichment if boredom and bickering are to be avoided. The internal furnishings of the cage are vital in this respect.

The concerns about transmission of disease, inflicting traumatic injuries on each other, competition and possible deprivation of food, water, shelter, the possibility of social housing interfering with research procedures, have to be weighed against the benefits of social housing, or conversely, the costs of solitary confinement. The provision of foraging opportunities in an adequate amount of space is a way of offering a socially sanctioned method of establishing the hierarchy that does not result in significant wounding and injury. The damage caused to an animal by individual housing may not be immediately apparent as the changes in behaviour may at first be very subtle but long term there may be self-mutilation and more obvious damage. The animal's individual experiences will modify its development since there is a dynamic process that determines its later behaviour. For example sucking and clinging, which should be directed towards the mother, may become directed towards other available objects or even the individual's own body. Although this does not provide the nutrition and contact that should come from the natural mother-directed behaviour, it continues to provide a state of a psychophysiological arousal. Thus, digit sucking or self-hugging will occur when an individual is anxious or distressed: the same circumstances in which an animal will return to the mother if reared by her. Stimulation-seeking behaviours will manifest themselves in a variety of ways depending on the available options afforded by the environment.

## NUTRITION

Primates will eat a variety of foods, including fruit, nuts, insects and commercially prepared feeds. The vitamin content is particularly important. Primates cannot synthesise vitamin C, and lack of it delays wound healing and predisposes to infections. Classical scurvy will develop, if deprived of vitamin C for long periods. It should be supplemented at 1–4 mg/kg bodyweight. Commercial diets with added vitamin C need to be used within 90 days of manufacture or the level of active vitamin declines.

Primates usually do well with a low dietary fat content, typically 5%. All dietary needs can be supplied with a commercial pelleted diet, but the addition of fruit and tit-bits will add to the richness of the environment. A small quantity of particulate food mixed with shavings and spread on the floor will keep monkeys occupied for considerable periods of time, and allows them to practise dexterity and discrimination skills.

## NEW WORLD MONKEYS

New World monkeys are increasingly used in the laboratory, yet many aspects of their biology and husbandry are poorly understood. There are many differences between outwardly similar species, and the different regimes encountered in captivity are likely to affect their responses in different ways. Animals may thrive in one captive environment, but exhibit poor reproductive capacity or ill health in another very similar environment, or even if moved to a different position in the same room. Social and environmental enrichment appear to play a particularly important role in maintaining the health of these small primates.

New World monkeys originate from tropical rain forests in Central and South America, where they are exclusively arboreal. Their native environment may be hot and humid, and the animals are exposed to sunlight. Since they are arboreal they climb well and if startled they flee upwards, not along the ground, so cages for these species should be taller and narrower to reflect this. The environment should be maintained at temperatures between 20°C and 28°C, with humidity of 55–65%. Ultraviolet light should be supplied if possible but, if not, vitamin $D_3$ must be added to the diet.

## Marmoset

The commonest New World species used in research is the common marmoset, *Callithrix jacchus*. Marmosets are small and relatively easy to keep in the laboratory. They are susceptible to many oncogenic viruses and infectious hepatitis, and they exhibit natural haematological chimerism, which makes them useful for immunological research.

### *Behaviour*

Wild marmosets live in family groups of three to eight animals or more, with a well-developed social structure. Males and females pair for life, and both parents care for the young. Individuals show a great deal of interaction, including play and mutual grooming. There is marked diurnal variation in their behaviour, and they are much less active at night.

### *Housing*

Caging for marmosets needs to reflect their behavioural needs. They are an arboreal species, and need tall cages. The stocking density within the room must be kept low,

**Table 15.2**  Useful data: marmoset.

### Biological data

| | |
|---|---|
| Adult weight (g) | 300–400 |
| Diploid number | 46 |
| Food intake | 20 g daily New World monkey pelleted diet |
| Water intake | Ad libitum |
| Natural lifespan (years) | 10–16 |
| Rectal temperature (°C)[a] | 38.6 (day) and 36.3 (night) |
| Heart rate/min[a] | 230–312 |
| Mean arterial pressure (mmHg)[a] | 65–100 (day) and 50–95 (night) |
| Blood volume (ml/kg) | 70 |

### Breeding data

| | |
|---|---|
| Puberty (months) | 8 |
| Age to breed (years) | 1.5–2 |
| Gestation (days) | 140–148, average 145 |
| Litter size | Usually dizygotic twins, can be 1–4 offspring |
| Birth weight (g) | 25–35 |
| Weaning age[b] | 6 months |
| Oestrous cycle (days) | 14–28, few overt signs of oestrus |
| Comments | Interbirth interval 154–178 days |

### Haematological data

| | |
|---|---|
| RBC ($\times 10^6/mm^3$) | 5.7–6.95 |
| PCV (%) | 45–52 |
| Hb (g/dl) | 14.9–17 |
| WBC ($\times 10^3/mm^3$) | 7.3–12.8 |
| Neutrophils (%) | 26–62 |
| Lymphocytes (%) | 30–67 |
| Eosinophils (%) | 0.6–4.2 |
| Monocytes (%) | 0.4–5 |
| Basophils (%) | 0.1–1.1 |
| Platelets ($\times 10^3/mm^3$) | 490 |

### Biochemical data

| | |
|---|---|
| Serum protein (g/dl) | 6.6–7.1 |
| Albumin (g/dl) | 3.8 |
| Globulin (g/dl) | 2.7–3.9 |
| Glucose (mg/dl) | 126–228 |
| Blood urea nitrogen (mg/dl) | 51.8 |
| Creatinine (mg/dl) | 0.9–1.2 |
| Total bilirubin (mg/dl) | 0.4–0.6 |

[a] Marked diurnal changes: heart rate, arterial pressure, activity and body temperature all fall at night.
[b] Young can suckle for longer, particularly if stressed.

since high-stocking densities and overcrowding are associated with increased levels of disease. Marmosets are usually housed in family groups composed of an adult pair and offspring. They are agile and like to climb, and so benefit from branches or other suitable perches within the cage. They will walk along branches on all four feet and use their tails to balance.

## *Feeding*

Marmoset diet must be palatable and carefully balanced nutritionally, to prevent any nutritional problems. Deficiencies in vitamin E, selenium and protein may lead to wasting marmoset syndrome. New World monkeys require vitamin $D_3$, which they normally produce during exposure to ultraviolet light. In the laboratory, it should be added at 1–2.5 i.u./g of diet. A deficiency in it will predispose to pathological lesions of the bones. Protein should be fed at 3 g/kg body weight daily. Diets for New World monkeys usually contain 20–25% protein. Marmosets will eat freshly milled New World monkey diet, but benefit from supplements, such as pieces of fruit or malt loaf. Drilled wood filled with gum provides good enrichment. Vitamins must be supplied as described above. Marmosets eat 20 g pelleted diet daily. Food hoppers and water bottles can be cleaned twice weekly. Water is supplied ad lib, using bottles or automatic systems. With bottles, vitamins can be added to the water.

## *Breeding*

Marmosets, as all New World monkeys, have oestrous cycles, whereas Old World monkeys have menstrual cycles. Sexual maturity is reached at 14 months, then the female is polyoestrous, having cycles every 14–28 days. However, no overt signs of oestrus are seen. If they are kept in large groups with more than one female, only the dominant female will breed. Mating results in gestation lasting 140 days, and twins are usually carried. The fetuses share a placenta with vascular anastomoses, so they share their blood supply and are natural chimeras. After birth, the young are normally weaned at 6 months and stay with their parents until sexual maturity. Typically, the males do much of the infant carrying. Females are mated again shortly after parturition and the interbirth interval is 154 to 178 days. Between 20% and 52% of pregnancies may result in triplets, and quads are not uncommon. With improved nutrition and health of marmoset colonies this percentage is increasing. Left alone, the weakest one will drop off at around the 3rd day and die, which raises ethical and welfare issues. The alternatives are rotational feeding, hand rearing or removing one infant for euthanasia. Each of these has certain disadvantages and the management method selected to deal with these extra offspring will depend on the individual circumstances of the colony.

## *Growth*

Marmosets reach their maximum bodyweight by 20 months of age (Figure 15.2).

## Biological data and useful reference data

See Table 15.2.

## OLD WORLD MONKEYS

Old World monkeys live in a variety of habitats in Africa and Asia, and are partly terrestrial and partly arboreal. Generally, they roam and forage on the ground, and sleep in trees, but the degree of time spent naturally on the ground or in the trees varies

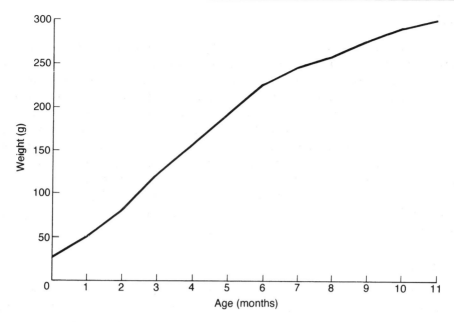

**Figure 15.2**    Typical marmoset growth chart.

depending on the species. The cynomolgus is more arboreal than the rhesus macaque. All macaques have calluses on their ischial tuberosities to facilitate sitting on narrow branches. Their housing usually provides much floor space with perching areas to reflect their habits. A wide variety of environmental conditions can be tolerated by these monkeys, but they thrive between 15°C and 24°C, with humidity at 45–65%. Draughtless ventilation providing 12–15 air changes per hour is adequate. The macaques are very wide ranging, and may be found in many different habitats extending from Gibraltar, Algeria and Morocco in the West to the Philippines and Japan in the East. The macaques range as far north as 42°N in Japan to 9°S in Indonesia. They are found from sea level to altitudes of over 3000 m, in locations where snowfalls and temperatures of −15°C occur in winter; to those where summer temperatures may be 50°C; from dry desert areas to those with annual rainfall in excess of 100 cm; from deeply forested areas to highly urbanised environments with a close relationship with humans. Some species, such as the lion-tailed macaque (*Macaca silenus*), have very specific requirements (rain forest), whereas others, such as the rhesus (*Macaca mulatta*), are found across the whole range of habitat conditions. Knowledge of the macaques' ecological requirements is helpful in managing captive populations, whether for research or breeding.

The species most commonly used in research are the rhesus monkey (*Macaca mulatta*), and the cynomolgus, long-tailed or crab-eating monkey (*Macaca fascicularis*). Rhesus monkeys are known for living near human habitations, which they raid for food. Cynomolgus monkeys are found more in coastal areas and will eat crustaceans. The cynomolgus monkey spends more of its time in the trees, whereas the rhesus is a ground-dwelling monkey that forages on the floor and takes to the trees for safety and to sleep.

## Behaviour

Macaques are quadripedal, but will walk upright if carrying infants or food. They are very sociable, and live in large groups. Macaque groups are composed of matrilines (female kin groups) and immigrant males that are unrelated to them. The matrilines have a rank order that is relative to one another such that the immature female of a high-ranking lineage will dominate the adult females from lower-ranking lineages. Intragroup activities, such as grooming will often be kin-related. Group size in the macaques ranges from 10 to 100; the adult sex ratio is female biased, although natal sex ratios are equal, due to the higher rate of mortality among males.

Juvenile macaques play together in age groups, where much social contact and mutual grooming tends to replace play as they get older. Playing and normal behaviour are essential preparation for adulthood, but some behaviour appears to be just for fun. The inability to play and express natural behaviour rapidly results in stereotypy, whatever the age of the animal. Marked behavioural differences may be seen between different species of macaques, and they also differ in their responses to environmental stressors. Cynomolgus macaques tend to be more stressed, even by minor procedures (such as routine capture), when compared with rhesus.

## Housing

Macaques can be kept in outdoor gang cages if well accustomed to a captive environment, but more usually are kept indoors in order to preserve the health status. Quarantine animals are often kept in smaller groups in cages to facilitate catching and observation. Compatible animals, such as a disease-free breeding colony, are kept together in large gang cages or rooms (Figure 15.3). Some cages are designed to be joined together, and great flexibility can be achieved using these. Care must be taken though in adding animals to established groups in case fighting occurs.

## Feeding

In the wild state, the gathering of food is the principal activity for primates, and yet is the most profoundly affected activity of a captive existence. Analysis of activity budgets in the wild has shown that up to 80% of time is given to this activity. The alteration in feeding imposed by captivity is not just on the feeding regime but also on the form and texture of the food. In the laboratory, food is generally provided in large quantities according to a set schedule leading to conditioned expectations, a potential social flashpoint and rapid consumption. The latter may have adverse effects on the digestive system, which is designed for a constant browsing intake of food, and will lead to boredom if the animal's daily time budget is not filled with some other activity.

Macaques require approximately 420 kJ/kg daily for maintenance, 525–630 kJ/kg if pregnant or lactating, and 840 kJ/kg if neonatal. Commercial Old World monkey diets are used providing a protein intake of 15–25%, with supplements of fruit and nuts. Foraging mix can be made up from a selection of peanuts in the shell, flaked maize, dog biscuits, locust beans, sunflower seeds, pine kernels, boiled eggs in the shell, and dog

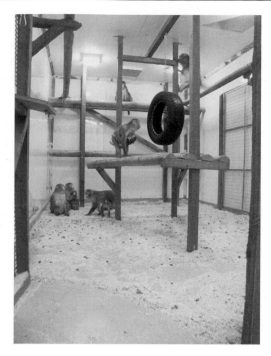

**Figure 15.3**   Group-housed rhesus macaques in an open-room environment.

chocolate drops. When mixed with substrate and scattered through the cage or placed in a tray, this adds interest to the diet as well as providing environmental enrichment.

## Water

Rhesus monkeys need 40–80 ml/kg/day. It is usually provided ad lib in bottles or automated systems.

## Breeding

The macaque menstrual cycle lasts around 30 days, some species being strictly seasonal breeders, others having an annual peak. Puberty occurs at 2–3 years for female rhesus monkeys, and 3–4 years for males. For cynomolgus monkeys, puberty occurs at 3–4 years in both sexes. Rhesus monkeys have a menstrual cycle lasting 28 days, and breed seasonally from September to January. Cynomolgus monkeys are non-seasonal breeders, with a menstrual cycle of 31 days. Captive macaques will copulate continuously whereas in wild populations, macaque females are sexually receptive during discrete intervals. This period of oestrus is indicated by changes in the female's behaviour, olfactory cues and swelling and reddening of the perineal skin may occur to a varying degree. Sexual activity peaks around the time of ovulation and the frequency of aggressive episodes also increases during mating periods. Mating occurs several times during the receptive period. Gestation lasts 164 days in the rhesus and 167 days in the cynomolgus; and one infant is usually born. Dependence on the mother for

**Table 15.3**   Useful data: macaques.

| | Rhesus macaque (*Macaca mulatta*) | Cynomolgus macaque (*Macaca fascicularis*) |
|---|---|---|
| ***Biological data*** | | |
| Adult weight (kg) | Male 6–11, female 4–9 | Male 4–8, female 2–6 |
| Diploid number | 42 | 42 |
| Food intake | 420 J/kg for maintenance, 525–630 J/kg for production, 840 J/kg for neonates | |
| Water intake | Ad libitum, 40–80 ml/kg daily | |
| Natural lifespan (years) | 20–30 | 15–25 |
| Temperature (°C) | 36–40 | 37–40 |
| Heart rate/min | 120–180* | 240 |
| Blood pressure (mm Hg) | | |
|    Systole | 125 | As rhesus |
|    Diastole | 75 | As rhesus |
| Blood volume (ml/kg) | 55–80 | 50–96 |
| Respiratory rate/min | 32–50* | |
| ***Breeding data*** | | |
| Age at puberty | Male 3–4 years, female 2–3 years | 3–4 years |
| Age to breed | Male 4–5 years, female 3–5 years | 4–5 years |
| Gestation (days) | 146–180, average 164 | 153–179, average 167 |
| Litter size | 1 | 1 |
| Birth weight (kg) | 0.4–0.55 | 0.33–0.35 |
| Weaning age | 12 months, can hand rear from birth | 12 months |
| Breeding cycle | Menstrual cycle 28 days | Menstrual cycle 31 days |
| Comments | Seasonal breeding – September to January | Non-seasonal breeding |
| ***Haematological data*** | | |
| RBC ($\times 10^6$/mm$^3$) | 3.56–6.95 | |
| PCV (%) | 26–48 | |
| Hb (g/dl) | 8.8–16.5 | |
| WBC ($\times 10^3$/mm$^3$) | 2.5–26.7 | |
| Neutrophils (%) | 5–88 | |
| Lymphocytes (%) | 8–92 | |
| Eosinophils (%) | 0–14 | |
| Monocytes (%) | 0–11 | |
| Basophils (%) | 0–6 | |
| Platelets ($\times 10^3$/mm$^3$) | 109–597 | |
| ***Biochemical data*** | | |
| Serum protein (g/dl) | 4.9–9.3 | |
| Albumin (g/dl) | 2.8–5.2 | |
| Globulin (g/dl) | 1.2–5.8 | |
| Glucose (mg/dl) | 46–178 | |
| Blood urea nitrogen (mg/dl) | 8–40 | |
| Creatinine (mg/dl) | 0.1–2.8 | |
| Total bilirubin (mg/dl) | 0.1–2 | |
| Cholesterol (mg/dl) | 108–263 | |

* Values determined under sedation.

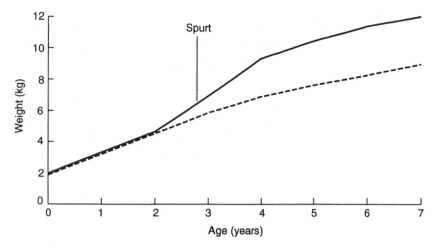

**Figure 15.4**  Typical rhesus growth curve. (——) Male; (– – –) female.

nutrition gradually wanes between 3 and 6 months of age and the infant becomes independent for foraging and travelling by about 1 year of age. However, psychological support and protective intervention from the mother will extend well into the juvenile years, so weaning (meaning the physical separation from the mother) should not occur until after 12 months of age.

## Growth

Old World monkeys show a prolonged period of development prior to adulthood. Their life can be divided into phases, for example, for rhesus monkeys:

- Fetal phase: 164 days.
- Infantile phase: 9 months.
- Juvenile phase: 1 year 9 months.
- Adult phase: 11 years plus.

This prolonged period of immaturity allows for a long period of learning, but with no sexual competition. Therefore, there is little discord in the group while the juveniles are learning from their parents. Both sexes show an adolescent growth spurt, particularly males (see Figure 15.4).

## HANDLING PRIMATES

Particular care must be taken when handling primates because of the danger of transmitting potentially zoonotic diseases. Appropriate protective clothing must be worn. For quarantine animals, this should include cap, gown, mask, boots and gloves. For other animals, gloves and protective gowns may be sufficient but there will be local safety rules for each institution, which must be followed. These rules will take into account the origin of the animal and the results of health screening.

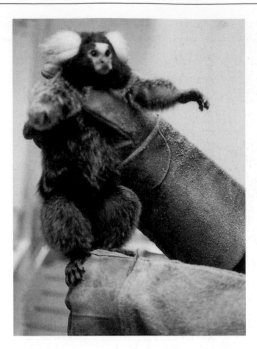

**Figure 15.5**    Holding a conscious marmoset.

Many experimental procedures require gaining access to the individual animal but since primates are smart they can readily be trained to provide researchers with the opportunity to gain access to them, even if they are living in social groups. Training is encouraged by the use of positive reinforcement, which may be in the form of a favourite food or drink that does not form part of their normal diet, so they are not habituated to it. Rhesus monkeys respond very well to being trained to co-operate using voice commands. In the USA, the pole and collar method is often used to handle larger primates. A special plastic collar with two hook holes is fitted around the monkey's neck. The monkey is trained to be caught using a special pole with a trigger-operated hook system. Initially, the animal may struggle as the two poles are used to restrain it, but it eventually gets used to the procedure and becomes compliant. Careful checks must be made to ensure that the collar does not become too tight as the animal grows.

In order to carry out a full examination of a primate it may be necessary to sedate it in order to reduce the risk of injury to the handler, to reduce the stress to the animal and also to enable the examination to be carried out thoroughly to yield the maximum possible information. For smaller primates, such as marmosets, manual restraint may be sufficient (see Figure 15.5), or may be used before then injecting a sedative by an appropriate route, usually intramuscularly (i.m.). Larger primates, such as the rhesus monkey, may need to be sedated prior to handling. A restraint cage may be used for this in which the back is pulled gently forward or the front pushed gently backwards. The animal may also be netted but this is a significant stress factor and most animals will not respond well to this method of capture. Much preferred is to spend time training the monkey to present its hindquarters for injection of seda- tive, which can then be carried out without stress to animal or handler. If a macaque

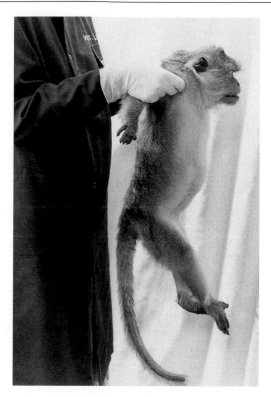

**Figure 15.6**   Holding a sedated macaque.

is sedated, then it should be held by the upper arms, to keep its face away from the handler (see Figure 15.6). Even better is to train the animal for manual capture and restraint as in Figure 15.7.

All primates can and will, on occasion, bite. They are very quick, surprisingly strong and will snatch and grab at such things as earrings, loose clothing and spectacles. Injuries can be prevented by knowledge of the particular species and the individual, and knowledge of the posture and expression of the animal. Primates communicate in a variety of ways with each other, and in the laboratory with humans, using sounds, facial expressions and postural changes. Many messages can be easily interpreted. For example, shaking a tree is a sign of aggression, which translates in a captive environment to rattling the cage. A low-grade threat can be communicated in some primates with a brief 'eyebrow flash' which in humans is an indication of recognition and may form part of ritualised flirting behaviour. Raised eyebrows combined with lip-smacking is used as social appeasement in macaques. Other facial expressions may communicate quite different meaning in non-human primates compared to humans. For example, the grimace, or silent bared-teeth face, indicates uncertainty or submission in many primates, but as a smile in humans can be seen as an expression of friendliness. Figure 15.8 shows a relaxed, but dominant, male monkey yawning as a threat to the cameraman and hence a statement of possession of the females in his group and therefore, indirectly, of his social status.

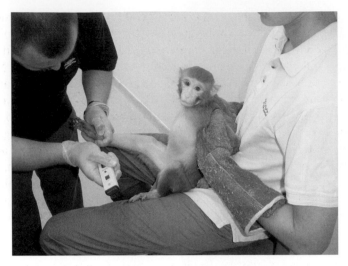

**Figure 15.7**    A rhesus macaque trained to sit while a blood sample is collected by heel prick, requiring only minimal restraint.

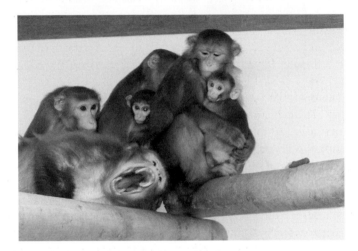

**Figure 15.8**    Exhibition of dominance in rhesus monkey.

## PAIN AND STRESS RECOGNITION

The welfare of primates will be maximised by keeping the animals in good health. This applies not just to their physical health but also to their psychological health. The health should be evaluated regularly, records kept and a programme to review and improve physical and mental health applied where necessary.

### Assessment of physical health

The first step in carrying out a clinical examination to assess the monkey's physical health is simply to observe the animal in its home cage and evaluate its appearance, behaviour and general demeanour. In order to do this it is vital that the observer has some experience of the animal (both the species and that individual) in order to be able to judge whether the animal is exhibiting a normal behavioural repertoire. Just like humans, some individual non-human primates will exhibit behavioural patterns that are specific for that individual, but do not necessarily reflect poor well-being. Note first the monkey's response to your presence. It may appear inquisitive or it may appear frightened or simply non-responsive. It may sit very still but be very aware of your presence and follow your every move with its eyes. A captive-bred macaque should interact well with its human carers and any changes in this behaviour should be investigated further.

Still without entering the cage, it should be possible to evaluate the animal's skin and fur condition. A loss of fur may indicate an underlying skin infection, which could be bacterial or parasitic or may be due to hair pulling. This over-grooming, either by conspecifics or self-inflicted, frequently indicates an inadequacy of the environment causing boredom to the animals. It may also indicate that there is some other stress factor, such as bullying by other animals in the area, which may be in visual or auditory, but not necessarily tactile, contact. A rough estimate of body condition can be evaluated from a distance, as can its ability to walk, run, jump and to use all four limbs without signs of lameness or imbalance. The monkey will usually look at the observer and chatter, which is an opportunity to examine head and eye movements and to look at the condition of the front teeth and nostrils. Note any abnormal discharges or any unevenness or swellings. Remember the cheek pouches in the macaque may be full of food and, therefore, uneven! Check again later to ensure the monkey has emptied them properly. If the monkey turns to present its hindquarters, this will give an opportunity to inspect the external genitalia. A full and careful observation of the animal requires time and patience and should not be hurried. Once this has been carried out, observe the animal's enclosure.

Notice the condition of any substrate material and whether the monkey has had diarrhoea, or indeed has passed any faeces at all. Check for evidence that the monkey has been playing with the substrate and the toys provided and that they do not appear to have been ignored showing that the animal is not, for some reason, exhibiting normal behaviour when you are not there. Check that the animal has food and drink provided and has been taking them. If there are traces of blood around, look to see if the monkey is menstruating; the regular carer should have details of her cycle.

Monkeys will often appear to show little reaction to pain. A monkey in pain will have a generally miserable appearance, and may adopt a huddled position or crouch with head forwards and arms across the body. It will have a 'sad' expression with glassy eyes. It may moan or grunt, and tend to avoid companions. Grooming may stop, and food and drink are usually refused. Ill monkeys may attract extra attention from cage-mates, varying from social grooming to attack. Acute abdominal pain may be shown by facial contortions, clenching of teeth, restlessness and shaking. Vocalisation is more likely to indicate anger than pain. Look at the monkey's companions. Are they all in a similar physical condition or is this one different in some way? A disease problem may be common to the whole group and all the animals may be affected in some way.

After completing the examination from a distance and noting the behavioural responses, only then should you catch the animal in order to look at it more closely. Catching it will markedly affect its behaviour whether or not sedatives are used, which is why it is important to make a full evaluation first, before you disturb it any more than simply by your presence.

## *Quantitative assessment of well-being*

Quantitative assessment of the animal's well-being can be usefully recorded with a general all-purpose clinical score sheet, such as in Figure 4.1. The animal should be reassessed at appropriate intervals in order to monitor its progress and check on the responses to any treatment given or changes in management that have been put in place. Often this type of general score sheet is too general to be sensitive enough to monitor these changes so it is necessary to modify this to provide more specific information. An example used to monitor a monkey with a neurological deficit is given in Figure 15.9. The general score sheet needs to be modified for each condition with which you are dealing, but once in place provides a very good way to monitor the animal. It is especially useful where more than one person is caring for the animal in order to achieve consistency between carers. For monkeys used experimentally, it also enables the setting of a humane end point by marking a score beyond which the animal will be euthanased in order to prevent or reduce suffering. Used in this way the clinical score sheet removes the variation in interpretation of clinical signs, which is frequently found between animal care staff and research staff; and the criteria for intervention are clearly defined before the animal's condition deteriorates.

## COMMON DISEASES AND HEALTH MONITORING

The potential of primates to carry fatal zoonotic diseases should not be underestimated (see Chapter 3, page 51). Captive-bred animals of known health status are less of a risk, and these should now comprise the majority of animals used. In addition, monkeys are susceptible to many diseases carried by humans, such as colds and flu, tuberculosis, measles, mumps, herpes simplex, hepatitis and many others. Therefore, if you are working with monkeys and are developing a cold, it is important to wear a suitable face mask to prevent the infection spreading to the monkeys. If in doubt, do not enter the monkey facility without consulting the Named Veterinary Surgeon (NVS), Named Animal Care and Welfare Officer (NACWO), or the Occupational Health Physician at your establishment. It is important to wear appropriate protective clothing and use good hygiene, to protect us from them, and them from us. Powerhoses promote the formation of aerosols, which may allow transmission of zoonotic diseases; so suitable protective clothing must be worn when operating these.

There are many diseases which should be included in a regular screening programme. *Herpesvirus simiae* (B-virus) can cause a fatal encephalitis in man, and filoviruses (Ebola and Marburg) have been implicated in outbreaks of fatal haemorrhagic fevers. Simian immunodeficiency virus and simian retrovirus D cause AIDS-like syndromes in monkeys, and little is known of their ability to infect man. Some workers have developed antibodies to these viruses, but so far without the development of signs. These should be screened for, as infection in the monkey can affect research as well as posing a risk for personnel.

Tuberculosis causes a chronic fatal disease in monkeys, and can pass from monkey to man and vice versa. This can be screened for using an intradermal skin test, and a common site for this is the skin of the eyelid (see Figure 9.4). The disease in monkeys can remain sub-clinical for 6 months or more, and indeed may be latent until the ani-

**Post Op Cranial Primate Score Sheet**

| Signs | | Score | | | | | | | | |
|---|---|---|---|---|---|---|---|---|---|---|
| | | **Date** | | | | | | | | |
| | | **Time** | | | | | | | | |
| **Signs** | | **Score** | | | | | | | | |
| Movements upon entering room | None | 3 | | | | | | | | |
| | Head only | 2 | | | | | | | | |
| | Walking sluggishly | 1 | | | | | | | | |
| | Normal | 0 | | | | | | | | |
| Head posture upon entering | Head pressing | 2 | | | | | | | | |
| | Lowered | 1 | | | | | | | | |
| | Normal | 0 | | | | | | | | |
| Provoked behaviour | None | 4 | | | | | | | | |
| | Blinking or frowning | 3 | | | | | | | | |
| | Head lifting | 2 | | | | | | | | |
| | Walks sluggishly | 1 | | | | | | | | |
| | Normal | 0 | | | | | | | | |
| Gait | Not moving | 4 | | | | | | | | |
| | Hind leg dragging | 3 | | | | | | | | |
| | Sluggish | 1 | | | | | | | | |
| | Normal | 0 | | | | | | | | |
| Ability to grasp | None | 4 | | | | | | | | |
| | Sluggish | 3 | | | | | | | | |
| | Normal | 0 | | | | | | | | |
| Grooming | No | 3 | | | | | | | | |
| | ≤once over 5 min | 2 | | | | | | | | |
| | Decreased but > once | 1 | | | | | | | | |
| | Normal | 0 | | | | | | | | |
| Wound | Discharge and swollen | 3 | | | | | | | | |
| | Discharge or swollen | 2 | | | | | | | | |
| | Sutures missing | 1 | | | | | | | | |
| | Normal | 0 | | | | | | | | |
| Eating | No | 4 | | | | | | | | |
| | Takes small bits only | 2 | | | | | | | | |
| | Takes larger bits | 1 | | | | | | | | |
| | Normal | 0 | | | | | | | | |
| Water consumption in the last 24 hours | None | 4 | | | | | | | | |
| | None to 50% | 2 | | | | | | | | |
| | >50% | 1 | | | | | | | | |
| | Normal | 0 | | | | | | | | |
| **Total score** | | | | | | | | | | |
| **Initials** | | | | | | | | | | |

Comments:

Total score possible: 31

Action points: more than 6: seek NACWO/NVS advice

Name:                                                                 Date of start of procedure:
PPL No./19b:
PIL Name/Contact:

**Figure 15.9**   Score sheet to monitor a primate with neurological impairment.

mal is terminally ill. To prevent the disease from entering the colony, all new animals should come with a health profile, which indicates they have been screened prior to arrival. Personnel intending to work with monkeys should be given the BCG vaccination or screened regularly for the disease. Any animal that has contacted a known human case should be effectively quarantined for at least 6 months until it is proved not to have contracted the disease.

Animals imported into the UK will need to be subjected to rabies quarantine, and any personnel intending to work with such animals will need to be vaccinated against rabies.

Old World monkeys are susceptible to measles, and may be vaccinated against this at weaning. Some immunology research programmes preclude this, in which case care must be taken that personnel do not bring this disease into the unit. Enteric disease may be caused by a number of factors including pathogenic organisms. Monkeys will pass loose stools if they are frightened, or if there are changes in their environment or diet. Stresses, such as these, can also cause sub-clinical infections to become clinical, so any case of diarrhoea should be investigated to eliminate infectious causes. Zoonoses (such as *Shigella*, *Salmonella*, *Campylobacter* and *Yersinia*) are common bacterial pathogens, and protozoa or helminth parasites may also pose a risk. Some of these organisms can cause explosive outbreaks of disease and death, if not controlled immediately. Regular screening and treatment will reduce the level of infection, and must be combined with strict hygiene and good husbandry to prevent transmission between animals and to personnel.

## Biological data and useful reference data

See Table 15.3.

## DOSES OF DRUGS FOR ANAESTHESIA IN PRIMATES

### Sedation

For smaller primates, such as marmosets, manual restraint may be sufficient to enable an intraperitoneal (i.p.) or i.m. injection of anaesthetic directly. Sedation may only be required in order to facilitate i.v. injection or administration of inhalation agents.

- *Ketamine* (5–25 mg/kg i.m.) is the drug of choice. Lower doses produce heavy sedation. Higher doses produce light anaesthesia. Peak effect is reached in 5–10 min and lasts 30–60 min.
- *Alphaxalone/Alphadolone* (12–18 mg/kg i.m.) is good for small primates, it produces heavy sedation. Additional doses (6–9 mg/kg) i.v. produce surgical anaesthesia. Peak effect is reached 5 min after i.m. injection and lasts 45 minutes. For larger primates the volume that has to be injected is too large for it to be used by this route.
- *Acepromazine* (0.2 mg/kg i.m.) produces sedation but insufficient for safe handling.
- *Diazepam* (1 mg/kg i.m.) also produces insufficient sedation for handling of larger primates.
- *Fentanyl/Fluanisone* (Hypnorm) 0.3 ml/kg i.m or *Fentanyl* 0.05–0.1 mg/kg subcutaneous (s.c.) or i.m. produce heavy sedation and good analgesia.
- *Medetomidine* can be used to produce moderate sedation which can be reversed with atipamezole. Use medetomidine at 50–100 µg/kg i.m.; reverse with atipamezole at 250–500 µg/kg i.m.
- *Atropine* (0.05 mg/kg i.m.) should be given to reduce bradycardia produced by neuroleptanalgesia, and to reduce salivary secretions, especially when ketamine is used.

# General anaesthesia

Primates should be fasted for 8 h prior to general anaesthesia and water withheld for 30 min. Prolonged withholding of water prior to anaesthesia is not necessary and indeed may be detrimental.

## *Injectable agents*

Intravenous (i.v.) injection can be performed in larger primates using the cephalic vein on the anterior forelimb or saphenous vein in the hindlimb. In marmosets, the lateral tail vein can be used. A butterfly needle or flexible over-the-needle cannula is recommended.

- *Alphaxalone/alphadolone* (Saffan) (6–9 mg/kg i.v.) produces good surgical anaesthesia with fairly rapid recovery. Prolonged periods of anaesthesia can be provided by administration of incremental doses every 10–15 min or by continuous i.v. infusion.
- *Propofol* 10 mg/kg i.v. for induction followed by incremental doses or continuous i.v. infusion.
- *Thiopentone* (15–20 mg/kg i.v.) produces 5–10 min of surgical anaesthesia. However, analgesia is poor and recovery from thiopentone will be prolonged in thin animals.
- *Ketamine* (10 mg/kg i.m.) with *xylazine* (0.5 mg/kg i.m.) produces surgical anaesthesia with good muscle relaxation lasting 30–40 min. *Ketamine* (15 mg/kg i.m.) with *diazepam* (1 mg/kg i.m.) or *ketamine* (5–10 mg/kg i.m.) with *medetomidine* (50–100 μg/kg i.m.) has similar effects. The medetomidine can be reversed with atipamezole.

## *Inhalational agents*

All common inhalational agents are suitable (e.g. *isoflurane, halothane*). Usually, anaesthesia is induced by injectable agents, then inhaled agents used for maintenance. For small primates, a face mask may be sufficient; but for larger primates, intubation is recommended. Anaesthesia can be maintained using the volatile agent with oxygen alone, or with nitrous oxide in addition.

# Doses of drugs used for analgesia in primates

## *Opioids*

- *Buprenorphine:* 0.01 mg/kg i.m. or i.v. Analgesia lasts 6–8 h.
- *Butorphanol:* 0.01 mg/kg i.v. lasts 3–4 h.
- *Pentazocine:* 2–5 mg/kg i.m. lasts for 4 h.
- *Pethidine:* 2–4 mg/kg i.m. produces analgesia lasting 2–3 h.
- *Morphine:* 1–2 mg s.c. or i.m. lasts for 4 h.

## NSAIDs

- *Carprofen:* 3–4 mg/kg s.c. daily for 3 days.
- *Naproxen:* 10 mg/kg orally lasts for 12 h.
- *Ketoprofen:* 2 mg/kg s.c. daily.
- *Flunixin:* 0.5–1.0 mg/kg i.m. daily.
- *Aspirin:* 20 mg/kg orally every 6 h.

## FURTHER INFORMATION

Altmann, S.A. (1962). A field study of the sociobiology of rhesus monkeys. *Annals of New York Academy of Science* 102, 338–435.

Bernstein, I.S. (1991). Social housing of monkeys and apes: group formation. *Laboratory Animal Science* 41, 329–33.

EUPREN UK Working Party (Owen, S., Thomas, C., West, P., Wolfensohn, S. and Wood, M.) (1997). Report on primate supply for biomedical scientific work in the UK. *Laboratory Animals* 31, 289–97.

FELASA Working Group on Non-Human Primate Health (Weber, H., Berge, E., Finch, J., Heidt, P., Kaup, F.-J., Perretta, G., Verschere, B. and Wolfensohn, S.) (1999). Health monitoring of non-human primate colonies. *Laboratory Animals* 33, S1: 3–18.

Fortman, J.D., Hewett, T.A. and Taylor Bennett, B. (2002). *The Laboratory Non-human Primate*. CRC Press.

Heath, M. and Libretto, S.E. (1993). Environmental enrichment for large-scale marmoset units. *Animal Technology* 44, 163–73.

Karl, J. and Rothe, H. (1996). Influence of cage size and cage equipment on physiology and behaviour of common marmosets. *Laboratory Primate Newsletter* 35, 10–14.

Kirkwood, J.K. and Stathatos, K. (1992). *Biology, Rearing and Care of Young Primates*. Oxford University Press.

Lindburg, D.G. (1991). Ecological requirements of macaques. *Laboratory Animal Science* 41, 315–22.

Luttrell, L., Acker, L., Urben, M. and Reinhardt, V. (1994). Training a large troop of rhesus macaques to cooperate during catching: analysis of the time investment. *Animal Welfare* 3, 135–40. http://www.awionline.org/Lab_animals/biblio/aw5train.htm

Mason, W.A. (1991). Effects of social interaction on well being: developmental aspects. *Laboratory Animal Science* 41, 323–28.

Napier, J.R. and Napier, P.H. (1985). *The Natural History of the Non-human Primates*. Cambridge University Press.

National Research Council (1997). *The Psychological Well-being of Non-human Primates*. National Academy Press. ISBN 0-309-05233-5.

Novak, M.A. and Suomi, S.J. (1991). Social interaction in non-human primates: an underlying theme for primate research. *Laboratory Animal Science* 41, 308–14.

Reinhardt, V. and Reinhardt, A. (2000). Social enhancement for adult non-human primates in research laboratories. *Lab Animal* 29, 34–41.

Reinhardt, V. and Seelig, D. (1998). *Environmental Enhancement for Caged Rhesus Macaques: A Photographic Documentation*. Animal Welfare Institute, Washington DC.

Reinhardt, V. (1990). Avoiding undue stress: catching individual animals in groups of rhesus monkeys. *Lab Animal* 19(6), 52–53. http://www.awionline.org/Lab_animals/biblio/la-avoid.htm

Reinhardt, V. (1990). *Catching Individual Rhesus Monkeys Living in Captive Groups* (Videotape with commentary). Wisconsin Regional Primate Research Center. Available on loan from Animal Care Audio-Visual Materials, WRPRC, 1220 Capitol Court, Madison, WI 53715, USA.

Roberts, R.L., Roytburd, L.A. and Newman, J.D. (1999). Puzzle feeders and gum feeders as environmental enrichment for common marmosets. *Contemporary Topics in Laboratory Animal Science* 38, 27–31.

Taylor Bennett, B., Abee, C.R. and Henrickson, R. (eds.) (1995). *Non-human Primates in Biomedical Research: Biology and Management*. American College of Laboratory Animal Medicine Series.

Wolfensohn, S.E. and Gopal, R. (2001). Interpretation of serological test results for Simian herpes B virus. *Laboratory Animals* 35, 315–20.

Wolfensohn, S.E. (1998). *Shigella* infection in macaque colonies: Case report of an eradication and control program. *Laboratory Animal Science* 48, 330–33.

Wolfensohn, S.E. (1997). Brief review of scientific studies of the welfare implications of transporting primates. *Laboratory Animals* 31, 303–305.

Wolfensohn, S.E. (1993). The use of microchip implants in identification of two species of macaque. *Animal Welfare* 2, 353–59.

# WEBSITE

CITES: www.cites.org.CITES/eng/what-is.shtml

# Chapter 16
# The larger domestic species

The larger domestic species used in research have all been domesticated for many thousands of years. The farm animal species (pigs, sheep, goats and cattle) belong to the order Artiodactyla (even-toed ungulates), while horses belong to the order Perissodactyla (odd-toed ungulates):

| Order | Family | Species |
|---|---|---|
| Artiodactyla | Bovidae | *Ovis aries* (Sheep) |
| | | *Capra hircus* (Goats) |
| | | *Bos taurus* (Cattle) |
| | Suidae | *Sus scrofa* (Swine) |
| Perissodactyla | Equidae | *Equus caballus* (Horses) |

## SUPPLY

With the exception of pigs and sheep that have been genetically modified, none of these species are included under Schedule 2 to the Animals (Scientific Procedures) Act (ASPA) 1996. Consequently, research establishments are free to purchase these animals from any source. The usual suppliers of farm animals for research in the UK are:

- *Specialist laboratory animal suppliers*: Some maintain mini-pig colonies of a defined type and known health status. However, these companies do not supply other farm animals in the UK.
- *Commercial pig-breeding companies*: These companies are the best source of standard pigs for research, as they generally have high health and welfare standards.
- *Individual farmers*: Local farmers can be good sources of the farm-animal species, but the health status of their stock will be variable and some may be reluctant to sell their animals for research.
- *Other research organisations*: Some larger UK research institutes maintain farms and sell animals surplus to their own requirements.
- *Markets and dealers*: These are generally a poor source of experimental animals, as they will be derived from a number of different farms with no medical or husbandry history. It is advised to purchase from a dealer only as a last resort.

The farm-animal species have several disadvantages when compared with the smaller laboratory species. First, they are an outbred population, with many different breeds and many cross breeds. Secondly, all of the species have gestation periods measured in months and not in days. Lastly, with the exception of pigs, they also have very small litter sizes. These factors make it extremely difficult to source large numbers of animals that are matched for breed, sex and age.

## Quarantine

In nearly all cases, farm animals are reared under conventional farm conditions and the husbandry and health of such animals can be extremely variable. The maxim 'caveat emptor' (buyer beware) applies. Whenever it is practicable, veterinary inspection and health screening of the animals should be undertaken on the farm of origin before transport to the research facility. Even if the health status of the animals is known, it is still advisable to isolate all animals on arrival for a period of at least 4 weeks. The following general rules should be observed whenever possible:

1. Purchase from as few sources as possible and as infrequently as possible.
2. Confirm that the source herd is free of pathogens of significance for that species.
3. Isolate incoming stock for as long as possible (4–6 weeks optimum).
4. During isolation, medicate for endemic pathogens, such as ecto- and endoparasites.
5. Screen for pathogens of significance at the end of isolation period.

## Biosecurity

To maintain the health status of an established large-animal facility, it is essential to impose a continuing high level of biosecurity. The following procedures are advised:

- Visitors should be kept to the absolute minimum and should not enter within 48 h of same species contact. A full change of protective clothing should be provided before entering the unit and wet-showering is often mandatory for high health status pig units.
- Use feed, bedding and equipment only from animal-free sources.
- Loading and unloading procedures must be strict. All livestock vehicles are a risk.
- The proximity of other animal units and major roads should be considered. Some airborne pathogens can be carried for several kilometres.

## PIGS

The various breeds of domestic pig are originally derived from the European wild pig, *Sus scrofa*, probably crossed with fast growing Asiatic pigs, such as *Sus vittatus* and *Sus indicus*. Pure breeds include the Large White and the Landrace, but the majority of breeding sows are now hybrids, produced by a small number of large pig-breeding companies. These sows can weigh up to 250 kg and have been developed for high fecundity and the rapid growth of their offspring for pork or bacon production. All commercial pig-breeding companies have pig herds free from significant disease, or at least of a well-defined health status, and pigs for research are best purchased from one of these companies.

*Miniature (mini-) pigs* are much smaller. Sows of the Yucatan and Göttingen mini-pig breeds only reach 50–70 kg adult weights. They are, therefore, easier to house and manage in a laboratory environment. Mini-pigs are available from some specialised suppliers of laboratory animals.

## Behaviour

Pigs are lively, intelligent, gregarious animals that are usually docile, although newly farrowed sows can be very protective of their litters and adult boars should always be treated with caution. They should be group housed wherever possible, and in a stable group they will develop a dominance hierarchy. If unfamiliar animals are placed together, they will normally fight and individual pigs must never be added to a stable group, as they will certainly be bullied and may be killed. It is always best to start with large groups and split these down in numbers as they grow. However, if mixing is unavoidable, then it is better to carry this out on neutral territory at feeding time or at dusk. Tranquillisers (e.g. azaperone) may be used in extreme cases.

Pigs rapidly become bored, and a barren environment will lead to stereotypic behaviour patterns, such as ear or tail biting, flank sucking or bar-biting. These vices may be minimised by environmental enrichment in the pen. Pigs have a very keen sense of smell and also well-developed rooting behaviour, hence their use to find truffles. If housed outside, they will rapidly turn a pasture into a mud bath by rooting for worms.

## Housing

Pigs may be kept outdoors, housed in simple arc-shaped huts with lots of straw bedding. However, such systems require free draining soil and light stocking densities (12–22 sows/ha) and management and handling difficulties make outdoor systems unlikely to be suitable for most pigs kept for research purposes.

The majority of pigs used in research are kept indoors, either in naturally ventilated or controlled environment buildings. There are many different designs of indoor accommodation for pigs, depending principally on their age. Careful design of pig housing encourages cleanliness, as will the provision of suitable bedding. Contrary to popular belief, pigs are naturally clean animals, and if provided with sufficient space will defecate only in the coolest, wettest areas, which can then be scraped out or hosed down daily, leaving their bedding area clean and dry. The lying area of the pen should be solid and insulated. It should preferably have bedding, such as sawdust, shavings or straw, to provide warmth, comfort and a substrate for rooting. Straw will be chewed and played with by the pig, aiding digestion and reducing boredom. If no bedding is provided, the ambient temperature must be higher and it is likely that more leg injuries will occur. The part of the floor where the pigs are fed and watered should remain unbedded, and the pigs will use this area for defecating. This can then be cleaned daily, without disturbing the lying area. It is possible to use a slatted area for this, but the design of slats is critical to avoid leg lesions. The specifications for slatted floors for pigs are now covered by European legislation protecting welfare.

Farrowing sows require special accommodation. There is a huge size difference between the sow and her piglets, and with litters of up to 16, it is not uncommon for a sow to inadvertently lie on one or more of her piglets. Devices, such as farrowing crates, have been designed to reduce this risk and may be used to house the sow until the piglets are weaned at 3 weeks of age. Newborn piglets require a temperature of 30–32°C, whereas the sow prefers a temperature of 18°C or lower. By restraining the sow in a farrowing crate, a heated 'creep' area can be provided within the pen for the litter. This should contain a heat lamp or heat pad and a creep feeder (see Figure 16.1).

## Feeding

Pigs are omnivorous single-stomached animals and will, therefore, eat a variety of foods. The vast majority of pigs are fed commercial diets, manufactured from ground cereals with added soya and/or fishmeal protein, vitamin and mineral supplements. These diets vary according to the age and physiological requirements of the pig. Young pigs are normally fed high-protein pellets ad lib from a hopper, whereas growing and adult pigs are fed restricted amounts of lower protein nuts or cobs in troughs. Pigs may also be fed directly from the floor in a clean environment, which has the benefit of allowing them to express natural rooting behaviour (see Figure 16.2). The concentrate food may also be purchased as a finely ground, unpelleted meal and fed with water in troughs as a gruel.

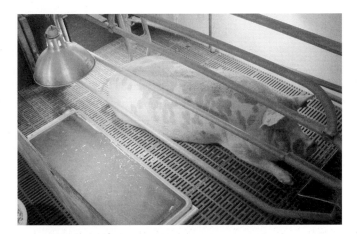

**Figure 16.1**   Sow in farrowing crate.

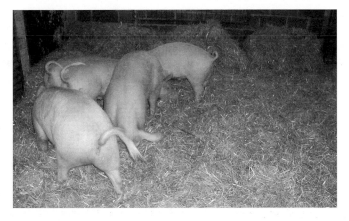

**Figure 16.2**   Pig rooting in substrate.

Pregnant sows require a ration containing 12–14% crude protein and will eat 1.8–2.3 kg daily, rising to 2.7 kg immediately before farrowing (more, if kept outside). Lactating sows should receive a 16–18% protein ration and may eat up to 10 kg daily. Piglets will begin to eat creep feed from 10 days of age, but it must be fresh to be palatable. Only offer small amounts to start with and clean out uneaten food daily. Creep feed usually has a protein level of over 20%. Following weaning at 3 weeks of age, creep continues to be fed ad lib until the piglets reach about 6 weeks. After this, lower-protein feeds are normally given ad lib until 12 weeks, following which the feed intake is restricted to improve the lean : fat ratio.

*Mini-pigs* have not been selected for any of the production characteristics of commercial hybrids (rapid growth, high lean : fat ratio and high fecundity) and, therefore, have different feed requirements, both in terms of quantity and quality. In particular, they are prone to excess fat and care must be taken not to overfeed them. Special commercial diets for mini-pigs are available.

# Water

Water is particularly important for pigs, and must be available at all times. *Water deprivation, even for short periods will cause a rapid increase in blood sodium levels (salt poisoning), which can be fatal.* Automatic watering systems are best as they provide ad lib water. This may be delivered in troughs or bowls (which tend to be dirty) or nipple drinkers (which are much cleaner). Troughs and drinkers need to be above ground to prevent contamination with faecal matter. Buckets and loose troughs are not suitable for pigs as they play with them and soon knock them over. As a general rule, adult pigs require 1 l/10 kg/day, while growing pigs and lactating sows need up to twice this amount. However, these figures are heavily dependent on temperature and feed, so ad lib water should always be provided.

# Environment

## *Temperature*

Pigs have very few sweat glands and find it difficult to lose heat in hot weather, leading to heat stress, which can often be fatal. The principal cooling mechanism available to pigs is evaporative heat loss, so outdoor pigs should always be provided with muddy wallows. Shade is also essential to prevent sunburn, which can be common in the summer months. Even indoor facilities without a cooling plant may find it difficult to prevent over-heating in the height of summer. In these buildings, cold water from a hose should be sprayed over the pigs if they show signs of heat stress. This can also be viewed as a form of environmental enrichment, as pigs love to play under a shower of cool water.

Although pigs have only a sparse hair covering, their subcutaneous (s.c.) fat deposits help them to keep warm. The optimum temperature for adults is 16°C, which is easily achieved providing the accommodation is well insulated and they have deep-straw bedding and shelter from draughts. Pigs kept outdoors can live and breed

**Table 16.1**  Temperature requirements for pigs (°C).

| | |
|---|---|
| Birth to weaning | 28–32 |
| At 20 kg | 22–24 |
| At 40 kg | 20 |
| At 60 kg | 18 |
| Over 80 kg | 16 |

perfectly well throughout the UK winter, providing they have a straw-filled hut to give warmth and shelter.

Piglets have a high surface area to body weight ratio and so need high ambient temperatures for the first few weeks of life. The ambient temperature should gradually be reduced as the pigs age, as shown in Table 16.1.

## Humidity

This should preferably be kept between 45% and 65%. However, adequate ventilation must be supplied to reduce the levels of ammonia and pathogens in the air and to dissipate the large amount of heat produced by the pigs. Air speed in lying areas should not exceed 0.2–0.3 m/s for adults and 0.1 m/s for piglets, or excessive cooling occurs.

## Environmental enrichment

Pigs easily become bored and develop stereotypic behaviours when confined in pens. It is mandatory under UK welfare legislation to provide some environmental enrichment for indoor pigs and a number of different devices are commercially available. These include heavy-duty plastic footballs, suspended chains, and a variety of plastic playthings. 'Feed-balls' are available, which distribute the daily feed ration only if the pig rolls the ball, which encourages activity and exploratory behaviour. Cheap but effective enrichment can be obtained by throwing empty feed-bags into the pen, when the pigs will spend some time tearing them to shreds. Pigs should be group housed where possible, but stable groups are essential to stop fighting. The provision of deep bedding encourages rooting behaviour. In hot weather, a cool shower from a hose tied high above a corner of the pen can provide entertainment and prevent heat stress.

## Breeding

Pigs are prolific breeders and will breed all year round, although they generally breed less well from May to September in the northern hemisphere. Large White pigs reach puberty at around 6 months of age and are normally bred from 8 months (180 kg). Maiden gilts can be triggered into oestrus by boar contact from 160 days of age. The oestrous cycle lasts 19–23 days (average 21). Sows normally return to oestrous 4–7 days following weaning, which takes place after 3–5 weeks lactation. Oestrus can be detected by pressing down on the sow's back – the 'back pressure test' – when she will stand to be mounted if in 'heat'. Other signs of oestrous are vulval swelling and vocalisation. Pregnancy may be confirmed by ultrasound scanning from 21 days or by the Doppler foetometer from 28 days. Pregnant sows are normally group housed until 7 days before farrowing, when they are moved to farrowing crates. Gestation lasts 114 days (3 months, 3 weeks, 3 days), and litter sizes vary between 3 and 18 piglets (average 10.5), dependent on the breed and age of the sow. Litter sizes are maximal for the fifth, sixth and seventh litters, then decline. Prolific commercial sows can produce up to 2.4 litters/year, and rear over 25 piglets/year.

*Mini-pigs* reach puberty at about 4 months of age and have an oestrous cycle of 19–20 days. They have smaller litters (average five) and the piglets seldom weigh more than 500 g. Weaning tends to be later (5–6 weeks). The inbred nature of these pigs, coupled with their tendency to become overweight, can lead to infertility problems.

## Growth

As with all farm animals, it is important for piglets to suck colostrum from the sow within 24 h, as no antibodies cross the placenta, and intestinal closure takes place after 24 h. If piglets are colostrum deprived, they gain no maternal immunity and are prone to diarrhoea and other diseases. Piglets are born with minimal body fat reserves, and need to suck frequently in the first 48 h of life to prevent the development of hypoglycaemia. Piglets born indoors, without access to soil, are prone to develop iron-deficiency anaemia, and should receive a single injection of an iron preparation within the first few days of life. The offspring of commercial hybrids grow very rapidly and should weigh 6–7 kg when weaned at 3–4 weeks. Daily weight gain following weaning is highly dependent on feeding and genotype, but can reach as much as 1 kg/day.

*Mini-pigs* have similar requirements as standard pigs, but obviously grow more slowly and only reach 50 kg by about 12 months of age.

## Handling

Pigs are easily startled and so should always be approached patiently and quietly. Any attempts at restraining or handling pigs are usually accompanied by loud squealing, which ceases only when the hold is released. Force should not be used to move pigs, since this will alarm them and cause them to become noisy, obstinate and dangerous. However, they are curious animals and will naturally explore their environment. This can be exploited since they will move along passages quite freely, and a rigid pig-board can be used to guide them, as pigs will turn away from solid surfaces (see Figure 16.3). Large pigs may be guided into a crate, or if this is not available, they can be restrained by using a rope snare (snatch), placed around the upper jaw, caudal to the canines. The pig pulls away from the snatch, causing the rope to tighten over the nose. Small piglets may be picked up, providing the abdomen is always supported. They should not be picked up by the hind legs alone. Larger piglets can be tucked under

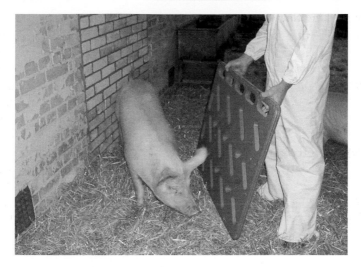

**Figure 16.3**   Moving a pig using a pig board.

one arm with the weight supported by the other arm placed under the belly. A foreleg can be held to provide additional restraint.

## Pain and stress recognition

Pigs in pain will show a decrease in their normal inquisitive behaviour, becoming listless and quiet, although they may show aggression on being handled. In white pigs, the skin may show marked colour changes (pallor or cyanosis) and there may be pilo-erection of the sparse hair coat. In a group, the sick pig will fail to thrive and may develop abnormal behaviour patterns, such as urine sucking.

## Common diseases and health monitoring

Pigs are prone to a number of diseases (Table 16.2), some of which are notifiable under the Animal Health Act 1981. The notifiable diseases include swine fever and foot and mouth disease, both of which were isolated in the UK in 2000–2001.

### *Zoonoses*

Many pig herds have sub-clinical infections of exotic *Salmonella* species, usually acquired through contaminated feedstuffs or birds. National Salmonella monitoring is now being conducted on pigs at abattoirs in an attempt to identify problem farms. It is sensible to obtain pigs from clean suppliers when these can be identified. In any event, faecal swabbing and culture for Salmonella should be undertaken in isolation facilities before studies are commenced. Meningitis caused by *Strepococcus suis* Type 2, can be seen in post-weaning pigs of 10–50 kg. *S. suis* Type 2 is classified as a zoonotic organism, although transmission to humans is rare. *Erysipelothrix rhusiopathiae* is a common cause of systemic disease in pigs. This organism can also cause a skin disease in man and care should be taken to cover and disinfect any wounds after contact with pigs.

**Table 16.2**    Diseases of pigs.

**Zoonoses**
*Salmonella* species
*Streptococcus suis* Type 2 (meningitis)
Influenza virus (swine influenza)

**Respiratory**
*\*Mycoplasma hyopneumonia* (EP – enzootic pneumonia)
*\*Actinobacillus pleuropneumoniae* (APP)
*Toxigenic *Pasteurella multocida* (AR – atrophic rhinitis)

**Enteric**
*Brachyspira hyodysenteriae* (swine dysentery)
*\*Clostridium* species
*\*E. coli*
Enteric coronavirus (TGE – transmissible gastroenteritis)

**Reproductive**
*Porcine parvovirus
*Porcine reproductive and respiratory syndrome (PRRS)
*Leptospira* species

**Other**
*\*Erysipelothrix rhusiopathiae* (erysipelas)
*\*Haemophilus parasuis*
Part-weaning multisystemic wasting syndrome (PMWS)
Mange (*Sarcoptes scabiei*)

*Vaccines licensed for use in pigs.

Swine influenza virus is closely linked to human influenza and has been recorded on occasions in humans.

## *Other conditions affecting research*

There are many infectious diseases that may affect the health of experimental pigs. Respiratory conditions are common and there are a number of pathogens of importance. It is essential to source pigs free of these organisms as well as the major enteric diseases, such as swine dysentery (*Brachyspira hyodysenteriae*). Macro endoparasites are not usually important in pigs, unless they have been reared outdoors, but ectoparasites, such as mange and lice, can be troublesome. Of particular note is a relatively new disease, Post-weaning multisystemic wasting syndrome (PMWS). This condition is seen in growing pigs of 10 weeks or older and is caused by *Circovirus* 2. It produces severe immunosuppression, with the result that sub-clinical diseases due to a range of pathogens manifest as clinical entities. *Circovirus* 2 infections have now become widespread in pig herds in the UK and mortality can be high in some herds. Sourcing pigs free of PMWS is currently very difficult.

Purchasing from sources of defined health status and applying rigid biosecurity measures will control most pig diseases. Providing the rules given in the introduction to this chapter are observed, a high health status for experimental pigs can be maintained.

# Anaesthesia in the pig

Anaesthesia in the pig is generally straightforward, but there are some unusual features that must be borne in mind:

1. They have a large covering of s.c. fat and care must be taken when giving intra-muscular (i.m.) injections that the agent is not injected into this. If so, absorption of the drug will be delayed and the expected effect will not be achieved. The usual site for i.m. injections is the musculature of the neck and an 18 G, 40-mm needle should be used in adult pigs. For ease of administration, the needle may be attached to the syringe by a long, flexible extension line to avoid the need for prolonged restraint.
2. Pigs lack easily accessible superficial veins and so intravenous (i.v.) injections may be problematical, especially in very small piglets. The marginal vein of the ear is the usual route of administration, the jugular vein being too deep in the pig to be certain that the needle is correctly placed. Local anaesthetic cream (e.g. EMLA, Astra) can be applied over the site of the ear vein for 45 min to provide desensi-tisation of the area. Less pain is caused if flexible cannulae are used in preference to rigid needles.
3. Respiratory depression and/or apnoea are common complications of surgical anaesthesia in the adult pig, especially if it is very fat. The head should be kept at as natural an angle as possible to prevent pressure on the larynx. If the pig is not intubated, it is essential to ensure that the airway is kept clear and laryngospasm is prevented. Applying pressure on the vertical ramus of the mandible, to push the jaw forward, and extruding the tongue will help to prevent obstruction. Adminis-tration of atropine (0.3–2.4 mg depending on the size of the pig) to dry secretions will also help.
4. Endotracheal intubation can be difficult in large pigs and a larnygoscope with a very long blade is required to visualise the larynx. The pig trachea is narrower than might be expected for an animal of its size and there is a pharyngeal diverticulum, which can cause confusion. An endotracheal tube size 8–10 is usually adequate for even the largest sow. The tube needs to be long and a rigid stylet is usually helpful.
5. Pigs have poor thermoregulation and can develop hyperthermia during prolonged anaesthesia. Some strains of pig also have an inherited biochemical myopathy known as porcine malignant hyperthermia. In these pigs, when anaesthesia is induced, a contracture of the muscles occurs, the pig becomes rigid and its tem-perature starts to rise. The strains affected are Poland–China, Pietrain and some lines of Landrace and Large White. However, genotyping has allowed breeding companies to select against this trait and they will normally be able to supply pigs free of this condition if requested.
6. Food should be withheld for 8–12 h before anaesthesia to prevent vomiting (1–3 h in neonates). Water must be available at all times up until the anaesthetic is given.

## *Sedation*

*Azaperone* (Stresnil), a butyrophenone, neuroleptic sedative, is the agent of choice and the only sedative licensed for use in pigs in the UK. *Azaperone* must be given strictly by i.m. injection behind the ear, using a 40-mm (1½ in.) needle. The dose is 1–2 mg/kg, with the higher doses used on more nervous or excitable individuals. Leave the pig undisturbed for 20 min following the injection or excitement may be provoked. *Azaperone* has no adverse effects on parturition, lactation, mothering instinct or food intake, but causes mild vasodilation and a slight fall in blood pressure.

Other (unlicensed) sedatives are *diazepam* (2.0 mg/kg i.m.) or *acepromazine* (0.1 mg/kg i.m.), or a combination of *droperidol* (0. 5 mg/kg) with *midazolam* (0.3 mg/kg).

## General anaesthesia

The most satisfactory method of inducing anaesthesia is the i.v. administration of an injectable agent to an already tranquillised pig. There are many anaesthetic agents available, although none of these are licensed for use in pigs.

## Injectable agents

- *Alphaxalone/alphadolone* (Saffan) is the injectable anaesthetic agent of choice for all ages of pig. Following *azaperone* sedation, a dose rate of 2 mg/kg (1 ml/6 kg) i.v., will give surgical anaesthesia for 10–15 min. For maintenance, the animal can be intubated and connected to a gaseous anaesthetic circuit. For short surgical procedures, or where gaseous anaesthesia is unavailable, incremental doses can be given. There is minimal respiratory depression with good muscle relaxation and recovery is smooth, provided that premedication has been used.
- *Propofol* can be used for induction of anaesthesia at 2.5–3.5 mg/kg i.v., but its duration of action is short. To maintain anaesthesia it may be infused i.v. at 8–9 mg/kg/h (4–8 mg/kg/h if premedicated). Significant respiration depression can occur and intubation and oxygen supplementation are advisable.
- *Thiopentone* is satisfactory for induction of anaesthesia, prior to intubation. Give 7.5 mg/kg of a 2.5% solution i.v. (4 mg/kg if a premedicant has been given). Incremental doses are cumulative and will result in prolonged recovery times.
- *Ketamine combinations* can produce satisfactory anaesthesia in pigs. Give 1 mg/kg xylazine i.m., followed 10 min later by 2–5 mg/kg ketamine i.v.

## Inhalation agents

The volatile agents, isoflurane, halothane and sevoflurane are all excellent agents for maintaining anaesthesia in pigs. Depending on the size of pig, a Bains, Magill or circle absorber should be used. For further details of these agents and anaesthetic circuits see Chapter 7.

## Doses of drugs for analgesia in the pig

### Opioids (none licensed for pigs in the UK)

- *Buprenorphine*: 0.005–0.02 mg/kg i.m. or i.v. – give 6–12 hourly.
- *Morphine*: 0. 2 mg/kg i.m. – give 4 hourly up to a maximum of 20 mg.

- *Pentazocine*: 2 mg/kg i.m. – give 4 hourly.
- *Pethidine*: 2 mg/kg i.m. – give 2–4 hourly up to a maximum of 1 g in large pigs.

### NSAIDs (licensed for pigs in the UK)

- *Ketoprofen*: 3 mg/kg i.m. – give daily
- *Tolfenamic acid*: 2 mg/kg i.m. – give once only. Will last for 72 h.

### NSAIDs (not licensed for pigs in the UK)

- *Flunixin*: 1 mg/kg s.c. – give daily.
- *Carprofen*: 1–2 mg/kg s.c. – give daily.
- *Asprin*: 10–20 mg/kg post operatively give 4 hourly.

## Useful data

For useful data see Table 16.3.

# RUMINANTS

Ruminants are kept worldwide for their meat, milk, skins and wool (sheep) or hair (goats). The ruminants most commonly used for experimental studies are sheep, goats and cattle. These are all members of the family *Bovidae* and have many anatomical, physiological and behavioural features in common.

## The ruminant digestive tract

All ruminants are herbivores and their digestive tracts have adapted to a diet of vegetable matter in a number of ways. They have no upper incisor teeth, but in their place possess a hard, ridged fibrous 'dental pad', against which the lower incisors bite. They have no canine teeth, leaving a gap, the diastema, between the lower incisors and the molar arcades. The molars are growing continuously and adapted for grinding fibrous food. The jaw is articulated to allow movement from side to side for efficient chewing.

The non-glandular fore-stomach has developed into three large chambers, the reticulum, the rumen and the omasum. The rumen and reticulum contain bacteria that digest cellulose, releasing fatty acids. Some of the rumen microflora also produce vitamins. Food from the rumen is regurgitated several times for extra chewing, in a process known as rumination. A side effect of the breakdown of cellulose is the production of large quantities of methane gas. This has to be removed from the rumen by frequent belching (eructation), which may occur as often as once every minute. If ruminants cannot release the gas produced (for instance, because of an oesophageal blockage or frothy rumen contents), the methane will accumulate to distend the rumen (bloat). In severe cases, the pressure of the distended rumen will cause circulatory disturbances and, unless relieved, death.

Food eventually passes from the rumen, through the omasum, which absorbs much of the fluid, to enter the abomasum, which is analogous to the true glandular stomach

**Table 16.3**  Useful data: pigs.

| | Large White | Yucatan |
|---|---|---|
| ***Biological data*** | | |
| Adult weight (kg) | 220–250 | 70–80 |
| Food intake | Needs vary with production status | |
| Water intake | 1 l/10 kg | |
| Natural lifespan (years) | 16–18 | 8 |
| Temperature (°C) | 38.7–39.7 | 38.7–39.7 |
| Heart rate/min | 50–100 | 50–100 |
| Blood pressure systole (mmHg) | 150 | 150 |
| Blood volume (ml/kg) | 56–69 | 56–69 |
| Respiratory rate/min | 10–16 | 10–16 |
| | | |
| ***Breeding data*** | | |
| Age at puberty (months) | 5–9 (average 7) | 4 |
| Age to breed | Male 9 months, female after third oestrus | Male 5 months, female 5 months |
| Gestation (days) | 113–115 (average 114) | 113–114 |
| Litter size | 8–12 | 6 |
| Birth weight (kg) | 1.3 | 0.56 |
| Weaning age | 3 weeks | 5 weeks |
| Oestrous cycle | 19–23 days (average 21) | 19.5 days |
| | | |
| ***Haematological data*** | | |
| RBC ($\times 10^6$/mm$^3$) | 5–7 | 5–10 |
| PCV (%) | 32–45 | 22–40 |
| Hb (g/dl) | 10–16 | As large white |
| WBC ($\times 10^3$/mm$^3$) | 7–20 | 4–10 |
| Neutrophils (%) | 30–50 | As large white |
| Lymphocytes (%) | 40–60 | As large white |
| Eosinophils (%) | 0–10 | As large white |
| Monocytes (%) | 2–10 | As large white |
| Basophils (%) | 0–1 | As large white |
| Platelets ($\times 10^3$/mm$^3$) | 350–700 | As large white |
| | | |
| ***Biochemical data*** | | |
| (for Yucatan and Large White) | | |
| Serum protein (g/dl) | 6–8.9 | |
| Albumin (g/dl) | 1.6–3.8 | |
| Globulin (g/dl) | 5.2–6.4 | |
| Glucose (mg/dl) | 100–500 | |
| Blood urea nitrogen (ml/dl) | 10–30 | |
| Creatinine (mg/dl) | 1–2.7 | |
| Total bilirubin (mg/dl) | 0–0.6 | |
| Cholesterol (mg/dl) | 36–54 | |

of other mammals. It is in the abomasum that absorption of nutrients takes place. In young animals the rumen is undeveloped and milk passes via a muscular groove (the oesophageal groove) to enter the abomasum directly, where it is digested. The rumen gradually develops in response to the ingestion of roughage, and is fully functional by about 8 weeks of age. All ruminants produce copious quantities of saliva. Vomiting does not occur in ruminants, but drooling and spillage of regurgitated rumenal contents may be seen.

## Housing

Ruminants are able to adapt to a number of different types of housing. They may be kept outdoors at pasture, or in covered or semi-covered yards, or in totally enclosed accommodation, which may or may not be environmentally controlled.

For ruminants kept outdoors, the fences must be robust and free of sharp projections that may cause injury. The enclosures should have protection from extremes of temperature, shade from the sun and shelter from wind and rain. Although outdoor housing has many advantages, it should be remembered that parasite control programmes will be necessary and such animals will be more liable to predator attack (from dogs or foxes) than those housed indoors.

For ruminants kept indoors, the walls and doors of the accommodation should be non-porous and easy to clean. The lying area must have a solid floor, which is usually of concrete, although in outdoor yards rammed chalk may be used, which gives better drainage. Bedding should preferably be deep straw to provide insulation and comfort, although under certain circumstances, wood shavings, sawdust or sand may be alternatives. Fresh clean, dry bedding should be added on a regular basis, until the height of the bed requires its removal. The pen should then be washed down and allowed to dry before re-bedding. Ruminants fed on silage will produce more urine and, therefore, require more straw, than those fed on hay. Part of the floor area (up to 20%) may be slatted with concrete, wooden or composite slats. These areas require no bedding and are, therefore, easy to keep clean. However, they are generally less welfare friendly to the animals. Specialist advice should be sought on the design of slatted floors for each species.

Male animals are usually housed separately from the females, although they should always be within sight and sound of other farm animals. Horned animals should not be close housed with polled animals.

## Feeding

Ruminants are normally fed on grass, or in the winter on conserved forage crops, such as hay, silage or straw. They need long-fibre roughage for efficient rumination, but under certain conditions (such as pregnancy and lactation), may require supplementation of the diet with higher energy foods. These are termed 'concentrate foods', because the energy and protein are concentrated into relatively low volumes. Concentrates are normally based on cereal products, such as wheat and barley, with an additional protein source, such as soya, together with added vitamins and minerals. If ruminants are kept indoors throughout the year, roughage should be permanently available in racks. If concentrate rations are fed, there must be sufficient room at the feed trough for all animals in the pen to feed at the same time. Where horned animals are kept, additional space allowance must be made at the feed troughs to avoid injuries.

# Behaviour

All ruminants are social animals and should, therefore, be housed in groups wherever possible. If individual housing is necessary for experimental reasons, they should always be within sight and sound of conspecifics. All ruminants are prey species and adapted to flight. However, entire males and females with young may be aggressive to humans, and adult bulls in particular cause several human deaths in the UK every year.

# Anaesthesia

There are a number of difficulties with general anaesthesia in ruminants and these, together with the placid and stoical nature of the species, have led to the widespread use of local anaesthetic techniques. Nonetheless, there are some procedures that require general anaesthesia and these difficulties must then be addressed. Note that the particular problems described below relate to adult ruminants only. Young ruminants below 8 weeks (before the development of the rumen) can usually be treated as if possessing a single stomach.

- *Pre-anaesthetic starvation*: Ruminants may generally be fed and watered up until 12 h before anaesthesia. Withholding food for longer periods has little effect on the volume of rumen contents, but may reduce the amount of gas produced, particularly if the animal has been out at grass.
- *Salivation*: All ruminants produce copious quantities of saliva. Under anaesthesia, this may pool in the mouth and once the swallowing reflex has been abolished, may be inhaled. It is always advisable to intubate ruminants and also to make sure that the head is lowered so that saliva may drain freely out of the mouth, to reduce this risk. The use of atropine is generally contraindicated in ruminants, as it renders salivary and bronchial secretions more viscous and harder to clear.
- *Regurgitation*: Regurgitation of rumen contents is always possible, making it essential that animals are intubated with a cuffed endotracheal tube as soon as anaesthesia is induced.
- *Bloat*: Microbial activity in the rumen continues throughout anaesthesia, leading to a build-up of gases. In lateral or dorsal recumbence, when eructation is impossible, the rumen will distend, leading to bloat. For prolonged anaesthesia, passing a stomach tube for the duration of the procedure will prevent this. If a stomach tube is passed, it is advisable to collect the rumenal contents into a bucket to prevent contamination of the operating theatre floor.
- *Rumen weight*: If ruminants are held on their back for long periods, the weight of the rumen will compress the posterior vena cava, compromising venous return to the heart. This can lead to circulatory collapse. In addition, the pressure of the rumen on the diaphragm may also restrict the lung capacity, causing respiratory embarrassment.
- *Intubation*: All ruminants possess a large dorsum to the tongue, which obstructs access and vision of the pharyngeal region. In order to pass an endotracheal tube into the trachea, it is necessary to use a laryngoscope in sheep, goats and calves. In adult cattle, it is possible to feed the tube into the trachea of an anaesthetised cow

by inserting a hand into the back of the mouth. A gag should always be in position between the molar arcades to prevent accidental closure of the mouth on the operator's arm during this procedure.

## Surgery

The rumen is a very large organ and occupies the whole of the left side of the abdomen. Paradoxically, abdominal surgery in ruminants is best conducted through flank incisions on the left side, directly over the rumen. This organ can then be pushed aside to reveal the area of interest (uterus, liver, etc.). If incisions are made in the right flank, the pressure of the rumen below forces the intestines out of the wound, making it very difficult to operate. Therefore, always perform laparotomies through the left flank of a ruminant, so the rumen will seal the hole and prevent the escape of intestines.

## SHEEP

It is believed that the numerous domestic breeds of sheep worldwide all originated from the wild Mouflon, which is still found in Asia and some parts of Europe. There are approximately 20 million breeding ewes in the UK and over 40 breeds. These vary in size from small native breeds, such as the Soay (25 kg adult weight), to the largest breeds, such as the Suffolk (90 kg). In the last 20 years, several continental breeds have also been introduced. Sheep can differ widely in temperament and fleece characteristics between breeds and may be either horned or naturally polled. The majority of sheep in the UK are kept for meat (lamb) production, with wool as a by-product. Several standardised hybrids have been developed with improved production characteristics, such as fecundity, growth rate and carcass conformation, but there are no commercial sheep-breeding companies.

In research, sheep are particularly useful for antibody production, since they are easily handled and large quantities of serum (up to 500 ml) can be harvested from them on a regular basis. They are the natural host of the agent that causes 'scrapie', a transmissible spongiform encephalopathy (TSE), and so are used for BSE and CJD research. They are also used in anaesthetic, cardiovascular and orthopaedic research.

## Behaviour

Sheep are normally docile and tractable. At pasture they spend a large part of the day grazing over wide areas, but they are timid and have very strong flocking instincts. If disturbed, they will rapidly flock together, which makes them relatively easy to drive. However, their well-developed flight reflex can easily turn into a headlong rush, in which injuries can occur. They will more readily move uphill, and away from dark towards light, and this should be born in mind when designing handling facilities. Sheep are flock animals that become distressed if separated from others. They should never be housed singly.

# Housing

Sheep can survive in a wide range of climates. Their thick lanolin-impregnated fleeces make them well adapted to severe weather conditions and they can remain outdoors throughout the year in the UK. However, for research studies that allow sheep to graze under natural conditions, shelter from wind and driving rain should be available. Fencing needs to be 1 m high, close meshed and robust. Sheep do not usually jump to escape, but will test the strength of fences by rubbing and pushing against them until they break.

Indoor accommodation may be either naturally ventilated or environmentally controlled. For sheep that are housed indoors, it is advised that they be kept in groups of no more than 30, matched by age and size to prevent bullying at feeding. Breeding ewes are usually housed in individual pens for a few days at lambing time. This ensures that the lambs receive colostrum and develop the maternal bond. After 24–48 h, ewes and lambs can be mixed with others in small groups.

# Feeding

Sheep are grazing animals and will nibble grass and vegetation at ground level. The optimum sward height for sheep is 2.5 cm, and they can have difficulty utilising very long grass. Grazing sheep will normally obtain sufficient nutrients from grass alone, but may require supplementary rations during the winter and at other times of the year if the grass quality or availability declines. This should take the form of long-fibre-conserved forage; either hay, silage or straw. For growing and pregnant animals, concentrate rations based on cereals may also be necessary. Approximately 125 g/head/day is fed daily from day 100 of pregnancy, and gradually increased to as much as 1 kg/head/day at parturition.

Mineral deficiencies may occur if the pasture or conserved foods are deficient in the trace elements copper, cobalt or selenium. Supplementary minerals may be advised in these circumstances, but great care is required in their formulation, as sheep are peculiarly susceptible to copper toxicity. Concentrate rations or minerals intended for cattle or pigs should never be given to sheep, because they contain added copper and can rapidly induce copper toxicity.

Poor dentition may be a problem in older sheep. Incisor teeth are frequently lost, particularly if they are eating root crops. However, the majority of sheep can maintain satisfactory body condition without incisor teeth. Of more importance are the molar teeth, which are essential for masticating food. Loose or infected molar teeth are a common cause of weight loss in older sheep.

Growing sheep are particularly prone to urinary calculi when fed high levels of concentrate. In male lambs (entire or castrated), where the urethra is narrower than that of the female, these calculi may cause a urethral blockage, with urine retention and fatal consequences. To prevent this, it is essential that the magnesium and phosphorus content of concentrate rations be restricted. Salt licks should always be provided to encourage drinking and urinary throughput, and urinary acidifiers may also be helpful.

# Water

Sheep must be provided with ad lib clean water at all times. Hill sheep prefer to drink from flowing water, although this may be difficult to achieve in practice. Static water tanks are acceptable, but care is required, because sheep can become cast in them and drown. Bowl drinkers are more satisfactory in indoor pens, but nipple drinkers are not generally suitable for sheep.

# Environment

Sheep will tolerate a very wide range of temperatures. The thermoregulatory neutral zone for sheep is −10°C to +30°C, but the extremes of this range depend on whether they have a full fleece or not. Sheep that are shorn are more susceptible to cold and should not be exposed to temperatures of less than +10°C. If winter shearing is practised, sheep must be housed for at least 2 months before they are turned outside, to allow some fleece re-growth. Conversely, unshorn sheep can suffer from heat stress, exhibiting panting and mouth breathing at temperatures over 20°C.

Sheep housed in environmentally controlled conditions will generally benefit from shearing and should be kept at between 10°C and 24°C. Adequate ventilation is essential to reduce the high risk of respiratory disease when this species is kept indoors. Extractor fans should remove $3\,m^3$ air/kg bodyweight/h to control ammonia levels and humidity levels should be kept between 45% and 60%.

Environmental enrichment can be difficult with sheep. Toys, such as balls or chains, as used for pigs, do not seem to be of interest to sheep. The provision of roughage and space to lie down to ruminate is probably the most important enrichment for housed sheep. Unchopped root vegetables, such as sugar beet, are well liked and give them something to gnaw at. They may be provided as a treat on a daily basis, although in the long term there is a risk of damage to the lower incisor teeth.

# Breeding

Sheep are seasonally polyoestrous, returning into oetrous every 16–17 days over the winter period (September–February). The onset of the breeding season is controlled by diminishing day length, but varies significantly between breeds. Normally, the hill breeds start later (October–November), than the lowland breeds (August–September). Dorset sheep are unusual in having a very long breeding season, extending from about June to March. This means that they may be mated every 8 months, allowing three litters in 2 years. Dorset breeds and their crosses, particularly the prolific Finn-Dorset, are popular research animals.

Under farm conditions, ewes are normally mated in the autumn months, to give birth in the spring. They run with the rams (tups) for a period of about 6 weeks, at a ratio of 1 ram:40 ewes (1:20 for ram-lambs). Ultrasound scanning at 50–90 days of gestation is widely practised to determine pregnancy and count fetal numbers. Ewes carrying multiple fetuses can then be grouped separately for differential feeding.

Gestation lasts approximately 147 days (142–150), although there are slight breed differences. Ewes carrying multiples normally have shorter gestations than those carrying singles, but as a rough guide, in the Northern Hemisphere, ewes mated on Guy Fawkes day (5th November) will lamb the following All Fools day (1st April). Ewes may be mated as lambs (ewe-lambs) in their first autumn, when they are 6 months of age, provided their body weight is 70% of adult weight for the breed. Alternatively, they may be left until the second autumn, when they are 18 months of age. Weaning normally takes place at 12–16 weeks, although there are management systems where weaning may be as early as 6 weeks, provided suitable concentrate rations are provided.

Advancing the breeding season: In most sheep breeds, the breeding season can be advanced by a number of methods. These include the use of progesterone-impregnated intra-vaginal sponges, melatonin implants or running vasectomised males with the flock. By advancing the breeding season in the UK to July or August, lambs can be produced in December/January.

Artificial insemination (AI) is possible in sheep using either fresh or frozen semen. Frozen semen is inseminated directly into the uterus by a laparoscopic technique. Fresh semen can be inseminated per vaginum. Embryo transfer may also be carried out by laparoscopy under general or local anaesthesia.

## Handling

Sheep are particularly easily startled and patience and gentle handling are required for success. They are inclined to follow one another, and will generally move away from humans, dogs or buildings towards open countryside. Where larger numbers are involved, a proper sheep handling system should be employed.

Where sheep are held indoors, carefully designed housing, consisting of holding pens leading through narrow walkways and races to smaller pens, will allow individuals to be caught with minimal stress. Where such facilities do not exist, the best method of restraint is to gradually restrict the sheep into a corner, using a number of hurdles. A trained handler can then restrain the individual sheep, by holding one arm under the neck and the other around the rump (see Figure 16.4). Sheep should never be caught by the wool, as grasping the fleece is painful and may result in handfuls of wool being torn out. It is also not advised that sheep be caught by their horns. It is an offence under welfare legislation to lift a sheep by its horns.

To cast a sheep, the handler stands on the left side of the sheep, grasps the muzzle with the left hand, and pushes the head round to the right to face the tail. This can be facilitated by placing the thumb in the diastema behind the incisor teeth. With the right hand, press down on the rump and the hind legs will collapse. The sheep can then be rolled over and sat onto its rump (see Figure 16.5). Alternatively, with smaller sheep, the handler may be able to reach over and grasp the fold of skin low down on the right flank. Using this fold, the sheep can be lifted up so that it comes to rest sitting on its rump.

## Pain and stress recognition

Sheep in pain appear dull and depressed with little interest in their surroundings. There may be drooping ears, a reluctance to rise and anorexia. However, sheep have

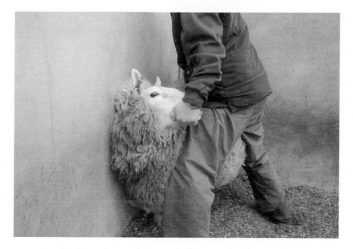

**Figure 16.4**    Restraining a sheep.

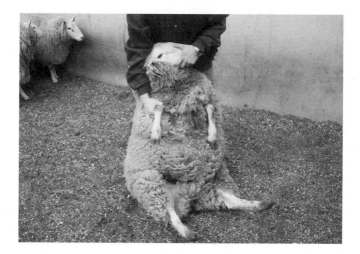

**Figure 16.5**    Casting a sheep.

a great ability to mask the signs of pain, and in the early stages, these may only be apparent to an experienced stockperson. In the later stages, separation from the group is a good indication of a sick sheep. Nasal discharge is a common sign of respiratory infection, and grunting or teeth grinding usually indicate abdominal pain. Lameness is a common problem with sheep and should never be ignored. Animals are not lame unless they have pain in the limb.

## Common diseases and health monitoring

Sheep are susceptible to a number of diseases, many of which are zoonoses (see Table 16.5). The majority of commercial flocks trade sheep regularly and so very few flocks are of a defined health status. It is safest to assume that all sheep are carrying all diseases and to thoroughly screen any that are purchased for research purposes. The rules for isolation and biosecurity outlined in the introduction to this chapter should always be followed.

## Zoonoses

Sheep suffer from a number of zoonoses and it is very important that steps are taken to minimise the risk to humans. Of particular concern are the numerous agents that may cause abortion (*Chlamydophilia, Toxoplasma, Campylobacter, Listeria, Coxiella* and *Salmonella*) and for this reason it is advisable that pregnant women do not handle ewes at lambing time. *Contagious pustular dermatitis virus* (Orf) is common in sheep, causing facial lesions in lambs and a painful skin condition in humans. Although a modified live vaccine is available, it should be used with caution, as it will significantly increase the virus burden in indoor situations. The protozoan parasite *Cryptosporidium* may cause enteritis in lambs and humans. *Brucella melitensis* does not occur in the UK, but is the cause of a serious infection in man, sometimes called Malta fever, in many parts of the world. It is usually contracted from drinking infected ewe or goat milk.

## Parasitic conditions

1. *Endoparasitic infections*. Parasitic gastroenteritis (PGE) is caused by a number of species of gastrointestinal nematodes and constitutes a major health threat to sheep. These parasites are endemic in grazing sheep and control can only be achieved by routine prophylactic anthelmintic treatment. However, their life cycle cannot be completed indoors, and so sheep born and reared indoors are very unlikely to suffer from these parasites. If grazing sheep are moved indoors, they should always be treated with an anthelmintic on housing. Liver fluke can also be a life-threatening parasite of sheep, although only if grazing pastures close to water or prone to flooding.
2. *Ectoparasitic infections*. Lice and psoroptic mange (sheep scab), cause irritation and wool loss in sheep. Treatment may be by spray or immersion in any of a number of parasiticides. Ticks and keds are important vectors of other diseases, particularly in the hill regions. Myiasis (fly strike) is seen in the summer and autumn months in the lowlands. Blue and green-bottle flies lay eggs on soiled wool, which rapidly develop into maggots. These proceed to eat their way into the flesh of the sheep, causing pain and irritation as well as releasing toxins. Undetected, such infections can prove fatal and prompt treatment is required.

## Bacterial diseases

Foot rot is a common bacterial disease of sheep, caused by *Dichelobacter nodosus*. Prevention is by foot trimming and foot bathing in antibacterial solutions, such as zinc sulphate. Foot rot can spread rapidly when sheep are housed indoors, so prophylactic treatment at housing should be undertaken.

*Clostridial* diseases are common and invariably fatal in sheep. These include diseases, such as tetanus, and the enterotoxaemias caused by *Clostridium perfringens*. Vaccines are available and should always be used. *Mannheimia haemolytica* and *Pasteurella multocida* are common commensals in the throat and nasal passages of sheep. Under stress, and particularly in conditions of poor ventilation and overcrowding, they can produce acute or chronic respiratory and systemic disease. Vaccines are available and should be routinely used in housed sheep. Other important bacterial conditions of sheep include *C. pseudotuberculosis* (caseous lymphadenitis) and *M. avium pseudotuberculosis* (Johnes disease).

## *Other*

- *Border disease virus* (BDV) is a pestivirus that can produce infertility and fetal abnormalities. All purchased sheep should be tested for this disease.
- *Maedi–Visna* (M–V) and *sheep pulmonary adenomatosis* (SPA) are both causes of chronic respiratory disease and may combine with *Mannheimia haemolytica* to produce acute disease. Infection with SPA was the cause of death of Dolly, the first cloned sheep, in 2003.
- *Scrapie* is a slow onset transmissible spongiform encephalopathy (TSE) of unknown aetiology, producing neurological changes in adult sheep. Resistance to scrapie is genetically controlled and a blood test to establish genotype can predict the susceptibility or resistance of sheep to infection.

# Drug doses for anaesthesia

Sedation may be used in combination with local or regional anaesthesia.
- *Acepromazine*: 0.05–0. 1 mg/kg i.m. produces good sedation, but no analgesia.
- *Diazepam*: 2 mg/kg i.m. (1 mg/kg slowly i.v.) or *midazolam,* (0.5 mg/kg i.v.) both produce good tranquillisation in sheep. They may be combined with *ketamine* to produce light anaesthesia.
- *Xylazine* or *medetomidine*: both of these must be used with extreme caution in sheep. They produce severe bradycardia and respiratory depression and several deaths have been reported. Give 0.1–0.2 mg/kg (xylazine) or 25 µg/kg (medetomidine). Both should be given i.m., when they will provide 30–35 min of heavy sedation with analgesia.

## *General anaesthesia*

### *Injectable agents*

- *Alphaxalone/alphadolone* (Saffan) is the injectable agent of choice for sheep. Given i.v. via the cephalic or jugular vein at a dose rate of 3 mg/kg (2 mg/kg, if sedated), this will give 15 min of surgical anaesthesia. Incremental doses of 1–2 mg/kg i.v., given every 15–20 min will produce stable long-term anaesthesia.
- *Propofol*: For very short procedures, propofol (4–5 mg/kg i.v.) can be used. Incremental doses can be given for maintenance, or an infusion at a rate of 0.4–0.6 mg/kg/min.

- *Thiopentone*: 10–15 mg/kg i.v. will give 5–10 min anaesthesia.
- *Ketamine combinations*: Diazepam (2 mg/kg i.v.), or midazolam (1 mg/kg) followed by ketamine (4 mg/kg i.v.), produces light anaesthesia. These combinations are preferable to ketamine and xylazine or ketamine and medetomidine, for the reasons given above.

### Inhalation agents

The volatile anaesthetic agents, isoflurane and halothane, are the agents of choice for the maintenance of anaesthesia following induction. Intubate with a size 8–12 endotracheal tube and use a Bain, Magill or circle anaesthetic system.

## Drug doses for analgesia

There are no analgesics licensed for use in sheep in the UK, but the following may be used safely.

### Opioids

- *Buprenorphine*: 0.005–0.01 mg/kg i.m. – lasts 4–6 h.
- *Butorphanol*: 0.5 mg/kg s.c. – lasts 2–3 h.
- *Morphine*: 0.2–0.5 mg/kg i.m. – total dose should not exceed 10 mg – lasts 2–3 h.
- *Nalbuphine*: 1 mg/kg s.c. – lasts 2–3 h.
- *Pethidine*: 2 mg/kg i.m. – lasts 2–4 h.

### NSAIDs

- *Flunixin*: 2.2 mg/kg i.v. or i.m. – once daily.
- *Carprofen*: 1.4 mg/kg s.c.or i.v. – once daily.
- *Ketoprofen*: 3 mg/kg i.v. or i.m. – once daily.

### $\alpha_2$-Agonists

*Xylazine* can be combined with a local anaesthetic and given by epidural injection. This will give prolonged analgesia of the perineal and pelvic regions.

### Useful data

For useful data see Table 16.4.

## GOATS

The ancestor of the modern domestic goat (*Capra hircus*), is the Bezoar, still found in the Middle East and Asia Minor. Selection for milk, meat or skins has led to the development of several breeds, of which the British Saanen, Toggenburg and Anglo-Nubian

**Table 16.4**    Useful data: ruminants.

|  | Sheep | Goats | Cattle |
|---|---|---|---|
| ***Biological data*** | | | |
| Adult weight (kg) male | 70–100 | 70–90 | 800–1000 |
| Adult weight (kg) female | 25–70 | 20–70 | 500–800 |
| Natural lifespan (years) | 10–15 | 9–18 | 15–20 |
| Rectal temperature (°C) | 39.0 | 38.5 | 38.5 |
| Heart rate/min | 60–120 | 70–135 | 40–100 |
| Blood volume (ml/kg) | 58–64 | 57–90 | 57–62 |
| Respiratory rate/min | 12–20 | 15–25 | 27–40 |
| ***Breeding data*** | | | |
| Puberty (months) | 7–12 | 3–8 | 12–15 |
| Age to breed (months) | First or second autumn | Second autumn | 15–24 |
| Gestation (days) | 144–150 (average 147) | 147–155 (average 151) | 274–291 (average 282) |
| Litter size | 1–3 | 2–3 | 1–2 |
| Birth weight (kg) | 3–5 | 2–4 | 25–45 |
| Weaning age (weeks) | 12–20 | 12* | 6* |
| Oestrus cycle (days) | 16/17 (September–February) | 19/20 (September–February) | 21 days (all year) |
| Post-partum oestrus | No | No | Yes |
| ***Haematological data*** | | | |
| RBC ($\times 10^6$/mm$^3$) | 8–13 | 12–14 | 5–10 |
| PCV (%) | 24–40 | 24–48 | 24–46 |
| Hb (g/dl) | 8–16 | 8–14 | 8–15 |
| WBC ($\times 10^3$/mm$^3$) | 4–12 | 5–14 | 4–12 |
| Neutrophils (%) | 20–40 | 20–40 | 6–45 |
| Lymphocytes (%) | 40–70 | 50–65 | 18–75 |
| Eosinophils (%) | 0–15 | 3–8 | 2 |
| Monocytes (%) | 1–12 | 1–5 | 1–7 |
| Basophils (%) | 0–1 | 0–1 | 0–1 |
| ***Biochemical data*** | | | |
| Serum protein (g/dl) | 6.6–8.1 | 5.4–7.5 | 5.3–7.5 |
| Albumin (g/dl) | 2.4–3 | 2.7–4.6 | 2.1–3.6 |
| Globulin (g/dl) | 3.5–5.7 | 1.5–2.8 | 3.5–5.5 |
| Glucose (mg/dl) | 100–500 | 75–150 | 2–3.2 mmol/l |
| Blood urea nitrogen (mg/dl) | 8–20 | 17–23.5 | 2–6.6 mmol/l |
| Creatinine (mg/dl) | 1.2–1.9 | 0.8–1.8 | 44–165 µmol/l |
| Total bilirubin (mg/dl) | 0.1–0.42 | 0.25–0.74 | 0–6.5 µmol/l |
| Cholesterol (mg/dl) | 52–76 | 35–53 | 1–3 mmol/l |

*Offspring weaned at 4 days of age in dairy breeds.

are the commonest in the UK. Some breeds, such as the Angora and Cashmere, have been developed specifically for fibre production (mohair and cashmere). Varieties of dwarf (pygmy) goats are also found that can weigh as little as 20 kg. Goats normally possess horns and may also have beards and wattles. The tail is naturally short and stands up when the animal is alert. They have strong smelling scent glands around the horns in both sexes and also under the tail in the male.

## Behaviour

Goats are inquisitive animals and tend to be more independent than sheep. They normally live in groups, but will cope well if they have other species, such as humans or sheep for companions. If disturbed, they will scatter, relying on their agility over difficult terrain to escape. This makes them impossible to drive. However, they can be led and will usually follow a handler, especially if they have food. They frequently stand on their hind feet to explore, and can easily reach to a height of 2 m, so this should be considered when suspending items near or above goat pens. Their curiosity causes them to lick or chew at any unusual material, which can lead to the ingestion of foreign objects and may be the cause of accidental poisoning or even electrocution from suspended electric cables.

Goats form a strong social hierarchy and the introduction of new members to a group may result in fighting. As many breeds are horned, this can lead to injuries. Males can be aggressive during the breeding season.

## Housing

Goats are less well protected from extremes of cold than sheep and should always be provided with shelter. They dislike rain and need a dry, draught-free bed. An open-fronted building will usually be sufficient, provided it backs into the prevailing wind. Goats are particularly agile and can leap over barriers several feet high; so all fences should be at least 1.5 m.

## Feeding

Goats are primarily browsing, rather than grazing, animals and will strip vegetation off trees to a considerable height. However, in the absence of trees, goats will graze and can be maintained on grass in paddocks. During the winter months, conserved forage, such as hay or silage, must be fed.

Lactating goats can produce as much milk/kg body weight as dairy cows and normally require supplementary concentrate feeds. They are less sensitive to the toxic effects of copper in the diet than sheep.

Goats are fastidious eaters, and will refuse food that has been soiled by faeces or urine. Feeding troughs must be clean and hayracks should be suspended well above the floor. This not only prevents soiling of the hay, but also allows the goats to perform their natural, browsing behaviour.

## Water

Goats are fussy drinkers and must be provided with ad lib clean water at all times. Water bowls must be regularly cleaned out. Lactating goats may drink 10 or more litres of water daily.

# Environment

Goats are more heat tolerant than sheep, but less able to stand extremes of cold. When housed indoors, they should be kept at temperatures between 10°C and 24°C and at humidities of 45–70%.

*Environmental enrichment*: Goats are natural climbers and so the provision of a raised area is advantageous, although this may be difficult to provide in an indoor pen. Owing to their natural inquisitiveness, goats will investigate objects, such as toys or chains, particularly if these are suspended above head height. The provision of roughage above head height, to allow natural browsing behaviour is also recommended. Goats readily become accustomed to contact with humans, and this should be encouraged during routine husbandry procedures and at other times.

# Breeding

Goats are seasonally polyoestrous, returning into oetrus every 21 days over the winter period. Puberty is reached at 5–7 months of age. As with sheep, the onset of the breeding season is controlled by diminishing day length, although the season can be advanced by the use of progesterone sponges and PMSG. Gestation length is 144–150 days and litter size is 1–3. Pregnancy can be confirmed by ultrasound scanning at 50 days. Some goats may suffer from a pseudopregnancy, showing increased abdominal and udder swelling over a period of months. This is normally resolved by the eventual discharge of copious quantities of uterine fluid (a so-called 'cloudburst'), at the expected time of parturition. Such animals may well breed normally in future years. Goats are unusual in that some maidens will come into lactation without any prior pregnancy or parturition.

Artificial insemination (AI) using frozen semen and embryo transfer techniques are both possible in goats, but not widely used.

Kids are normally weaned at 5–6 months of age, although if the dam is producing milk for human consumption, the kid will be artificially reared from 4 days of age.

# Handling

Goats are usually horned, which can be dangerous for the handler, but they are generally less nervous than sheep and can be caught quite easily with a little patience. Goats should not be caught or restrained by the horns, but by holding the hands either side of the head, behind the lower jaw. Goats are not suitable for casting, and examination of the feet or udder is usually performed in the standing position, as for a cow.

# Pain and stress recognition

Goats are usually more vocal than sheep, although they too have an ability to mask the signs of pain. Dullness, drooping ears, reluctance to rise, anorexia and separation from the group are all indicators of pain or distress.

# Common diseases and health monitoring

Goats suffer from all of the diseases of sheep and similar precautions and treatments are required (see Table 16.5). The major differences between the species can be summarised as follows:

- There are only two licensed vaccines available for goats – both against *Clostridial* diseases. Other sheep vaccines are not licensed for use in goats and should only be used under veterinary direction.
- Goats are more susceptible than sheep to infections with mycobacteria (Johnes disease and tuberculosis (TB)). They should be routinely tested for TB, especially if they have been in contact with cattle.
- The *Maedi–Visna virus* produces arthritis, encephalitis, pneumonia and mastitis in goats, where it is known as *caprine arthritis and encephalitis virus* (CAE). This is commoner in the US than in the UK. Serological tests are available to detect infected animals.
- Goats do not usually suffer from fly strike, because their short-hair coat is kept cleaner than the long wool of sheep.

**Table 16.5**   Diseases of sheep and goats.

**Zoonoses**
*Chlamydophilia psittaci* (Enzootic Abortion of Ewes – EAE)
*Toxoplasma gondii* (Toxoplasmosis)
*Parapox virus (Contagious pustular dermatitis – Orf)
*Listeria monocytogenes*
*Campylobacter*
*Coxiella burnetti* (Q Fever)
*Salmonella* species
*Brucella melitensis*

**Respiratory**
*Mannheimia haemolytica*
*Pasteurella multocida*
Lentivirus (Maedi–Visna in sheep – Caprine arthritis encephalitis in goats)
Jaagsiekte retrovirus (SPA)

**Enteric**
Parasitic gastroenteritis (PGE)
*Mycobacterium avium paratuberculosis* (MAP – Johnes disease)

**Other**
†Clostridial diseases
*Dichelobacter nodosus* (Foot rot)
Border disease virus
*Corynebacterium pseudotuberculosis* (Caseous Lymphadenitis)
Scrapie
Ectoparasites (sheep scab, lice, ticks, blowfly strike)

*Vaccines licensed for use in sheep.
†Vaccines licensed for use in goats. Other sheep vaccines should only be used in goats following veterinary advice as to their safety and effectiveness in this species.

- In order to facilitate future handling, most goat kids have their horn buds removed at about 4 days of age (disbudding). If this procedure is delayed beyond a week, there is a danger of incomplete removal and re-growth. This procedure must be carried out under general anaesthesia by a veterinary surgeon.

## Drug doses for anaesthesia and analgesia

The anaesthetic and analgesic agents and doses used for goats are identical for those given for sheep on page 347. ACP or diazepam is the sedative of choice. Goats are extremely sensitive to *xylazine* and this must be used with extreme caution at doses half those indicated for sheep. Alphaxalone/alphaladone is the injectable anaesthetic agent of choice for goats of all ages and isoflurane is the inhalation agent most suitable for maintenance.

## CATTLE

The domesticated cattle of the world are nearly all derived from two major species: *Bos taurus*, which includes all of the European breeds, and *Bos indicus*, which includes the Asian and African cattle. By selection, a number of different breeds have developed. Some of these are kept primarily for meat production (beef breeds) and some for milk production (dairy breeds).

In the UK, the Holstein–Friesian is the predominant dairy breed, although Jersey and Guernsey breeds remain in the Channel Islands and areas of the West Country. Holstein–Friesians are the largest dairy breed, weighing over 600 kg (bulls over 1000 kg), while Jerseys are the smallest (400 kg).

Beef breeds include the native Aberdeen Angus and Hereford, as well as continental breeds, such as the Charolais, Simmental and Limousin. Dairy cows are frequently mated to bulls of the beef breeds, to produce hybrid calves with greater growth potential and better carcass conformation than the pure Friesian.

Cattle are not widely used in research, because of their large size and expense. However, they are the species of choice for certain zoonotic infections (*Escherichia coli* 0157, BSE and TB) and also for studies on ruminant physiology.

## Behaviour

Dairy cows are normally docile and creatures of habit. They rapidly become accustomed to the regular routines involved in twice daily milking and are habituated to close human contact. Calves are easily handled up to about 12 weeks of age (100 kg), but as they grow, their increasing weight can make them potentially dangerous to humans.

Beef breeds are generally less amenable than dairy breeds, because they are handled less regularly. All bulls are unpredictable and cause several human deaths each year. They should always be handled with extreme caution.

## Housing

Cattle can survive outdoors in a very wide range of climates. However, it is customary to bring milking cows and most beef breeds inside for the winter months in the UK.

During the grazing season (usually April–October in the south of England), fields should be enclosed by wire fencing approximately 1.5 m high. A simple plain wire fence can be sufficient to restrain all but the most determined cattle. Electrified fencing is frequently used to subdivide paddocks for more efficient utilisation by dairy cows.

Beef cattle and calves that are housed over winter are normally bedded on deep straw, over a base of concrete or rammed chalk. Slats may also be used. Groups should be matched by age and size and horned breeds should not be mixed with polled breeds to prevent injuries.

Dairy cows may be housed for long periods over winter in a variety of accommodation, including straw yards, cowsheds, kennels and cubicle systems. Cubicles may be bedded with straw, wood shavings, sand or lined with rubber mats. For ease of feeding, dairy cows are normally grouped according to their date of calving and milk yield.

## Feeding

Beef breeds normally graze during the summer months and are fed conserved forage (hay, silage or straw) over winter. They receive little in the way of concentrate feeds and their calves are naturally weaned at 6–7 months of age. Dairy cows require additional concentrate rations throughout lactation, and the feeding of these has become a science in itself. Dairy calves are normally removed from the dam at 2–4 days of age and reared on milk replacers. There are many different systems for artificially rearing calves, ranging from twice daily bucket feeding of warm milk, to fully automatic milk dispensers. Hay and concentrate rations should be made available after 2 weeks and weaning normally takes place at 6–7 weeks, at which time the calves should be eating in excess of 1 kg concentrate/head/day.

## Environment

Calves artificially reared in calf houses are prone to enteric and respiratory diseases. They require temperatures above 15°C, a clean, dry bed of straw and good ventilation, without exposure to draughts.

Weaned calves housed indoors remain particularly prone to respiratory infections and good ventilation (either natural or forced) is essential. Temperatures should be above 10°C and humidity 45–70%. Wide fluctuations in temperature and humidity, as may occur in the autumn, can predispose cattle to pneumonia.

Adult cattle are able to withstand considerable variations in temperature and are normally kept at ambient temperature in sheltered buildings.

Environmental enrichment for cattle has not been well defined. Where cattle have to be kept in sterile environments, group housing, comfortable bedding and ad lib provision of roughage are probably the most important aspects. The provision of toys and similar does not appear to elicit much interest.

## Breeding

Cattle are polyoestrous throughout the year, although they are generally less fertile during the winter months. The oestrous cycle is every 21 days, but can be manipulated by the use of various hormones (progesterone, GNRH and prostaglandins). Mating may be by bull service or AI. Pregnancy can be confirmed per-rectum by manual palpation or ultrasound scanning from 35 days. Progesterone assay at 21 days can also be used as a test for pregnancy, although this is less reliable. Gestation length is 280 days ($\pm 10$ days), although there are breed variations. Cows normally have a single calf, although twins are not uncommon. They will normally return to oestrus within 42 days of calving and are usually mated at approximately 85 days, to achieve a 'calving index' of 365 days.

AI is widely practised in dairy cattle. Commercial AI centres hold stocks of frozen semen from genetically superior sires and supply a daily insemination service to farms.

Embryo transfer is also commercially available for cattle, using stored, frozen embryos.

## Handling

Cattle are generally docile and easily handled, but their large size makes a good handling system essential. In research establishments, cattle may be trained to feed through a neck yoke, so that they can be restrained and haltered at any feeding time. A cattle crush is necessary to carry out examinations and procedures (foot trimming, blood sampling, AI) and a number of different models are commercially available.

Calves less than 70 kg can usually be restrained by two handlers. One should hold the head, putting a hand across the bridge of the nose (taking care not to obstruct the nares), and turning the head towards them, while the other restrains the rear end. For cattle over 100 kg, a halter should be used to restrain the head or the animal placed in a crush (see Figure 16.6).

## Pain and stress recognition

Cattle show the same signs of pain as sheep. They may appear dull and depressed with little interest in their surroundings. There may be drooping ears, a reluctance to rise and anorexia. In later stages, separation from the group and grunting or teeth grinding may be heard.

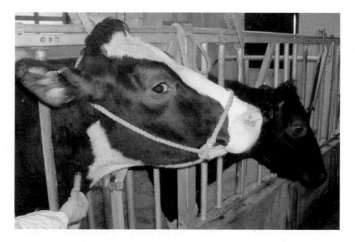

**Figure 16.6**    Restraint of a cow for blood sampling.

# Common diseases and health monitoring

## Zoonoses

Cattle suffer from several important zoonoses, including BSE, TB, salmonellosis, leptospirosis (*Leptospira hardjo*) and *E. coli* 0157, all of which are potentially fatal to man. In addition to these, ringworm is commonly transmitted from cattle to handlers. *Brucella abortus*, which causes undulant fever in man, has been eradicated from the UK but remains an important zoonosis in many parts of the world.

## Parasitic infections

Parasitic infections are generally less important in cattle than sheep, although calves grazing for their first season can occasionally become badly affected. Very few of the nematodes that cause parasitic gastroenteritis (PGE), transmit between sheep and cattle, so cross grazing between the species may be safely practised. Liver fluke may cause disease in cattle grazing pastures liable to flooding, and coccidiosis can be a problem in calves. With the exception of liver fluke, parasite control measures are generally only required in growing calves under 2 years of age.

**Table 16.6**    Diseases of cattle.

**Zoonoses**
*Salmonella* species
*E. coli*
*Trichophyton* and *Microsporum* (ringworm infections)
*Leptospira hardjo*
*M. bovis* (tuberculosis – TB)
Bovine spongiform encephalopathy (BSE)
*Brucella abortus*

**Respiratory**
*Respiratory syncytial virus (BRSV)
*Infectious bovine rhinotracheitis (IBR)
*Parainfluenza 3 virus (PI3)
*Mannheimia haemolytica*
*Pasteurella multocida*
*Dictyocaulus viviparus* (lungworm)

**Enteric**
*Mycobacterium avium paratuberculosis* (MAP) – Johnes disease
*Rotavirus and coronavirus
Parasitic gastroenteritis (PGE)

**Other**
*Clostridial diseases
*Bovine virus diarrhoea (BVD)
Ectoparasites (sheep scab, lice, ticks, blowfly strike)

*Vaccines licensed for use in cattle.

## *Respiratory diseases*

Three respiratory viruses are common in cattle. Bovine respiratory syncytial virus (BRSV) is endemic in the UK, while Parainfluenza 3 virus (PI3) and Herpesvirus 1 (infectious bovine rhinotracheitis – IBR) are both widespread. They often produce disease in association with bacterial agents, such as *Mannheimia haemolytica*, *Mycoplasma bovis* and *Haemophilus somnus*. In addition, *Mycobacterium bovis*, the cause of TB in cattle, is on the increase in the UK. Regular skin testing for this disease is mandatory under DEFRA, but all purchased cattle should additionally be privately tested before introduction to a research establishment. Lungworm, due to *Dictyocaulus viviparus*, can be the cause of pneumonia in all ages of cattle, but there is a vaccine available for use in calves that gives lifelong protection.

## *Enteric infections*

Salmonellosis, due to a variety of *Salmonella* species, is a common cause of diarrhoea in neonatal calves, particularly if they have been traded through a market. All purchased calves should be tested on arrival. *E. coli* infections, either enteric or systemic are also common in calves. Enterohaemorrhagic *E. coli* 0157 can cause a very serious disease in humans. Rotavirus and coronavirus infections are also common in neonatal calves, while *M. avium paratuberculosis* is seen occasionally in adult cattle over 2 years of age.

## *Other infections*

Bovine virus diarrhoea (BVD) is a very common disease in the UK. When first infected, cattle will show few signs of disease and recovery will be complete. However, if infected during pregnancy, the fetus may subsequently be aborted, or mutated, or persistently infected with the virus. Persistently infected calves, are immunosuppressed and are, therefore, unsuitable for use in research. They also act as a source of BVD infection for other cattle and will cause severe fertility problems in a herd. All purchased cattle should be tested for their BVD status before arrival. *Leptospira hardjo* can be carried asymptomatically by cattle and transmitted to man via splashes of infected urine. A vaccine is available and should be used routinely.

BSE was common in adult cattle from 1985 to 2000, but has now been virtually eradicated from the UK by a government slaughter policy. Calves frequently suffer from 'ringworm' a fungal skin disease that is transmissible to humans. They may also suffer from lice infestations, but do not suffer from 'blowfly strike', as sheep do.

## Drug doses for anaesthesia

By virtue of their placid nature and large size, cattle are particularly suited to regional nerve blocks, such as epidural and paravertebral, using lignocaine or procaine. There are no licensed agents for general anaesthesia in cattle. Many of the agents used for sheep and goats would probably be suitable, but there is little information about their use.

## *Sedation*

*Xylazine* is the sedative of choice for cattle. Give 0.05–0.3 mg/kg i.m., according to the depth of sedation required. At the higher dose rates, the animal will become recumbent and may remain sedated for several hours. It is possible to intubate cattle under deep sedation using xylazine.

## *Anaesthetics*

- *Injectable agents*: Give 10 mg/kg of a 5% solution of *Thiopentone*, i.v. in an unsedated animal. 50% of the dose should be administered as rapidly as possible, while the second half is given more slowly and to effect. Thiopentone 5% is extremely irritant and it is vital that no solution is given perivascularly, so it is best to administer this through an indwelling catheter. Thiopentone will only give surgical anaesthesia for approximately 5 min, sufficient for intubation, prior to maintenance on halothane or isoflurane. Premedication with *xylazine* will reduce the total dose of *thiopentone* by half.
- *Inhalation agents*: Halothane is the usual volatile anaesthetic agent for cattle, and anaesthesia can be safely maintained for several hours using this. A circle absorber is normally used to reduce the wastage of oxygen and halothane.

## Drug doses for analgesia

### *NSAIDs*

NSAIDs are the normal analgesics used in cattle. They may be safely given to animals sedated with xylazine. There are three licensed preparations in the UK.

- *Flunixin*: 2.2 mg/kg given i.v., repeated at 24-h intervals for up to 5 days.
- *Ketoprofen*: 3 mg/kg given i.v. or i.m., repeated at 24-h intervals for up to 3 days.
- *Tolfenamic acid*: 4 mg/kg i.v. will provide 72 h of pain relief.

### $\alpha_2$-*Agonists*

*Xylazine* has analgesic properties at the higher-dose rates (0.2–0.3 mg/kg).

### *Opioids*

There is little information on the effectiveness or suitability of opioid drugs in cattle.

## EQUINES

Members of the family Equidae all possess a single functional digit. They include horses, asses (donkeys) and zebras. The modern horse (*Equus caballus*) has been used by man for work, pleasure, war and sport over many millennia. There are many breeds of horse, varying in size from the Shetland (30 in. high at the withers) to the Shire (72 in.).

In recognition of their long and close association with man, the use of horses in research requires special justification under ASPA. Their principal use is for the donation of blood for various blood products, and also for studies directly benefiting other equidae, such as equine reproduction, sports sciences and orthopaedics.

## Behaviour

Horses are normally very well adapted to humans and the majority are trained to human commands. However, they are easily startled, and their large size and powerful hind limbs make even the quietest of them a potential danger. Stallions are particularly unpredictable.

## Housing

Horses are mostly kept outdoors during the summer months. Some hardy pony breeds may be kept outside throughout the year, but the majority of breeds are stabled during the winter. Stables should have concrete floors and all walls and doors should be easily cleaned. It is usual to stable horses individually, although they should always be within sight and sound of other equidae. Horses kept outdoors without the companionship of other horses, will benefit from the company of sheep or donkeys.

Fencing for horses needs to be at least 1.5 m high and preferably made of wooden rails. Barbed wire is not suitable for horses as they easily become tangled in it and can suffer severe lacerations.

## Feeding

Horses are herbivorous and rely on grass during the season and conserved forage, such as hay, during the winter. However, many horses suffer from chronic obstructive pulmonary disease (COPD), which is an allergic condition, caused by allergens in hay and straw. For these animals, stable management must be of the highest order. The hay may need to damped with water before use and the horse bedded on paper, shavings or peat to reduce dust. Modified feeds that are low in allergens (i.e. horsehage) are available. Silage is generally too rich in protein for horses and is not used.

At pasture, horses are very selective grazers, and will leave unpalatable grass, especially if contaminated by faeces. Collecting the horse faeces from the pasture is a daily task in well-managed pastures. Due to the uneven grazing of pastures by horses, it is frequently advantageous to graze other species, such as cattle, in the same field.

Over winter, most horses are fed concentrate rations in addition to hay. This may continue throughout the year if horses are working or performing (sport) but must be restricted to prevent them becoming too over-exuberant. Some horses are prone to laminitis (inflammation of the laminae of the feet, causing lameness), if they are fed a diet too high in protein. Grass alone may be too rich for some ponies at certain times of the year.

## Water

Horses must be provided with ad lib clean water at all times. This is usually from a tank at pasture, or from a bucket in the stable.

## Environment

Horses will tolerate a wide range of temperatures and many breeds can be out-wintered in the UK providing some wind shelter is available. Additional protection in the form of a 'rug' is often used. With some of the thinner-skinned breeds, such as thoroughbreds, rugs may be used throughout the year, even in stables.

*Environmental enrichment*: Close association with man over many millennia has made horses very accustomed to the company of people and this should be an essential part of any environmental enrichment. Grooming and exercise should be given daily. They are also very partial to nutritional treats, such as carrots, and there are several commercial products available.

## Breeding

Mares come into oestrus every 3 weeks throughout the year. The gestation length is 340 days (330–350), and only one foal is born. Twins are, sometimes, conceived but nearly always aborted before full term. Foals are normally suckled for 6 months before weaning. The mare will come into oestrus again within 3 weeks of foaling (the foaling heat) and may be mated again at this time. Pregnancy is normally determined by ultrasound scanning at 21 days, which is carried out per-rectum.

## Handling

Most horses are trained to a halter or head-collar and can be led without difficulty. If greater control of the head is required, a bridle and bit may be used. A snare (twitch), tightened over the loose skin of the nares will give a greater degree of restraint and is used by some for minor procedures, such as injections. Great care is required in the application of the twitch and such a device must be used only as a last resort and for the minimum length of time necessary. Sympathetic handling and training should make the use of a twitch unnecessary. For most procedures, and certainly for fractious horses that may present a hazard to their handlers, purpose built stocks should be used.

## Pain and stress recognition

Horses are notable for their low tolerance to pain, and they can be vocal in their recognition of it. Abdominal pain (colic) usually results in looking at the flanks, adopting a hunched stance, straining, kicking and in severe cases rolling on the ground. In systemic disease or generalised pain the head is normally lowered, and the ears droop. There may be reluctance to rise.

# Common diseases and health monitoring

## *Zoonoses*

There are no serious zoonotic diseases of horses in the UK (Table 16.7). Ringworm, due to *Microsporum* or *Trichophyton* fungal infections, may occasionally be seen, although much less commonly than in cattle.

## *Parasitic diseases*

Horses kept outdoors will become infected with gastrointestinal nematodes and must be regularly treated with anthelmintics on a control programme drawn up with veterinary advice. Ectoparasites, such as lice are relatively common, but easily eliminated by treatment.

## *Respiratory diseases*

There are a number of respiratory diseases of horses. Equine influenza is common and, as with human influenza, tends to appear in epidemics every few years. There are a number of different strains, but vaccines are available and should always be used. Strangles, caused by *Streptococcus equi*, is a serious disease of the upper respiratory tract of young horses. Newly purchased horses should be isolated from others for several weeks to prevent the spread of this highly infectious condition. A number of other virus conditions may also cause respiratory disease. In addition to these, many adult horses suffer from COPD. This is an allergic condition that requires very careful management (see earlier under feeding).

## *Other diseases*

Horses are peculiarly susceptible to the soil organism *Clostridium tetani*, which causes tetanus. All horses must be vaccinated against this invariably fatal disease.

**Table 16.7**   Diseases of horses.

**Zoonoses**
Trichophyton and Microsporum species
  (ringworm infections)

**Respiratory**
*Myxoviruses (several strains) Equine influenza
*Streptococcus equi* (Strangles)
Equine herpes virus

**Enteric**
Parasitic
*Salmonella* species

**Other**
*\*Clostridium tetani* (tetanus)
Ectoparasites (lice and mange)

*Vaccines licensed for use in horses.

## Drug doses for anaesthesia

Local anaesthesia is commonly used for regional anaesthesia (nerve blocks) in the limbs of horses and can also be used for some minor procedures, such as suturing superficial skin wounds or collection of blood samples. In conjunction with deep sedation, more invasive procedures may also be undertaken under local anaesthesia. However, abdominal surgery will always require general anaesthesia. The large size of horses makes the induction and recovery phases particularly hazardous for all concerned. The horse may injure itself when falling, or when attempting to rise postoperatively. Consequently, it is essential to perform these operations in a padded room, or if this unavailable, then outdoors on clean pasture. Handlers must be very careful to keep well clear of flailing legs, which can inadvertently cause considerable damage. If the horse is shod, it is advisable to remove the shoes before anaesthesia. Food should be withheld, but not water, for 4–8 h before anaesthesia.

For long operations, the weight of horses can induce pressure ischaemia of tissues. The brachial nerves may become trapped and venous congestion can occur in the upper hind limb. Support for these limbs should be given (i.e. rest on a straw bale). The head and eyes must be protected by appropriate padding. In prolonged anaesthesia, respiratory acidosis may develop and assisted ventilation may be required.

### Sedatives

There are a number of excellent sedatives for horses.

- *Xylazine*: 0.6–1 mg/kg by slow i.v. (2.4–3 mg/kg i.m.).
- *Detomidine*: 10–80 μg/kg i.v. or i.m.
- *Romifidine*: 40–120 μg/kg i.v. only.
- *Acepromazine*: 0.03–0.1 mg/kg i.v. or i.m.

The degree of sedation is dose related, hence the wide ranges given above. Veterinary advice should always be sought.

### Anaesthetics

### Injectable

- *Thiopentone*: Following sedation with ACP, thiopentone at 10 mg/kg i.v. will produce anaesthesia for 5 min.
- *Ketamine*: Following sedation with xylazine, detomidine or romifidine, 2. 2 mg/kg of ketamine i.v. will produce short-term anaesthesia of horses, suitable for minor surgical procedures. This anaesthesia can be prolonged by the use of *Guaiphenesin* as an i.v. infusion, where inhalation anaesthesia is unavailable.

### Inhalation

Volatile agents, such as halothane or isoflurane are the anaesthetics of choice for maintenance of anaesthesia in horses. Intubation is normally carried out blindly. Advance the tube into the pharynx and rotate as it touches the larynx. The trachea is wide and a cuffed tube of size up to 30 mm can be passed.

# Drug doses for analgesia

## Opioids

- *Butorphanol*: 0.1 mg/kg i.v.
- *Pethidine*: 1 mg/kg.

## NSAIDs

- *Flunixin*: 1.1 mg/kg given i.v., repeated at 24-h intervals for up to 5 days.
- *Ketoprofen*: 2.2 mg/kg given i.v., repeated at 24-h intervals for up to 5 days.
- *Phenylbutazone*: 4.4 mg/kg i.v or orally, daily or every other day.

## $\alpha_2$-Agonists

*Xylazine*, *Romifidine* and *Detomidine* all have analgesic properties at the higher-dose rates.

## Useful data

For useful data on horses see Table 16.8.

**Table 16.8**    Useful data: horse.

| Biological data | | Haematological data | |
|---|---|---|---|
| Adult weight (kg) | Up to 500; much breed variation | RBC ($\times 10^6$/mm$^3$) | 7–14 |
| | | PCV (%) | 29–47 |
| Food intake and breed | Depends on work | Hb (g/dl) | 10–16.9 |
| Water intake | Ad lib | WBC ($\times 10^3$/mm$^3$) | 4.1–10.1 |
| Natural lifespan (years) | >30 | Neutrophils (%) | 14–85 |
| Rectal temperature (°C) | 37.6–38.2 | Lymphocytes (%) | 14–77 |
| Heart rate/min | 23–70 | Eosinophils (%) | 0–7 |
| Blood volume (ml/kg) | 75 | Monocytes (%) | 0–2 |
| Respiratory rate/min | 8–12 | Basophils (%) | Rare |
| **Breeding data** | | Platelets ($\times 10^3$/mm$^3$) | 120–360 |
| Puberty (months) | 12–18 | **Biochemical data** | |
| Age to breed (years) | 2–3 (depends on use) | Serum protein (g/dl) | 6–7.3 |
| Gestation (days) | 321–362 (average 336) | Albumin (g/dl) | 2.5–3.8 |
| | | Globulin (g/dl) | 3–4.8 |
| Litter size | 1 – twins do not survive | Glucose (mmol/l) | 2.5–5.5 |
| Birth weight (kg) | Depends on breed | Blood urea nitrogen (mmol/l) | 2.5–7 |
| Weaning age (months) | 6 | Creatinine ($\mu$mol/l) | 50–147 |
| Oestrous cycle | Seasonal polyoestrous May–November Cycle 13–25 days (average 21) | Total bilirubin ($\mu$mol/l) | 17–34* |
| | | Cholesterol (mmol/l) | 2.3–3 |
| Post-partum oestrus | Yes (not used) | | |

*Horses have no gall bladder, hence high circulating bilirubin.

# FURTHER INFORMATION

## Swine

Straw, B.E., Allaire, S.D., Mengeling, W.L. and Taylor, D.J. (1999). *Diseases of Swine*. Iowa State University Press. ISBN 0-8138-0441-8.
Hu *et al*. (1993). A simple technique for blood collection in the pig. *Laboratory Animals* 27(4), 364–67.
Muirhead, M. (1981). Blood sampling in pigs. *In Practice* 3(5).
Potter R.A. (1998). Clinical conditions of outdoor pigs. *In Practice* 20(1).
Rispat *et al*. (1993). Haematological and plasma biochemical values for healthy Yucatan micropigs. *Laboratory Animals* 27(4), 368–73.

## Ruminants

Allen and Borkowski (1999). *The Laboratory Small Ruminant*. CRC Press LLC. ISBN 0-8493-2568-4.
Dunn, P. (1994). *The Goatkeepers Veterinary Book*. Farming Press. ISBN 0-85236-279-X.
Evans, G. and Maxwell, W. (1997). *Salamon's Artificial Insemination of Sheep and Goats*. Butterworth.
Henderson, D.C. (1990). *The Veterinary Book for Sheep Farmers*. Farming Press. ISBN 0-85236-189-0.
Martin, W.B. and Aitkin, I.D. (1991). *Diseases of Sheep*. Blackwell Science. ISBN 0-632-05139-6.
Scott, P. (1996). Caudal analgesia in sheep. *In Practice* 18(8).
Taylor, P.M. (1991). Anaesthesia in sheep and goats. *In Practice* 13.

## Equine

Johnston, A.M. (1994). *Equine Medical Disorders*. Blackwell Science. ISBN 0-632-01684-1.
Urquart, K. (1981). Intra-venous catheterisation of the horse. *In Practice* 3(5).

## General

FELASA (2000). Recommendations for the health monitoring of experimental units of calves, sheep and goats. *Laboratory Animals* 34, 329–350.
The Management and Welfare of Farm Animals (1999). *UFAW Handbook*. Baillière Tindall, London.
Dougherty, R.W. (1981). *Experimental Surgery in Farm Animals*. The Iowa State University Press.
Gordon I. *Controlled Reproduction in Farm Animals*. CABI Int. ISBN 0-85199-118-1.
Turner, A.S. and McIlwraith, C.W. (1982). *Techniques in Large Animal Surgery*. Philadelphia, Lea and Febiger.
Department of Environment, Food and Agriculture Publications: *Operations on Farm Animals* (1991); *Summary of the Law Relating to Farm Animal Welfare* (1992); *Codes of Recommendations for the Welfare of Livestock: Pigs, Sheep, Goats, Cattle* (1990–2000).

# Chapter 17
# Birds

## INTRODUCTION

Birds constitute a very diverse group of animals. There are more species of living bird (about 9600) than there are mammals (4500), reptiles (6000) or amphibia. Birds have highly developed sensory systems and considerable cognitive abilities; therefore, they should be considered to be able to experience discomfort and pain, and treated appropriately in the laboratory. Different species of birds have different requirements with regard to housing, husbandry and care, and it is essential to be familiar with the specific requirements of the species being used. It is important to consult specialist texts and discuss the exact requirements with those experienced in the care of birds prior to beginning any studies.

Birds, like mammals, are able to control their temperature by physiological means (homeothermic), but otherwise they differ from mammals in several ways, being more closely related to the cold-blooded reptiles than mammals. Birds possess many evolutionary adaptations in their anatomy and physiology, which enable them to fly. These adaptations and features have many implications for research, in that they affect the responses of birds to handling, stresses generally, anaesthesia and surgical techniques, and drug administration. All birds are anatomically similar, since the adaptations for flight are somewhat restrictive, although the digestive tract may vary in size and morphology, depending on the diet of the bird. Birds range in size from tiny humming-birds weighing no more that 2 g, to the ostrich, which can weigh as much as 120 kg. The upper weight limit for flying birds, however, is about 12 kg.

## ANATOMICAL FEATURES

The *skeleton* of the bird has to be light and strong in order that the animal is able to fly. To achieve this, the medullary cavities are often filled with extensions of air sacs, and many bones are fused or deleted to retain strength. However, the cortices of the bones are thin and susceptible to trauma.

Many of the vertebrae are fused. The lumbar and sacral vertebrae have fused to form the structure called the synsacrum (see Figure 17.1), which gives the vertebral column strength. At the end of the column is the pygostyle. This is composed of several fused bones, and the tail feathers originate from it. The pygostyle can rotate, which is important in enabling the bird to change direction and slow down during flight.

The ribs have two parts, both bony, contrasting with the bone and cartilage structure found in mammals.

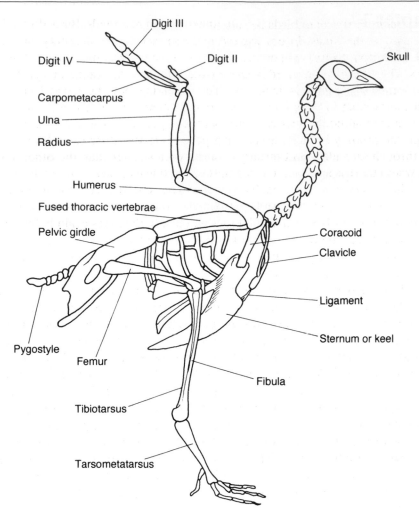

**Figure 17.1**   The simplified skeleton of a bird.

The limbs are derived from the basic vertebrate structure, but the hind limb has adapted for locomotion on land, and the fore limb has adapted to become the wing. There is a single bone in the upper limb (humerus or femur in fore and hind limbs, respectively), followed by two bones in the lower limb. In the hind limb, the tibia is fused with the top row of tarsal bones, producing a tibiotarsus, and the second row of tarsals is fused with the metatarsals, producing tarsometatarsals. In the fore limb, the 'hand' has adapted so many of the carpals and metacarpals are fused, and only digits II, III and IV are present. The third digit is elongated, forming the leading edge of the wing from which the main flight feathers originate.

The pectoral girdle and sternum of a bird are well developed, to accommodate the large pectoral muscles, which are needed to move the wings up and down for flight. Both the muscles that draw the wing down and those which pull it up again are situated on the front of the chest.

The *respiratory system* of birds is quite unlike that of mammals. Birds do not have a diaphragm, so the lungs do not expand and contract due to diaphragmatic movements. The respiratory system of birds consists of the trachea and bronchi, lungs, and air sacs. The air sacs are derived from six pairs, although the cranial two pairs usually fuse to form a single interclavicular sac. The remaining sacs, the cervical, cranial and caudal thoracic, and abdominal, usually remain paired, resulting in a total of nine individual sacs, although this can vary between species. On inspiration, air passes through the primary bronchi. Some then passes into the more caudal air sacs, and some through secondary and tertiary bronchi, each smaller than the other, into the lungs, where there is an anastomosing network of tiny passages, namely the air capillaries, where oxygen is extracted. The air then goes through from the lungs into the cranial air sacs. On expiration, stale air from the cranial air sacs passes straight to the outside, but fresh air from the caudal sacs passes into the lungs again before passing out of the nares, giving the lungs another chance to extract oxygen. The avian lung is considerably more efficient than the mammalian lung, which only gets one chance to extract oxygen from the air in each breath.

Birds have *feathers*, and the structure of the feather is such as to insulate the bird against the cold and provide the wings with the properties required for flight. Feathers also insulate the bird, and their colour may help camouflage the bird or be used to signal to other birds. There are two basic types of feathers, namely contour feathers and down feathers. Contour feathers give shape to the plumed bird. These have a flat vane on each side of a central shaft, the rachis. Barbs project laterally from the rachis, and thread-like barbules attach to the barbs. Barbules have hooks on one side and grooves on the other: the hooks on one barbule engage the grooves on the barbules from the adjacent barb, holding the vane of the feather firm (see Figure 17.2). This strong interlocking structure allows the wing to force air down during the downstroke to produce uplift. The feathers can rotate in their follicles though, so reducing resistance on the upstroke during flight. Regular grooming results in the feathers being covered with an oily secretion from the preen gland, rendering them waterproof.

Down feathers have long, fine barbules, which do not interlock. These feathers are found beneath the contour feathers and particularly over the breast, and keep the bird insulated. Birds will often pluck their own down feathers to line their nests and keep hatchlings warm.

The *gastrointestinal tract* of birds consists of the mouth, oesophagus, crop in some species, gizzard (muscular stomach), glandular stomach, small intestine, paired caeca (which may be large or small) and rectum. Birds do not have lips or teeth. The paired *kidneys* are located dorsally in the abdominal cavity, closely adherent to the body wall. The main excretory product is uric acid, which is deposited as the white emulsion seen in guano. The ureters open with the genital and intestinal tracts into a common chamber, the cloaca, which opens to the outside through the vent.

In the female of the majority of species, only the left *ovary* and oviduct are functional, the latter being specialised for the formation of the white and shell of the egg, which are deposited around the yolk as it passes through the oviduct. Male birds have internal testes. The vasa deferentia end in the cloaca, where there is an erectile copulatory organ in some species.

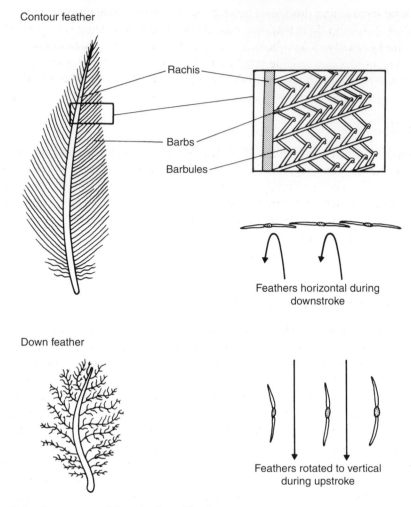

Contour feather

Rachis

Barbs

Barbules

Feathers horizontal during
downstroke

Down feather

Feathers rotated to vertical
during upstroke

**Figure 17.2**    Structure and functioning of feathers.

# PHYSIOLOGICAL FEATURES

Many physiological adaptations which facilitate flight must be considered when planning procedures on birds. In order to produce sufficient energy to fly, birds have an efficient food conversion rate, very high basal metabolic rate (BMR), high body temperature and the flight muscles have a high proportion of red fibres, capable of sustained exercise. Small birds have a higher BMR than larger ones: a hummingbird weighing 3.5 g has a BMR of around 6,720 kJ/kg/day, whereas a swan weighing 9 kg has a BMR of around 200 kJ/kg/day. This high metabolic rate renders birds prone to hypoglycaemia if starved even for only a few hours. The heart is relatively large and beats very fast, and birds will readily develop acute cardiovascular failure if stressed. The red blood cells are nucleated. The body temperature is often 41°C (105°F or 106°F) or more, which allows the rapid metabolism required, but which also renders birds prone to hypothermia. Body temperature is regulated by physiological and behavioural means, and this varies between species depending on their natural habitat. Birds will fluff up their feathers, take shelter and shiver when it is cold, but they have limited capacity to lose heat if it is warm. They do not possess sweat glands; therefore, heat loss can only be effected by panting or gular fluttering, which is the rapid movement of the thin floor of the mouth and upper area of the throat.

## BEHAVIOUR

The behaviour of different species of birds varies widely. Some are solitary, others are gregarious. Some come together only to roost at night or to breed. Some birds are migratory, and if kept in captivity may show restlessness or repeatedly try to move in the direction in which they would migrate, particularly if exposed to external cues such as the sun or stars, which indicate in which direction to fly. Different species of birds spend different amounts of time performing different activities, such as foraging, resting and maintaining their territories.

## HOUSING AND HUSBANDRY

The needs of each species of bird vary, so specialist texts should be consulted to determine what is required. Housing for birds should be secure to prevent escapes or ingress of predators, and must be large enough to allow the birds to exercise and fly, and as a minimum, there must be sufficient space for the bird to stretch its wings fully. Ideally, the captive environment should provide for all the birds physiological and behavioural requirements. This in turn requires a detailed knowledge of the particular species. Environmental enrichment can, however, be easily achieved for many species by simple means. For example, some species like to rest on perches rather than the floor, so several perches at different heights can provide a suitable environment. Many species of birds forage for food, so rather than providing all their food in a bowl, it could be scattered through bedding. This allows the birds to perform natural foraging behaviour to a similar extent to that which would be done in the wild. The provision of a secluded area in the cage gives the birds somewhere in which to feel safe. Some birds like to bathe in water, others in dust baths. The type of flooring used depends on the species and the need for hygiene. Dirt or gravel floors may allow birds to forage, but solid floors may be more hygienic. The requirement and siting of nest boxes depends on the species. Different types of cages may be required depending on the circumstances. Isolation cages may be needed which are away from other birds, cages for stock animals may need to hold a large number of birds together, breeding cages may need to provide numerous nest boxes with secluded areas, and cages for experimental birds may need facilities for observation without disturbance to the birds.

The environmental temperature should be between 15°C and 20°C for most species, although newly hatched birds will need higher temperatures. The light cycle is important, since it can influence breeding performance and behaviour. Birds produce a lot of dust and dander, so good ventilation is vital to keep dust levels to a minimum. There should be at least 10 air changes per hour.

# FEEDING

The diets of birds vary greatly between species, but the nutritional requirements are less varied. If possible, diets similar to the bird's natural diet should be fed, but if this is not known, it can be difficult to supply adequate nutrition, and deficiencies are common in captive birds, particularly calcium deficiency. Many texts describe diets, which have been used for species of captive birds (see Further reading). Some commercially prepared diets are available. Containers used for food and water should be sanitised frequently.

# REPRODUCTION

Most birds do not reproduce until they have finished growing, or indeed in some species several years thereafter. Birds have many different mating systems and courtship rituals, depending on the species. Some may mate for life, for example pigeons and magpies, whereas others are polygamous, having several mates during one mating season, for example dunnocks. Consult specialist texts for more details. Fertilisation is internal, and eggs are incubated by one or both parents. In birds, the sex of offspring is determined by females, which are the heterogametic sex, whereas males are homogametic. Incubation periods range from about 14 days to 2 months. In chickens, the incubation period is 21 days; in pigeons, it is 17–18 days. Eggs are protected under the Animals (Scientific Procedures) Act 1986 from halfway through incubation, although procedures begun before this point with consequences which extend beyond it, are also covered (see Chapter 2). After hatching, there is a variable period of parental care by one or both parents or even other adult birds, until the fledgling can fend for itself. Birds grow more rapidly than mammals of the same size: birds which are helpless at hatching tend to grow more rapidly than those which are more developed.

# HANDLING

Birds are very susceptible to stress, particularly small species, and excessive exertion can result in respiratory collapse or hypoglycaemic episodes. These problems can be reduced by ensuring the bird has fed recently, by handling them slowly and deliberately, and by ensuring that movements of the sternum are not restricted. Also, injuries may occur as the birds flap their wings to try to escape, so gentle restraint of the wings is vital. All birds are disoriented by sudden darkness, so handling can be facilitated if the lighting is subdued. This can also be achieved by covering the head with a cloth or bag, or in a small bird with a yoghurt pot. Large birds should generally be approached from above, with the base of the wings held in a naturally folded position without flapping. Gloves, tissue or a cotton cloth should be used to prevent the feathers coming into contact with perspiration from the hand, since this can reduce waterproofing and interfere with insulation. Assistance may be required to restrain the heads of large birds with long necks.

## Psittacine and passerine birds

It may be easier to catch small birds using a soft net or by covering them in a soft cloth before removing them from the cage. They can then be held with the back

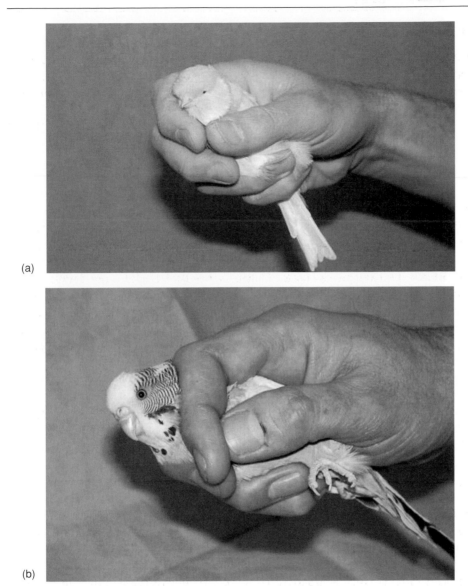

(a)

(b)

**Figure 17.3**   Holding a small bird.

against the palm of one hand. Place the thumb and index finger or index and middle fingers each side of the head to prevent the bird from turning and biting the handler, and wrap the other fingers around the body to restrain the wings and legs (Figure 17.3).

Larger birds should be allowed to grip the perch or cage. Approaching the bird from behind, place a cloth around its neck and wrap the fingers gently around the neck. Use the other hand to place the cloth over the animal's head and wrap it lightly around the wings to prevent flapping. Then, release the legs from the perch or cage, holding them with a finger between them.

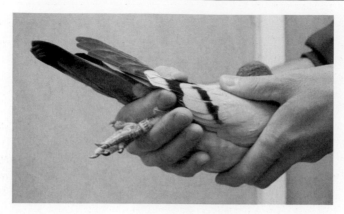

**Figure 17.4**    Holding a pigeon.

## Pigeons

To catch pigeons, grasp them from above, placing one or both hands around the body and closed wings. To hold the animal in the hand, hold the feet side by side between the index and middle fingers of one hand, place the other fingers beneath the body, and place the thumb over the primary flight feathers to keep the wings closed (Figure 17.4).

Due to the potential health risks from handling birds, handlers should wear appropriate protective clothing, including gloves and a face mask as a minimum, to handle birds. Cuts and grazes should be protected, and hands and arms washed thoroughly in disinfectant afterwards.

## PAIN AND STRESS RECOGNITION

As in any species, pain and distress may be recognised by disturbances to their normal appearance and behaviour, clinical signs such as changes in heart and respiratory rates, or a reduction in food and water intake. Typical signs of distress include ruffled feathers, lethargy or increased sleep time, dyspnoea or noisy breathing, and nasal or ocular discharges.

## COMMON DISEASES AND HEALTH MONITORING

The range of diseases likely to be exhibited depends on the species of bird; therefore, relevant information should be obtained prior to the design of any health-monitoring programme. There are several potentially *zoonotic diseases*, which may be caught from birds. Bacteria including *Listeria, Salmonella* and *Campylobacter* can be isolated from chickens and other birds quite frequently, and many bird species can carry avian tuberculosis. Psittacine birds may carry *Chlamydophilia*, which causes the respiratory disease psittacosis in people. Some birds may carry parasites, such as *Taenia* (tapeworms) or ectoparasites. West Nile virus is found in several species of birds in Africa, Asia and parts of Europe, and recently in North America. It can be transmitted to people via infected mosquitoes, and causes encephalitis.

Common *subclinical or clinical diseases* in birds include parasite infestations and dietary deficiencies. Wild birds caught, in particular, may have infestations with endo- or ectoparasites. For example, *Trichomonas gallinae*, a protozoan, causes canker, which can cause death in young pigeons due to asphyxiation. *Syngamus trachea* is the gapeworm, which inhabits the trachea and can cause asphyxiation, particularly in small birds. Intestinal parasites and ectoparasites such as lice or mites may cause ill thrift or more distinct clinical signs, particularly in birds which are stressed by scientific procedures. Parasites can be controlled by paying attention to the husbandry, and by the careful use of drugs as prescribed by the veterinary surgeon. It is important to disinfect housing and food and water receptacles, since parasites may be transmitted if these are unclean. Many parasites have intermediate hosts such as worms or slugs, and controlling these in the aviary will reduce transmission.

Many non-infectious diseases of birds are associated with poor management. Nutritional deficiencies are common, particularly in wild birds, since their exact needs are often unsure. These can lead to problems such as neurological abnormalities or nutritional bone disease. Birds may require supplementation with vitamins or minerals to maintain health; and if in doubt, these should always be provided. Feather plucking is also often noted in captive birds, and may be related to an inadequate environment.

There are some viral diseases which occur in birds, such as fowl pest (Newcastle disease) of chickens, which is a notifiable disease under the Animal Health Act 1981. Paramyxovirus in pigeons is caused by a similar virus, and is also notifiable. Both of these can be controlled by good management, reducing overcrowding and vaccination.

## ANAESTHESIA

Several aspects of their behaviour, anatomy and physiology require consideration when giving an anaesthetic to a bird. They have a very high BMR compared to mammals and a higher body temperature (40–44°C). This means there is a high rate of food conversion resulting in rapid onset of hypoglycemia when a small bird is deprived of food. Fasting is generally only required in birds which possess a crop, to ensure it is empty, for example chickens. This takes from 1 to 2 h in a chick, up to overnight in some adult birds. Fasting is not needed in other birds.

The difference between ambient temperature and body temperature will be great, and thermoregulation is less efficient and less adaptable in birds than in mammals. Prevention of heat loss is, therefore, vitally important during avian anaesthesia. A heat source should be provided, insulation provided (such as bedding or wrapping in aluminium foil), a minimum of plumage removed (with due regard for maintaining sterility), and as little water or alcohol based products as possible used in skin preparation to prevent cooling. In-flowing gases should be warmed and the rectal temperature of the bird monitored.

The rapid heart rate is subject to profound alteration in response to stress. Acute cardiovascular failure may occur, especially in small birds, from postural hypotension if the bird is maintained on its back for long periods or if sudden alterations in posture are made. Damage to the brachial or lumbo-sacral plexuses due to over-extension of wings or legs, or due to struggling will also cause cardiovascular failure. All movements of the bird must be made slowly and gently.

## Injection sites for anaesthesia

- *Intraperitoneal (i.p.)*: These are given in the midline, halfway between the cloaca and the sternum. A 25 G needle is inserted at a shallow angle directed cranially, so the point lies parallel to the abdominal wall. Care must be taken to avoid the air sacs.
- *Intramuscular (i.m.)*: The pectoral muscles, or the thigh in a larger bird, are used. Care is needed not to hit a blood vessel.
- *Intravenous (i.v.)*: For larger birds, the brachial veins are used. The walls are quite fragile.

If possible, weigh the bird prior to injection, but without increasing the stress by excessive handling. For example, placing it in a suitable narrow bag will aid restraint for this purpose.

## Injectable anaesthetic drugs

### Ketamine combinations

For poultry or wildfowl, 15–50 mg/kg will give light surgical anaesthesia. It may be given in incremental doses of 5 mg/kg at 5 min intervals and can be used to maintain light anaesthesia/sedation for several hours.

For small birds, mix 0.1 ml ketamine (100 mg/ml) in 0.9 ml sterile water. Give 1 mg (0.1 ml)/bird i.m. This will produce sedation in 3–4 min and recovery in about 20 min. At 2 mg/bird, there is light surgical anaesthesia for 5–12 min and recovery in 30 min. At 3 mg/bird, there is 5–20 min of anaesthesia and recovery in 60 min.

Ketamine may be used alone for induction prior to using volatile agents for longer procedures, but is most useful when used in combination with other drugs.

For deeper anaesthesia for surgical procedures where some relaxation of the muscles is required, ketamine at 20 mg/kg i.m. may be combined with midazolam (4 mg/kg i.m.), or diazepam (1.5 mg/kg i.m.), or xylazine (2–10 mg/kg), or acepromazine (0.5 mg/kg i.m.). The combination with midazolam provides the best level of analgesia. With xylazine, there is marked respiratory depression and bradycardia.

### Saffan

This may be used i.v. in larger birds; 10–14 mg/kg will give about 5–10 min of surgical anaesthesia and further incremental doses may be given.

### Barbiturates

These agents are not satisfactory for avian anaesthesia because of their narrow safety margins.

### Propofol

Due to their high BMR, this drug only lasts for a very short while, and may not provide time for intubation.

## *Other drugs*

If required, diazepam at 0.5–1.5 mg/kg i.v. or i.m. can be used for premedication. Atropine may be administered to decrease secretions, which may block the airways. The dose is 0.05 mg/kg i.m. For respiratory depression, use doxapram 5 mg/kg i.v.

## Inhalation anaesthesia

The inhalational anaesthetic of choice for birds is isoflurane, as very little is metabolised, so recovery is very rapid. It is a good analgesic, so a lower plane of anaesthesia is necessary than with halothane, with improved muscle relaxation and less respiratory depression. If halothane is used for induction, extreme care must be taken since the induction is very rapid (awake → asleep → dead in a small bird may take just 45 s). Following induction, the bird may be intubated and maintained on $O_2/N_2O/$ isoflurane or halothane, preferably via a T-piece system. Gas-flow rates should be high, about three times the minute volume. For example:

- *chicken*, body weight: 2.5 kg = 770 ml minute volume
- *pigeon*, body weight: 300 g  = 250 ml minute volume
- *cage bird*, body weight: 30 g  = 25 ml minute volume.

The airway is easily obstructed and care must be taken to keep it clear. Even short periods of apnoea can result in severe hypoxia, especially in small birds. A small plastic tube placed in the oesophagus will draw up fluid by capillary action and prevent it being aspirated into the glottis. Gases may be given directly into the interclavicular air sac by catheterisation, but the trachea will be unguarded and aspiration may occur.

Following gaseous anaesthesia, oxygen must be administered to flush anaesthetic from the air sacs as it is released from the circulation. If the bird is not properly ventilated and this is not cleared, it will be reabsorbed and could result in fatal overdose.

## POST-OPERATIVE CARE

For small birds, a quiet, dark, recovery box should be maintained at 40°C, and the bird adequately monitored. The wings should be fixed (taped to the back with micropore tape or the bird wrapped up in a towel and then taped) to prevent damage from flapping during the excitatory part of the recovery phase. Fluids should be administered at the rate of 5 ml/kg/h. Isotonic or dextrose saline should be given subcutaneously to small birds or i.v. to larger ones. Haemorrhage may be significant in a small bird, whose blood volume is 60–100 ml/kg. A 20 g bird, therefore, has a maximum blood volume of 2 ml. Losing five drops of blood will represent a 15% blood loss, which will decrease venous return causing hypotension and cardiac arrest. The bird should be encouraged to eat as soon as possible and isoflurane induced/maintained birds will eat more rapidly than others, who may be left very depressed post-operatively. Milupa baby food is a useful food to give to convalescent birds. Perches should be removed or lowered for birds in the recovery phase to avoid injury.

# ANALGESICS

- *Butorphanol*: 3–4 mg/kg is the opioid analgesic of choice.
- *Morphine*: 15–30 mg/kg.
- *Codeine*: 2.5–30 mg/kg.
- *Carprofen*: 2 mg/kg i.m.
- *Ketoprofen*: 2 mg/kg daily i.m.
- *Flunixin*: 1–5 mg/kg.
- *Xylocaine*: may be used for local analgesia.

# USEFUL DATA

Useful data for birds are provided in Tables 17.1–17.4.

**Table 17.1**    Domestic fowl: *Gallus gallus domesticus*.

| | |
|---|---|
| ***Biological data*** | |
| Adult weight (kg) | 1.3–4 |
| Diploid number* | 78 |
| Food intake (g)† | 85–150 |
| Water intake | Ad lib (200–300 ml) |
| Natural lifespan (years) | 5–8 (can live up to 30 years) |
| Rectal temperature (°C) | 41.5 |
| Heart rate/min | 200–400 |
| Blood pressure systole (mmHg) | 71–95 |
| Blood volume (ml/kg) | 60–90 |
| Respiratory rate/min | 15–30 |
| ***Breeding data*** | |
| Sexual maturity (weeks) | 19–24 |
| Age to breed (weeks) | 20–23 |
| Incubation (days) | 20–22 |
| Clutch size | 1–14, if eggs removed, birds lay daily for up to 1 year |
| Weight at hatching (g) | 50–70 g |
| ***Haematological data*** | |
| RBC ($\times 10^6$/mm$^3$) | 2.5–3.5 |
| PCV (%) | 22–35 |
| Haemoglobin (g/dl) | 7–13 |
| WBC ($\times 10^3$/mm$^3$) | 12–30 |

*Birds have a number of macrochromosomes that are of normal size, and also microchromosomes which are of reduced size and are difficult to count. This figure includes 60 microchromosomes.
†Chicks require a diet with metabolisable energy of 12.13 MJ/kg diet, which is best fed as crumbs. Layers need 11.5–11.7 MJ/kg diet.

Notes: Domestic fowl come in several varieties, including meat and egg producing varieties, and strains with defined susceptibilities to certain diseases. They are used for studies of immune function, and in studies of diseases, such as avian leucosis. Naturally, they are ground dwelling, living in groups of 4–12 females with a dominant male, and their offspring. Groups form stable hierarchies, with males being dominant. The introduction of new individuals leads to fighting. Males kept in all male groups can become aggressive.

**Table 17.2**    Japanese quail: *Coturnix japonica*.

*Biological data*

| | |
|---|---|
| Adult weight (male) (g) | 100–250 |
| Adult weight (female) (g) | 120–300 |
| Diploid number | 78 |
| Natural lifespan (years) | 2–3 |
| Rectal temperature (°C) | 38.5–41.5 |
| Food intake (g) | 100 |
| Heart rate/min | 265–548 |
| Blood pressure systole (mmHg) | 120–165 |
| Blood volume (ml/kg) | 65 |
| Respiratory rate/min | 40–85 |

*Breeding data*

| | |
|---|---|
| Sexual maturity (weeks) | 5–6 |
| Age to breed (weeks) | 8–9 |
| Breeding life (days) | 120 |
| Incubation (days) | 19–20 |
| Clutch size | 1–14 |
| Weight at hatching (g) | 6–12 |

| *Haematological data* | *Male* | *Female* |
|---|---|---|
| RBC ($\times 10^6$/mm$^3$) | 4.1 | 3.8 |
| PCV (%) | 52–54 | 45–48 |
| WBC ($\times 10^3$/mm$^3$) | 108–126 | 115–149 |

Notes: Japanese quail were domesticated as early as the twelfth century, possibly being kept for their song, and then bred for egg and meat production in the early part of the 20th century. However, many of these lines were lost during the war. The species was reconstructed after the war from a few remaining birds, from which all commercial and laboratory birds are derived. Quail are widely used in the laboratory for studies of behaviour, development, genetics, growth, nutrition, physiology and in many other areas. Quail form dominance hierarchies in the laboratory, dominant birds gaining priority access to resources. Aggression may be seen if resources are scarce, or if new birds are introduced to established groups.

**Table 17.3**    Domestic pigeon: *Columba livia*.

*Biological data*

| | |
|---|---|
| Adult weight (g) | 250–600 |
| Diploid number | 80 |
| Natural lifespan (years) | Up to 30 |
| Rectal temperature (°C) | 41 |
| Food intake (g) | 25–100 |
| Water intake (ml) | 40–50 |
| Heart rate/min | 115 (increases to 600 during flight) |
| Blood pressure systole (mmHg) | 135 |
| Blood pressure diastole (mmHg) | 105 |
| Respiratory rate/min | 25–30 |

*Breeding data*

| | |
|---|---|
| Sexual maturity (months) | 6 |
| Breeding life (years) | 8–10 |

*(Continued)*

**Table 17.3**    *(Continued).*

| Incubation (days) | 16–18 |
|---|---|
| Clutch size | 2 |
| Weight at hatching (g) | 20–50 |

Notes: Pigeons and doves constitute a range of species with variations in size, colour, habitat and feeding habits. The domestication of pigeons may date back to Ancient Egypt. Domestic pigeons may be the most common birds used in research, being used for comparative studies between classes of animals. Navigation and orientation are particular areas of interest, since pigeons can home from remarkable distances, sometimes over 500 km. They are also used in studies of cognition and learning. Pigeons usually live in loose flocks, and are monogamous, although females will mate with other males, if their partner fails to breed or dies. Pigeons can be kept in single sex groups, but are usually housed in mixed groups to prevent aggression. Pigeons need sufficient perches for all individuals to rest, and must have room to be able to stretch and flap their wings at least twice daily. Pigeons can reach speeds of up to 65 miles per hour (104 km/h) in flight.

**Table 17.4**    Zebra finch: *Taeniopygia guttata.*

| *Biological data* | |
|---|---|
| Adult weight (g) | 10–16 |
| Natural lifespan (years) | 5–12 |
| Rectal temperature (°C) | 40–42 |
| Heart rate/min | 850–1200 |
| Respiratory rate/min | 140–200 |
| BMR (kJ/h) | 0.8–0.88 |
| *Breeding data* | |
| Sexual maturity (days) | 90 |
| Age to breed (months) | 9 |
| Incubation (days) | 14 |
| Clutch size | 4–6 |
| Weight at hatching (g) | 0.7 |

Notes: The zebra finch is a small passerine bird from the Australian grasslands. They are popular in the laboratory because they are readily available and breed easily. They are used in behavioural, neurobiological and physiological research, such as studies of imprinting and sperm competition. Zebra finches are active, curious and gregarious birds, which gather in the wild in flocks of up to 1000 individuals in appropriate conditions. Breeding animals congregate in colonies of between 5 and 25 pairs. They are monogamous and form lifelong pairs. They should never be housed singly: stock birds are best housed in large single sex groups, breeding birds in pairs or small groups. They are not territorial, but if they are overcrowded or held in mixed groups with a biased sex ratio, there may be aggression. They can be housed in indoor or outdoor aviaries. They are very active, and need lots of perches of different sizes in their cages, which should not impede their flight.

# FURTHER INFORMATION

BVAAWF/FRAME/RSPCA/UFAW Joint Working Group on Refinement (2001). Laboratory birds: refinements in husbandry and procedures. *Laboratory Animals* 35(Suppl. 1).

Harrison, G.J. and Harrison, L. (1986). *Clinical Avian Medicine and Surgery.* W.B. Saunders Co., Philadelphia.

Kirkwood, J.K. (1991). Energy requirements for maintenance and growth of wild mammals, birds and reptiles in captivity. *Journal of Nutrition* 121 S29–S34.

Kirkwood, J.K. (1996). Nutrition of captive and free living wild animals. In *BSAVA Manual of Companion Animal Nutrition.* (eds. N. Kelly and J. Wills). BSAVA, Cheltenham.

Petrak, M.L. (ed.) (1982). *Diseases of Cage and Aviary Birds.* Lea and Febiger, Philadelphia.

Poole, T.E. (ed.) (1999). Birds. In *The UFAW Handbook on the Care and Management of Laboratory Animals (7th edn). Vol. I: Terrestrial Vertebrates.* Blackwell Science Publications, Oxford; pp. 661–826.

# WEBSITE

http://animalscience.ucdavis.edu/Avian/Coturnix.pdf

# Chapter 18
# Amphibia

## INTRODUCTION

Amphibians are used in a variety of research studies in the laboratory, including demonstrations of anatomy and physiology, experiments using nerves and muscles, and reproduction and hormone studies. The external development of their eggs makes them particularly suitable for studies of developmental biology. The amphibia are primitive vertebrates, which originated from fish approximately 350 million years ago, and exist between aquatic and terrestrial life. Most amphibian species today are either totally aquatic, or semi-terrestrial, needing to return to the water for breeding. The word 'amphibious' is based on the Greek, and means 'living a double life'. Amphibia have a moist, glandular skin, which secretes a mucous layer to protect against abrasions and osmotic changes, and is permeable to toxins and water, and through which they obtain a large proportion of their oxygen needs. It is vital that the skin is kept moist for gas and water exchange, and that they are not exposed to dirty conditions, where there may be toxins or bacteria.

The quality of the water is the major determining factor in the health of these animals, and should be monitored periodically. Water quality can be affected by many factors, including geographical location, source, method of transport, and type of food. Pipes for aquatic systems should not be galvanised or copper, since heavy metals can leach from such pipes and may be toxic. Water that is over-saturated with dissolved gases may cause bubbles under the skin and in the toe webs, so water should stand for several hours before use to allow dissolved gases and chlorine to dissipate and to adjust to the current room temperature. Water pH outside the range 6.5–8.5 can cause sudden death of an entire colony. Water quality standards for fish can be applied to anurans.

Amphibia are poikilothermic, which means they are unable to regulate their body temperatures by physiological means. Thus, they will be at the same temperature as their environment. This has effects on their metabolic rate – they move faster when kept in warm surroundings – and consequently on the breakdown of drugs such as antibiotics and anaesthetics. It also means that particular care must be taken to prevent unnecessary variation due to temperature fluctuations, although enclosures should provide some temperature gradients, to allow the animals to move within the gradient and regulate their body temperature behaviourally as needed. A constant temperature can cause stress. The environmental temperature has marked effects on behaviour, affecting reproduction and stress responses. All species have a preferred body temperature (PBT) range at which they function optimally. Tadpoles prefer slightly warmer temperatures. The critical maximum temperature is approximately 40°C, beyond which terrestrial amphibia may pant to try to reduce body temperature.

Many species of amphibia hibernate in the winter, and can be kept in the refrigerator for this period provided they have been well fed beforehand, and they are kept moist.

The amphibia can be divided into three groups: the Anura, which comprises the frogs and toads; the Caudata or Urodela, which comprises newts and salamanders; and the Apoda, which are little known and have no legs. The majority of amphibia used in research are Anurans, frogs and toads, but some Caudata are used as well. Some laboratory animal suppliers provide amphibians for research purposes, however, if wild caught animals are to be used it may be necessary to obtain licences under other legislation (e.g. Wildlife and Countryside Act) for their acquisition and use.

## ANURANS

Anurans are tailless amphibians (only larval stages have tails), which have well-developed hindlimbs and are good at jumping. The head and trunk are fused and the toes are webbed. Anurans do not drink, they absorb water through an area of specialised skin in the pelvic region. Respiration is largely carried out through the skin, the lungs of adults having only a minimum of lung vesicles. As frogs lack ribs, air is pumped into the lungs by muscles in the floor of the mouth. Larval stages absorb oxygen via gills, which degenerate after metamorphosis.

In anurans, the tongue is important for securing prey. It is usually muscular, flexible, and can be sticky. In most species, the tongue is attached at the front of the mouth and folded back, and can be protruded rapidly to catch prey. *Xenopus* are an exception, with the tongue completely attached to the floor of the mouth.

The commonest species of amphibians used are *Xenopus* (*X. laevis* and *X. borealis*), which are totally aquatic, and *Rana* (*R. pipiens* and *R. temporaria*), which are mainly terrestrial. These two families require different conditions in the laboratory. For both, a 12 : 12 h light : dark cycle is preferred. For successful breeding, it may be necessary to block out all outdoor lighting cues. Lights should include UV frequencies in order to maintain proper vitamin D levels and calcium/phosphorous balance. The Home Office recommendation for humidity is 70%.

## Xenopus

*Xenopus* are members of the family Pipidae, which are totally aquatic, and will desiccate after several hours if removed from water. *X. laevis*, the South African Clawed Toad, is the largest and most widely distributed of its genus. The common name comes from the presence of small, black claws on the inner three toes of the hind feet. They originate from sub-Saharan Africa, where their natural habitat is murky ponds. They are extremely hardy: *X. laevis* have been known to migrate between ponds during the rainy season, and they should *not* be released into local ponds or rivers because they will outcompete the native species. They have character traits in common with frogs and toads, and may be referred to either way. Their skin is speckled pale to dark grey or green dorsally with an off white underside, and will change colour to a certain extent to blend into the environment. It will also become pale if the animal is under stress. They absorb oxygen through the skin, and rise to the surface to breathe only occasionally. In the laboratory, *Xenopus* can live for up to 25 years.

**Table 18.1** Biological data for *X. laevis*.

| *Biological data* | | *Breeding data* | |
|---|---|---|---|
| Adult length (cm) | 5–10 (male), 8–15 (female) | Sexual maturity (months) | 12–14 (7.5 cm) |
| | | Age to breed (years) | 2 |
| Diploid number | 36 | Breeding life (years) | 6 |
| Lifespan (years) | 6–25 | Clutch size | 1–5000 |
| Heart rate/min | | Time to independent | 10 |
| (at 25°C) | 40–60 | feeding (days) | |
| (at 2°C) | 8 | | |
| Preferred temperature range (°C) | 15–18 | | |

Smaller species, including *X. borealis* and *X. tropicalis* are often available and require similar care to *X. laevis* (Table 18.1).

## Biological data

See Table 18.1.

## Housing and environmental conditions

*Xenopus* can be kept in glass or polycarbonate tanks measuring $30 \times 100$ cm. The water level should be up to 40 cm, to ensure all animals are covered with water. Twelve to twenty animals can be kept in one tank of this size (i.e. approximately 6–101 of water per animal): females are larger than males and fewer can be held in one tank. The tank should be connected to a warm water supply, containing fresh water at 15–18°C. If the temperature is too high, breeding performance may decline, whereas if it is too low, frogs will not eat and their metabolism will be slow. It is not necessary to aerate the water, but the animals benefit if the water is dechlorinated, since chlorine attacks the protective mucus layer over the skin and can predispose to infections. A wire or nylon mesh lid should be used to prevent the animals from jumping out of the tank. If the water is filtered and circulated, then cleaning out is only required infrequently. If the water is static, the tank should be cleaned out 3–5 h after feeding, that is, about three times a week. Regurgitation of food may occur if the frogs are disturbed too soon after eating. Cleaning the cage after feeding removes uneaten food that would otherwise rot. Frogs are sensitive to small changes in water temperature and fresh water should be at the same temperature as the existing water.

Amphibians can be identified in a number of ways. They shed their skin, so tattooing or branding need to be repeated after a few months to a year. Toe clipping is not an acceptable method, and in any case toes can regenerate. The best methods are documenting skin patterns (via drawings or photographs), or microchip implants. Coloured plastic or glass beads of appropriate size can also be sutured into the toe webs. Leg banding should not be used, since bands either slip off or cause necrosis of the limb.

## Behaviour

*Xenopus* spend most of their time lying motionless below the surface of the water. Captive *X. laevis* can become quite tame and may take food from a person's fingers.

Frogs will stand on their hind legs, protrude their heads from the water and may even chirp, particularly in the evenings.

## Feeding and nutrition

Frogs and toads are carnivorous. *Xenopus* naturally feed from the bottom of the lake or pond they inhabit, and in the laboratory will readily eat pelleted food, which is normally consumed within 30 min. Alternatively, they can be fed beef heart from which any tough tissue has been removed, and given supplements with vitamins. Two or three strips of heart per animal two or three times weekly is sufficient. Individual animals should be monitored to ensure they are feeding: animals 'off' feed should be noted as they may be sick. The tank should be cleaned out a few hours after feeding, to remove any debris from the water, unless a circulating filtered water system is in use. Care must be taken not to disturb the animals unduly however, as this can lead to regurgitation of the food.

## Breeding

*Xenopus* are seasonal breeders in the wild, but can be bred in the laboratory all year. Sexual maturity is reached between 12 and 14 months, and they should be bred from 2 years. Female *X. laevis* are much larger in body size than adult males of the same age, and have much larger ventral flaps, called anal papillae, located immediately above their cloacas. Males have black, spinulose nuptial surfaces (pads) on the inner arms and enlarged 'thumbs' to hold onto the females during breeding season.

Females should spawn approximately every 3 months. This avoids atresia of the eggs, but allows the female to recover between spawnings. In the laboratory, gonadotrophic hormones are usually required to initiate spawning. By altering the time of the hormone injections and the temperature of the water, the time of spawning can be regulated. A typical protocol for breeding is as follows:

- Day 1: Check the male for sexual activity, by looking for black thumb pads. If these are absent, inject 25 IU HCG per 10 g bodyweight into the dorsal lymph sac.
- Day 2: Inject 50 IU HCG per 10 g into both male and female. Place the pair into a small tank with a grid floor and a tray beneath. The water should be at 10°C. After several hours, gradually increase the water temperature to 23°C, and maintain it at this level. Eight hours later, eggs can be collected from the tray. Eggs are laid throughout the day and can continue to be collected.

## Growth of larvae

Good nutrition and water quality are essential for normal development. The speed of egg development is affected by temperature and they are generally kept at 18–22°C. The water should be aerated and direct sunlight should be avoided. Initially the water should be changed daily, then from about 10 days old they begin feeding on suspended food particles such as algae, so only half the water needs changing daily. They are herbivorous filter feeders but may also begin to eat smaller tadpoles as they grow. They hang, head down at a 45° angle, using their tails to produce a current in the water to bring microscopic food to them. Strained baby food (green beans or peas), liquefied fish food or commercial tadpole food can be added at a rate of 1 drop per 100 ml of water, if required. Food should only be added when the previous batch of food has been consumed.

*Xenopus* tadpoles have two long tentacles on their heads and are quite large, and may need to be re-accommodated several times before they metamorphose. At 2 months old they can be transferred to a standard adult tank, and metamorphosis begins at 4 months. There is gradual resorption of the tail and development of legs. This is controlled by the thyroid hormones, thus the larvae require a source of iodine. After metamorphosis, they are carnivorous and need live prey such as daphnia or mosquito larvae. Tadpoles have a high calcium requirement and in addition to their diet, absorb calcium through their gills and skin.

## Rana

*Rana* spp. are semi-terrestrial frogs, living on land in damp places and returning to water only to breed or during a drought. They are very sensitive to changes in humidity, and should have an area of water within their accommodation. Females are larger than males. *R. temporaria*, the common frog, is found in Europe and North East Asia. They are 7.5–8 cm long, and are varying shades of brown, with grey, olive, yellow or pink tones. *Rana pipiens*, the Northern Leopard frog, is native to North America. They may grow to 8 or 9 cm in length. They may be varying shades of green or brown, with round black spots scattered randomly about the back and on the sides, with a plain white belly.

### *Housing and environmental conditions*

Naturally, *Rana* spp. are found in ponds, rivers or streams, and they may move considerable distances from water especially in wet grasslands or damp woodlands. *Rana* should be kept in tanks with one third of the area covered by water 4–12 cm deep. A dry area can be created either by sloping the tank, or by providing a flat raised area. Rocks, logs, floating and submerged vegetation in the tank provide areas for the animals to warm themselves, hide, or gain access to the water. Six animals can be kept in a tank measuring 60 × 30 cm, which should have a lid if less than 60 cm in height. The animals should be provided with shelters in the dry area, where they can hide, and they may benefit if the floor is rough so they can grip it easily. If possible, a trickle of water should be allowed to flow over the dry area into the water, to remove any waste, and the whole tank should be cleaned thoroughly at least once weekly. Tap water is acceptable for terrestrial species. The temperature should be between 15 and 20°C, but may vary for different species.

### *Hibernation*

These frogs need to hibernate for up to 3 months. Naturally, they may hibernate in deep or running water that does not freeze, in muddy holes, or under rocks, sunken logs, or vegetation. In the laboratory, hibernating frogs should be kept in *dechlorinated* water in a cold room (3–4°C), and the water changed every 2 weeks. Frogs respire percutaneously during hibernation, and the presence of chlorine will be fatal. The frog may be maintained this way for 2–3 weeks. For longer periods of hibernation they need to be kept in circulating filtered and aerated water, with light restricted to less than 10 h daily.

## Behaviour

Most frogs are sluggish animals, often staying immobile for long periods of time. The characteristic croaking of frogs is used to establish individual territories and attract females. Frogs tend to hide in damp places during the day, but often wander far from standing water. They search for food during the night or on rainy days.

## Feeding and nutrition

Tadpoles and froglets are herbivorous, feeding on algae and other plant matter. The mature frogs are carnivorous, eating insects, earthworms, and other invertebrates depending on the time of year. Terrestrial anurans like *Rana* only take active prey: they may starve to death if their food does not move. Individuals can be trained to take meat from forceps, but for large numbers it is necessary to obtain live prey. Crickets are a good food source – 10 crickets dusted with a multivitamin powder can be fed to an adult frog once weekly, although a variety of foodstuffs is preferred. Large species of amphibia may take neonatal mice, slugs, or earthworms.

## Breeding

Frogs are seasonal breeders, and most frogs do not breed until 3–4 years old. They may stray far from water, but must return to open water to breed. There is a complex courtship ritual under hormonal control during which the males and females select suitable mates. Mating is by means of external fertilisation and takes place in water. The male climbs on the back of the female and grasps her body with his specialised thumbs, and releases his sperm as she lays her eggs. The eggs are in gelatinous envelopes and are laid in thick groupings. After mating, the frogs abandon their eggs.

In the wild, *R. temporaria* breed in warmer lowlands in February and March and in cooler places as late as June. The breeding period is short in this species: in three nights they lay about 400 eggs, which hatch in approximately 30–40 days. *R. pipiens* spawn annually between March and July. A single female may lay 3000–5000 eggs in a round mass, which hatch in 10–20 days. *R. temporaria* are difficult to breed in captivity, *R. pipiens* are easier. The optimal time to spawn is soon after hibernation ends, at the start of the breeding season. Place the male and female together in shallow water 8 cm deep at 10–15°C, and they should spawn in a few days.

## Growth of larvae

Eggs and tadpoles require warm (preferably 18–28°C), shallow water. Tadpoles metamorphose in about 3 months. Thereafter, the larvae require an area of dry land or they will drown. *R. temporaria* reach maturity in about 3 years, *R. pipiens* at 12 months. Temperature will affect the speed and type of development: at 10°C the young may develop into females, at 25°C they may develop into males.

## Common diseases and health monitoring

Few viruses have been isolated from amphibia.

Bacterial infections are a common cause of death in laboratory anurans. The causative agents are usually opportunists that cause infections in animals, which are stressed. Anurans may suffer from 'Red Leg', a septicaemia caused by normal water flora such as *Aeromonas, Proteus, or Pseudomonas*, with high morbidity and mortality. Sudden death is common. This is frequently associated with poor water quality, and is more common if the water is not dechlorinated. *Salmonella* is frequently isolated from the faeces of healthy anurans, and can also be pathogenic.

Fungal infections are common in amphibians and are often secondary to stress, trauma or other immunosuppressive factors.

Parasites may cause problems in animals under stress. Quarantine procedures for newly acquired animals should include routine antihelmintic therapy.

Dehydration is potentially lethal for amphibians. Care should be taken to avoid desiccation from heat sources. The delicate nature of aquatic amphibian skin predisposes them to trauma of all kinds. Any wound becomes a potential entry point for pathogenic organisms. Amphibia are particularly susceptible to toxic chemicals in their water.

If they do not have exposure to ultra violet light, amphibia may develop rickets.

## CAUDATA (URODELES)

The only member of this group found commonly in the laboratory is the Mexican Axolotl, *Ambystoma mexicanum*, which belongs to the group of salamanders known as mole salamanders. Axolotl are only found naturally in Lake Xochimilco, Mexico, where they inhabit underwater caves in clear water. They are threatened in the wild and are on CITES list II. They are characterised by the phenomenon known as persistent neoteny, in which the animals reach adulthood without metamorphosis, retaining the aquatic nature and gills of the larval form. Thus, the normal adult has gills, and these require particular care as they are susceptible to fungal infections. Metamorphosis may be induced by a number of manipulations however (see below).

Laboratory stock differ from the naturally occurring variety, but both types are highly inbred. There are several strains of axolotl available and selective breeding has allowed the accumulation of at least 35 mutant genes.

The adult wild type has brownish/black skin with black dots and diffuse grey/brown spots, although albinos are common. Animals that are ill or old become grey. They may reach 30 cm in length, and have three pairs of well-developed external gills. The sexes cannot be distinguished until they are sexually mature, at about 1 year. Adult males have relatively straight bodies and large glands about the cloaca (vent). The female has a plumper body, and a flatter cloaca without the conspicuous glands. Their natural lifespan is 8–10 years, although they rarely survive more than six under laboratory conditions.

In young axolotl it is possible to induce metamorphosis by:

1.  Feeding or injecting thyroxine, iodine or pituitary extract.
2.  Immersion in thyroxine solution.
3.  Gradual adaptation of the animal to terrestrial life.

After metamorphosis, the adult must be provided with a terrestrial environment or it will drown. The gills disappear and the tail becomes rounded. The skin becomes smooth and grey with yellow spots and there is frequent sloughing. The haemoglobin changes from larval to adult form.

## Housing and environmental conditions

Water quality is extremely important for successful husbandry. Hard water helps to maintain the integrity of the skin, which provides defence against infection. Chlorine, chloramines, or ammonia must be removed from the water. Tap water should be left standing for several hours before use to allow the gases to come off, otherwise it may cause skin damage. Salts may be added to the water, to restore hardness after water treatment and help maintain the animals' health by discouraging parasites and fungi. Extra salts are not essential, however, if husbandry is good and the water is hard and free of chemicals and heavy metals. The pH should be between 6.5 and 8.

Adult axolotl may be kept individually or in groups of up to 10, in a depth of 35–40 cm of water, which is necessary to protect the gills. High walls are required to prevent the animals from jumping out. Half the container may be covered to provide a dark area. The tank should have a large surface area to allow for gas exchange. Aeration can be beneficial. Rapidly moving water may damage the skin, so if the system used circulates the water, the rate of circulation should be as slow as possible. Still aerated water, which is partially changed two to three times weekly, is best. If gravel is used, this should be coarse to prevent the axolotl from ingesting it.

Containers for axolotl must be kept very clean, to prevent the growth of bacterial scum along the bottom and sides of the container, which may cause sores to develop on the toes and feet.

Axolotl may be given natural or artificial light, but should be kept out of direct sunlight. Some light promotes the formation of algae, which remove harmful nitrates from the water, but the growth should not be allowed to become excessive. A light cycle of 14:10 light dark is acceptable. The temperature should be kept between 15 and 20°C. Prolonged temperatures above 22°C should be avoided.

## Behaviour

Axolotl spend the bulk of their time lying nearly motionless at the bottom. They can be aggressive toward one another, and will bite off each other's gills, feet, and tails, although lost body parts will regenerate.

## Feeding

In the wild, axolotl eat worms, tadpoles, insect larvae, crustaceans and small fish. In the laboratory, they can be fed a similar diet to *Xenopus*. They should be given strips of beef heart, liver, or pelleted fish food three to four times weekly. The tank should be cleaned 1–2 h after feeding to remove any debris, or it will rot in the tank. If insufficient food is given, the animals may exhibit cannibalism. Overfeeding causes regurgitation however, and should be avoided.

## Breeding

Sexual maturity is reached in the larval stage. Adults that have metamorphosed will temporarily become amphibious again to breed. Axolotl are able to breed from 18 months of age, but are best left until 2 or 3 years. In their native habitat, axolotl breed seasonally from December to mid-July, although in captivity they may breed all year. The male and female should be kept apart, except for spawning, which should be permitted twice during the season at three monthly intervals. The animals should be kept separately for 7 days at 22°C, then placed in a tank together at 12°C, as the drop in temperature induces spawning. The tank should have a dark area for oviposition, and have a textured bottom or contain rocks to which the male can attach his spermatophores, which are mucoid packets containing spermatozoa. The male courts the female by nudging her with his snout, then there is a short mating dance. Pheromones from the female stimulate the male to deposit several spermatophores. The female is attracted to these by male pheromones, and takes one up into her cloaca. Fertilisation is internal. The male and female can be returned to separate tanks within 24 h. The female usually begins to lay eggs 12–20 h after mating. Between 200 and 600 eggs are laid in several clumps over a period of 1–2 days, and the female attaches them to plants or rocks with her back legs. The eggs or the adults should be moved before the eggs hatch, or the adults will eat the hatchlings. The eggs hatch in 2–3 weeks. At 2 weeks of age they begin swimming in search of food.

## Growth of larvae

Eggs and larvae can be reared in dishes of water at 14–18°C. These must be kept clean, and rotten eggs removed immediately. The temperature must be stable, and the eggs not exposed to sunlight. After hatching, axolotl may be kept in plastic containers with lightly aerated water. The larvae are susceptible to water pollution, and water quality must be maintained to a high standard. Larvae can be fed soon after hatching, with Daphnia or similar prey, but no uneaten food should be left which can rot in the bowl. Water should be changed daily. Once they reach 4 cm in length, they can be given the adult diet in addition, gradually increasing in proportion. Once they reach 8–10 cm, they need only the adult diet. Larvae must be fed daily until 16 cm long to prevent cannibalism. The rate of growth depends on temperature, frequency and amount of food, and the number of animals per bowl. Larvae should be about 2.5 long by the time they are 2 months old. As they grow, the number per tank should be gradually reduced. Larvae grow at different rates, so when they are divided, they should be sorted according to size, or larger ones will try to eat the smaller ones. In any case, young axolotl housed together tend to lack toes or feet, because the larvae will snap at anything that moves. Lost toes will regenerate.

# Common diseases and health monitoring

Axolotls that are properly cared for and kept in clean water are hardy animals with few diseases. If stressed, they are vulnerable to opportunistic bacterial infections such as *Pseudomonas* or *Aeromonas*. The delicate gills are a common site of fungal infection, and wounds frequently become mouldy. Disease spreads readily once it enters a colony, so meticulous hygiene is essential. Axolotls about 1-year old that are just reaching sexual maturity are most prone to illness. Ill axolotl exhibit loss of appetite and deterioration of the gills. There may be anaemia. As disease worsens there may be jaundice and open skin sores, ascites or severe oedema.

# HANDLING

Amphibia do not like to be handled, and so should only be handled if absolutely necessary. As their skin is moist and permeable, the hands should be moistened and thoroughly cleaned before handling. Ideally personnel handling animals should always wear gloves, as traces of chemicals on the hands may be very harmful. Most amphibians secrete a mucus covering and are slippery, so restraint can be difficult. They should be gripped gently but firmly, and a soft damp cloth can be used to increase grip. In some species the mucus covering is acrid, and gloves are best worn for such species. A good way to hold most frogs is to cup the body in the hand, with the hind legs facing away from the handler, between the fingers (Figure 18.1).

Wearing gloves and/or normal handwashing is usually sufficient to prevent the transmission of any diseases from amphibians to humans. However, care should be taken not to rub the eyes after handling frogs until the hands have been washed: secretions can be very irritating to the conjunctiva.

# ANAESTHESIA

Anaesthesia in amphibians is assessed by loss of righting reflexes and respiratory effort. As the level of anaesthesia deepens, abdominal respiration is lost, followed by slowing of gular movement, which stop as surgical anaesthesia is reached. At low temperatures cutaneous respiration provides sufficient oxygen to support life.

Agents intended for fish can be used in amphibians. The absorption and metabolism of anaesthetic agents are directly affected by environmental temperatures. Therefore, amphibian anesthetic dosages are frequently listed with environmental temperatures.

MS222 (tricaine methanesulphonate) can be injected or administered by immersion. For injection, the powder must be diluted in water and sterility cannot be guaranteed. The dose is 50–150 mg/kg. Immersion in a buffered solution of 300–500 mg/l in water usually results in anaesthesia within 5 min. The animal can be removed from the solution once immobile. The animal will recover within 15–30 min when placed in clean water, and will recover more quickly if the water is aerated.

Benzocaine (ethyl *p*-aminobenzoate) is similar to MS222. It requires dissolution in alcohol before use. A solution of 200–300 mg/l is needed for adults, 50 mg/l for larvae.

Volatile anaesthetic agents can also be used. In aquatic species, halothane or similar agent can be bubbled through the water, and for terrestrial species, these can be anaesthetised in a chamber, taking particular care as the agents can be irritant to the skin.

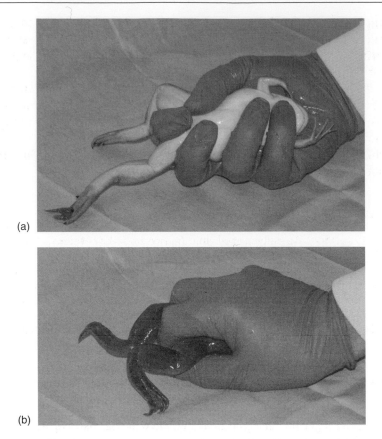

(a)

(b)

**Figure 18.1**    Handling frogs.

Some injectable agents may also be used. Ketamine can be given at 50–150 mg/kg by i.m injection, although animals may remain sensitive to pain. It can also be given with xylazine.

While the animals are anaesthetised, it is essential that they are kept moist, by regular spraying with sterile water or saline, and by keeping on a damp towel. The temperature should be below 21°C. Adult axolotl and larval forms, which have gills, will die if kept out of water for more than 5 min, so procedures on these must be short.

Hypothermia may appear to result in anaesthesia, since the animals become immobile, but there is no evidence that analgesia is produced by cooling, so potentially painful procedures, such as entry into a body cavity, must be carried out using one of the anaesthetic methods outlined above.

## TECHNIQUES

Intramuscular injections can be given into the muscles of the thigh.

Anurans have subcutaneous lymph spaces that connect with the vascular system. A common site for intravenous injections is the dorsal lymph sacs, which are actually paired lymph hearts located dorsally on either side of the last vertebrae. A long fine needle should be inserted at a shallow angle with the animal suitably restrained.

Intraperitoneal injections should be given into the groin area with the frog held on its back with its head directed downward.

Blood collection in amphibians is often difficult because of low body weight and poor access to vessels. Blood samples can be collected by cardiac puncture under general anaesthesia, or small samples may be collected by clipping a nail or toe web after using some local anaesthetic.

Amphibian blood contains nucleated erythrocytes, leukocytes and thrombocytes. Amphibian erythrocytes are the largest of all vertebrate erythrocytes.

## FURTHER INFORMATION

Crawshaw, G.J. (1993). Amphibian medicine. In *Zoo and Wild Animal Medicine*, 3rd edn (ed. M. Fowler). Saunders, Philadelphia, pp. 131–39.

Halliday, T.R. (1999). Amphibians. In *The UFAW Handbook on the Care and Management of Laboratory Animals,* 7th edn (ed. T.B. Poole). Longman, London; pp. 90–103.

Mattison, C. (1983). Anura-frogs and toads. In *The Care of Reptiles and Amphibians in Captivity*, 3rd edn (ed. C. Mattison). Sterling Publishing Co., New York; pp. 121–27.

O'Rourke, D.P. (2002). Reptiles and amphibia as laboratory animals. *Lab Animal Europe* 2(6), 37–41.

## WEBSITES

http://www.images/leopardFrog.jpgimages/leopardFrog.jpg

http://www.aquatic.uoguelph.ca/amphibians/amphib/accounts/ranidae/leopard/account.htm

http://allaboutfrogs.org/info/species/leopard.html

http://www.indiana.edu/~axolotl/axolotls/shortguide/guide.html

http://www.ahsc.arizona.edu/uac/iacuc/xenopus/ref.shtml University of Arizona Learning Module on Amphibia.

www.ukans.edu/~ssar/SSAR.html Society for the Study of Amphibians and Reptiles

# Chapter 19
# Wild animals

## GENERAL CONSIDERATIONS

There are particular considerations when dealing with wild animals. Since they are not bred specifically for the laboratory and are not used to being handled, they are likely to be more stressed by the presence of humans and by procedures than standard laboratory species. Captivity will induce particular stresses; and in many cases, their exact biological needs will be unknown. All these features will contribute to the overall costs of acquiring and keeping such animals for research, and should be taken into account when performing the cost–benefit analysis on the project licence application. The Code of Practice (CoP) for the housing and care of animals used in scientific procedures specifies minimum standards of care for the common laboratory species, and at least the same degree of care should be given to wild species. Researchers should familiarise themselves in advance with the needs of their particular species, and techniques to minimise the distress caused to the animals during captivity.

## Legislation and guidance

Many wild species will be covered by legislation other than the Animals (Scientific Procedures) Act 1986 (ASPA) (see Chapter 2). For example, some endangered or threatened species are covered by the Convention on International Trade in Endangered Species (CITES) of flora and fauna. Wild animals, including birds, reptiles and amphibians, are protected by the Wildlife and Countryside Act 1981. Badgers, seals, deer and fish are afforded additional statutory protection. In some cases, permission from DEFRA may be required.

For work done in the UK, it will be necessary to take account of the following:

- The Protection of Animals Acts 1911–1988.
- The Animal Health Act 1981.
- The Welfare of Animals in Transit Order 1997.
- The Abandonment of Animals Act 1960.
- The Wild Mammals Protection Act 1996.
- The Wildlife and Countryside Act 1981.
- The CITES.
- A range of species-specific legislation (e.g. the Badgers Acts, the Deer Act 1991).

The trapping of wild animals for use in research should be humane and may only be undertaken by competent personnel. If pharmacological restraint is required, it should be given under veterinary supervision. Relevant professional or local guidance must be followed at all times. This will include, as appropriate:

- guidance from expert bodies (such as the British Trust for Ornithology or Nature Conservancy)
- Codes of practice set by professional journals and learned societies (e.g. Association of the Study of Animal Behaviour, Mammal Society)
- guidance from site owners/wardens
- guidance from sponsors
- health and safety advice
- welfare guidance.

No one may work with animals in any capacity without having satisfactorily completed appropriate training. For example, if licences are required under the ASPA, licensee training will be needed. In the case of research on wild birds, training will be required in the netting and ringing of birds (from the BTO); for the trapping of mammals, training from the Mammal Society may be needed and training in relevant health and safety issues may be necessary. The supervisor of the programme must ensure competence in any necessary handling of the species, and the researcher must be sufficiently familiar with the habits and biology of the species to detect major departures from the normal state. Veterinary or animal welfare advice must be sought and taken in any case where the health or welfare of an animal gives rise to concern. Adequate time must be allocated to allow aptitude to be developed with adequate training, then assessed and the required standards achieved. For netting birds, 6-months training is typically advised.

## Project planning

Before beginning a project involving the use of wild species, plan the project carefully. Consider the following points:

- Consult a statistician at an early stage, to ensure that the minimum number of animals consistent with the aims of the project is used, and that animals are not wasted by having a sample that is too small. This is of course true for all projects involving animals, but is particularly important when dealing with endangered or threatened species.
- Review the literature, to become familiar with current techniques and husbandry methods. Ignorance of these may cause undue distress and is unacceptable.
- Ensure familiarity with the biology of the species involved. Avoid disturbances at times when interference may have a great impact on the species as a whole, such as breeding times, nesting, late pregnancy, parturition and neonatal periods.
- Avoid causing disturbances to other species in the area, which are not being studied, and minimise damage to the habitat.
- Ensure maximum use of samples and material obtained from the study.
- When trapping animals, the trap must keep the animal alive, uninjured and in a comfortable microenvironment. An open-sided wire mesh trap is unlikely to fulfil this requirement, since the animals will be uncomfortable and may feel exposed

and vulnerable. Traps should be designed according to the biology of the species, and should avoid trapping non-target species.

- Anaesthetics and analgesics suitable for the species and procedure should be used, which allow the animal to make a rapid return to consciousness. Animals should only be released when they have recovered sufficiently from the procedures to be able to cope with hazards in the environment.
- Since there may not be the opportunity to check on the animals post-operatively, surgical procedures must be performed to a particularly high standard, using strict aseptic techniques and good surgical and suturing methods.

## CONSIDERATIONS UNDER THE ANIMALS (SCIENTIFIC PROCEDURES) ACT 1986

Much research in the wild does not come under ASPA, but any scientific procedures that may have potential to cause pain, suffering, distress or lasting harm will be regulated and may only be carried out as approved. The Home Office Inspectorate can advise on a case-by-case basis and must be consulted wherever a question arises as to whether or not a particular programme of work requires regulation under ASPA. Capture and handling are not in themselves currently regarded as coming within the definition of a regulated procedure, but best practice is essential to ensure that trapping does not cause pain, suffering, distress or lasting harm. Best practice will include careful attention to the choice of trap, its layout, siting and positioning; and appropriate supply of food and bedding. Extra care will be needed in hot or cold weather or where traps may be in the presence of predators. Traps must be checked sufficiently frequently that stress to captured animals is minimised. Equal care is required on release to ensure animals have not been unduly compromised in their chances of survival. Consideration must be given to their ability to re-establish themselves within their own community and to find sources of food and water, and that they are not unreasonably exposed to predators. The netting and ringing of birds is also not regulated under ASPA, but is covered by controls drawn up by the British Trust for Ornithology on behalf of the Joint Nature Conservancy Council, English Nature and other bodies, under the Wildlife and Countryside Act 1981. Anyone wishing to work in an area that requires the capture of wild birds must be familiar with these controls and have received the necessary training.

It is important to bear in mind the potential consequences which interventions may have on animals other than those captured; for example on dependent young (lactating females should be promptly released from traps). Relevant issues should be discussed with the Home Office Inspectorate since regulation under ASPA may be required if a project has potential to cause distress to, for example, animals dependent on those captured.

## Release of animals back to the wild

Animals which have been taken into captivity and subjected to scientific procedures may need to be released back into the wild at the end of or during the procedures.

The release of animals under these circumstances, however mild the procedures, requires the prior consent of the Home Office. The ASPA requires that animals on which regulated procedures have been performed are killed at the conclusion of the series of regulated procedures, unless a veterinary surgeon or other competent person determines that they are not suffering or likely to suffer as a result of the procedures. In addition, if the animal is to be released at a place which is not a designated establishment, a veterinary surgeon must certify that the animal will not suffer if it is released in that place. However, such work may be undertaken at remote sites (e.g. nature reserves), where it is not practicable for a veterinary surgeon to be in constant attendance. In such situations, it may be necessary to rely on observance, by suitably trained and qualified persons, of a written protocol, which is not expected to cause lasting harm if followed correctly. The veterinary surgeon may then be assured that an animal will be fit, if the protocol is carefully followed by these trained and competent individuals.

If animals are to be released to the wild in the course of regulated procedures, for example in studies where individuals are captured, measurements are made, then the animals are released and recaptured at intervals, additional safeguards must be put in place. Under Section 10.3 of the Act, the Secretary of State will need to be satisfied that 'the maximum possible care has been taken to safeguard the well-being of the animal; that its state of health allows it to be set free; and setting it free will pose no danger to public health or the environment.' These issues should all be addressed in Section 18d of the project licence. The Secretary of State will require the project licence holder to obtain certificates of fitness from a veterinary surgeon or other suitably qualified person that the animals are indeed fit for release.

In addition to ensuring that the requirements of other relevant legislation have been met, it is equally important to ensure the well-being of animals released into the wild after capture, even if they have been used for purposes not regulated under ASPA. In the case of research on farms or other partially protected sites, it may be possible to exercise a degree of supervision after their release. Where possible, there should be appropriate monitoring of the animal for unexpected adverse effects. The animals should not find themselves at a biological disadvantage as a result of the procedures performed or of their captivity. Regard should also be paid to the welfare of other individuals (e.g. the offspring of those captured). The following considerations should apply:

- Animals should not be released in such a way as unreasonably to expose them to risk (e.g. of predation, thirst or hunger).
- Animals should be released at a suitable site, normally within their home range.
- The timing of the release should take account of the animal's normal daily and seasonal activity patterns and other relevant factors.
- Where animals have been injured or found to be injured or unwell, account must be taken of relevant veterinary advice and welfare considerations.
- The duration of capture should be the minimum consistent both with the object of the experiment and with humane release.
- Thought should be given to the consequences of the release of animals into the food chain.

# HEALTH AND SAFETY CONSIDERATIONS

Chapter 3 covers general health and safety aspects of animal use. However, there are particular problems associated with the use of wild species. They are more likely to bite, scratch or otherwise injure the handler than domestic species. There may still be risks from allergies, the health status is unknown, and they may be harbouring potentially zoonotic diseases. In addition, in the case of dangerous species, steps need to be taken to protect the public from the hazards associated with the animals. All personnel working with wild animals should be appropriately trained in their care, and familiar with the action to be taken in the event of injuries, escapes or disease problems.

# IDENTIFICATION OF WILD ANIMALS

The ringing, tagging or marking of an animal for the sole purpose of identification is not regulated under ASPA, if it causes only momentary distress and no lasting harm. Best practice must none the less be followed, as prescribed, for example, by the British Trust for Ornithology, and account taken of the ways in which identification techniques may compromise an animal's ability to function. Individual animals may be identified by their unique features, or by methods as used in other laboratory species. Leg rings, ear tags or wing tags, freeze branding, tattoos, collars and microchips are all suitable methods depending on the species. Methods which involve physical alteration of the animal such as ear notching or toe clipping are not recommended, since they can affect the animal's behaviour or ability to survive once released back into the wild.

# ANAESTHESIA OF WILD ANIMALS

## General considerations

Particular success for a wide range of wildlife species has been noted with the use of isoflurane, either alone or in combination with injectable agents. For larger species, such as badgers, otters and foxes, induction of anaesthetic is generally by injectable agents. These are administered through the mesh of the trapping cage, using a crush cage (see Figure 19.1) or by means of a blowpipe. However, many commonly used injectable combinations include non-reversible agents with associated prolonged recovery times. This is generally undesirable in the field: facilities are unlikely to exist to provide warm, stable temperatures; it is difficult for personnel to monitor the recovery of more than a few individuals, thereby limiting productivity; and animals are prevented from resuming normal activities (e.g. hunting for food or protecting young). It is also important to note that controlled anaesthesia is important for the operator: an animal suddenly recovering from anaesthesia is likely to bite and so present a risk of injury and zoonotic disease transfer.

Although fieldwork presents particular challenges, many of the procedural refinements used in the laboratory or surgery can be transferred. A folding 'wallpaper pasting table' covered in thick polythene sheeting and disposable paper covers functions well as an operating table, which can readily be disinfected between animals (see Figure 19.2). Some of the problems encountered in the trapping and subsequent

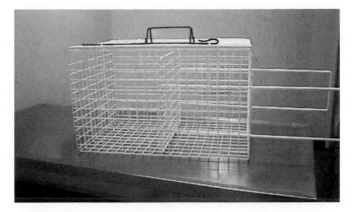

**Figure 19.1**    Crush cage for use with small wild animals.

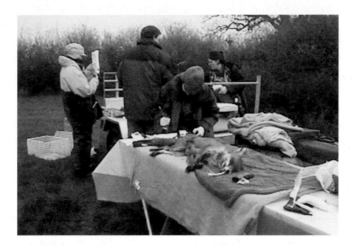

**Figure 19.2**    The field laboratory for wildlife anaesthesia.

anaesthesia of small wild animals are due to their very small size. Their high ratio of surface area to body weight is such that they lose heat rapidly and hypothermia must be prevented. All animals should, therefore, be placed on a hot-water bottle covered in veterinary bedding during anaesthesia. Portable gel heat-pads or hot-water bottles should be used during recovery where appropriate. All animals must be placed in sheltered positions, provided with food, and their holding cages covered with blankets or bubble wrap for this period. Death rates in traps are known to be high for shrews, possibly because their very high metabolic rates and thermal requirements mean that they are in poor condition at the start of the procedure.

## Inhalational anaesthesia

Apparatus for inhalational anaesthesia in the field is simple in concept and light enough to be portable in a simple backpack. A vaporiser, which weighs approximately 7 kg, is attached to a portable oxygen cylinder (see Figure 19.3). It is important to note

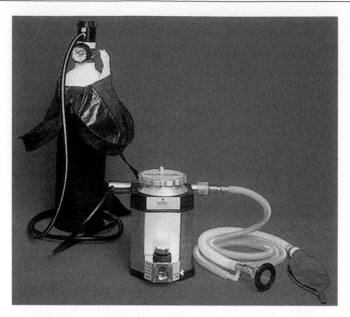

**Figure 19.3**   Isoflo apparatus for use in the field.

even with a temperature-compensated model, prolonged exposure to temperatures below 10°C (e.g. overnight storage in a vehicle in winter) will adversely affect the calibration for some time after air temperatures have risen again. This is due to the slow rate at which the vaporiser is designed to expand and contract. This problem can be overcome in the field by protecting the vaporiser from protracted exposure to low temperatures using an insulated box, if necessary supplied with hot-water bottles. The vaporiser is connected using standard circuitry to a portable 230L medical oxygen cylinder (weight 2.9 kg). The cylinder can be refilled from a standard-sized canister using a recharging adaptor. The cylinder should be fitted with a regulator permitting flow rates of 1–15 l/min.

The protocol used for induction depends on the size of the animal. Small mammals caught in metal box Longworth traps can be gently tipped with their bedding into a transparent polythene bag. This bag then serves as an induction chamber, with the neck of the bag being held closed around the anaesthetic gas tube (see Figure 19.4). Larger species caught in wire mesh traps, such as squirrels, rats and rabbits, can be anaesthetised as above, except the whole trap is placed inside a polythene bag. Larger animals such as badgers and foxes are better given short acting reversible injectable anaesthetic for induction (Figure 19.5). All species are then transferred to a face mask or intubated for maintenance (see Figures 19.6 and 19.7). Since fieldwork is often conducted out of doors, there may be no need for a scavenging system to be included in the circuit. The main advantage of this inhalation system is its safety for the animal, despite their unknown health status at induction. In addition, the animals recover very quickly from isoflurane, most are fit for release within 20 min of the end of anaesthesia and can be returned to the wild with less disruption to them and to their population than using injectable methods alone.

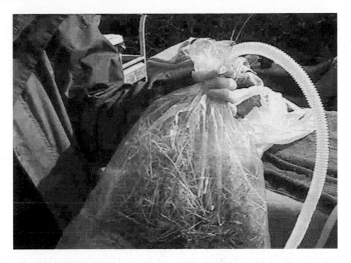

**Figure 19.4**    Induction of inhalation anaesthesia in small rodents in the field.

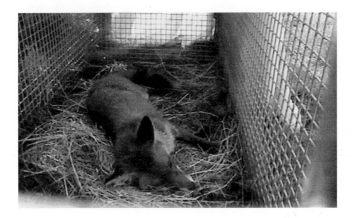

**Figure 19.5**    Fox given injectable induction agents.

# Drug doses and body size

When administering drugs to wild animals, it is common to extrapolate doses from other species where the dose rate is known. However, since smaller animals have a relatively higher basal metabolic rate, the dose required is not dependent on the body weight ($W$, kg), but on the metabolic body weight, which can be obtained by $W^{0.75}$, and the energy group to which the animal belongs. Animals can be divided into five energy groups depending on the mean core temperature range (see Table 19.1). Hainsworth identified constants for each group, and when the metabolic body weight is multiplied by the Hainsworth constant, the product can be used to set up ratios for scaling pharmacokinetic or physiological parameters from one species to another. This process is known as allometric scaling.

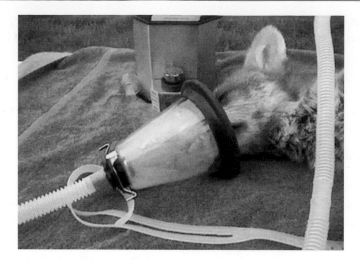

**Figure 19.6**    Fox with inhalation maintenance agent via face mask.

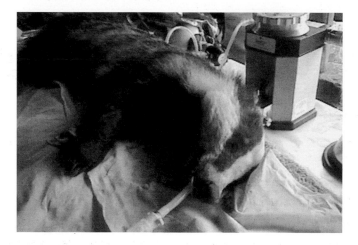

**Figure 19.7**    Badger with an endotracheal tube.

**Table 19.1**    Hainsworth's energy groups.

| Group | | Constant ($K$) | Mean core temperature (°C) |
|---|---|---|---|
| A | Passerine bird | 129 | 42 |
| B | Non-passerine bird | 78 | 40 |
| C | Placental mammal | 70 | 37 |
| D | Marsupial mammal | 49 | 35 |
| E | Reptile | 10 | 37* |

*Requires body temperature to be held artificially at 37°C.

To extrapolate dose rates or frequencies from one species to another, the animal's specific minimum energy cost (SMEC) must be calculated. This is given by

$$\frac{K(W^{0.75})}{W} = K(W^{-0.25})$$

Then to calculate the test dose or frequency by extrapolating from a known dose rate or frequency:

$$\frac{\text{Control dose or frequency}}{\text{Control SMEC}} = \frac{\text{Test dose or frequency}}{\text{Test SMEC}}$$

For example, if the dose of a drug for a 10 kg dog is 10 mg/kg twice daily, the dose $D$ and frequency $F$ for a 20 g mouse can be calculated by

$$\frac{10}{70 \times (10^{-0.25})} = \frac{D}{70 \times (0.02^{-0.25})} \quad \text{therefore} \quad D = 47.3 \text{ mg/kg}$$

$$\frac{2}{70 \times (10^{-0.25})} = \frac{F}{70 \times (0.02^{-0.25})} \quad \text{therefore} \quad F = 9.4$$

So, a mouse needs 47.3 mg/kg of the drug 9.4 times daily, or every 2½ h.

These formulae can be used to calculate reasonable, effective dose regimes for any species of warm-blooded animal, ranging from the smallest birds to large ungulates.

## Drug doses for wild animals

The following regimes may be used as guidelines for injectable anaesthesia of some particular species of wild animals:

### Rats, mice, voles and rabbits

The doses described in Chapter 12 may be used remembering that the health and condition of the animal may not be as robust as an animal in the laboratory.

### Squirrel

*Medetomidine* (Domitor) 250 µg/kg + *Ketamine* (Vetalar) 60 mg/kg administered together intramuscularly (i.m.). For a 700 g squirrel, use 0.2 ml Domitor + 0.4 ml Vetalar.

Reverse with *atipamezole* (Antisedan) at 1 mg/kg subcutaneously (0.15 ml Antisedan for a 700 g squirrel).

### Hare

- *Medetomidine* (Domitor) 0.25 ml/kg. i.m. Adjust according to response. For a 3 kg hare, start with a dose of 0.75 ml Domitor.

- Reverse with *atipamezole* (Antisedan), starting dose 0.1 ml Antisedan (for 3 kg hare). Adjust according to response. May need up to 0.75 ml Antisedan. Try a low dose and give more if necessary after 3–5 min.
- *Ketamine* (Vetalar) may be used if medetomidine does not prove successful. Use a starting dose of 0.25 ml Vetalar/kg (0.75 ml for 3 kg hare).
- If respiratory failure occurs, give *doxapram* (Dopram V) 1 ml intravenously (i.v.) if possible, or if not i.m., repeat after 5–10 min if necessary.

## Hedgehog

*Ketamine* (Vetalar) at 20 mg/kg produces sedation with recovery in 30 min. For general anaesthesia, use ketamine 20 mg/kg with *xylazine* (Rompun) at 0.2 ml/kg, given i.m.

## Badger

*Ketamine* (Vetalar) at 15–20 mg/kg i.m. produces immobilisation, and at 30 mg/kg produces deep tranquillisation. This lasts for about 45 min, but will take much longer to work if the environmental temperature is low.

For general anaesthesia: 20 µg/kg *medetomidine* (Domitor) with 4 mg/kg *ketamine* + 0.8 mg/kg *butorphanol* is an excellent combination. Alternatively, 2.0 mg/kg (0.1 ml/kg) *xylazine* (Rompun) with 7.0 mg/kg (0.07 ml/kg) *ketamine* i.m. or 0.05 ml/kg *medetomidine* (Domitor) with 0.1 ml/kg Hypnorm i.m. Reverse with 0.05 ml/kg *atipamezole* (Antisedan) and 0.1 ml/kg *naloxone* (Narcan) i.m., or 70–80 µg/kg *medetomidine* with 3.5–4 mg/kg *ketamine* i.m. Reverse with 350–400 µg/kg *atipamezole* i.m.

## Beaver

*Ketamine* 20 mg/kg + *acepromazine* 2.5 mg if it weighs under 18 kg, 4 mg if it is over 18 kg, top up with 50–80 mg *ketamine* if necessary.

## Otter

*Medetomidine* 40 µg/kg + *ketamine* 4 mg/kg administered via a blow pipe to produce heavy sedation, then 30 µg/kg *medetomidine* + 3 mg/kg *ketamine* given i.m. will produce 40 min anaesthesia and can be reversed with 350 µg/kg *atipamezole*.

## FURTHER INFORMATION

Association for the Study of Animal Behaviour (1996). Guidelines for the treatment of animals in behavioural research and teaching. *Animal Behaviour* 51, 241–46.

Brooman and Legge (1997). *The Law Relating to Animals*. Cavendish.

Fowler, M.E. and Miller R.E. (1999). *Zoo and Wild Animal Medicine: Current Therapy*. Saunders

Hainsworth, F.R. (1981). *Animal Physiology: Adaptations in Function*. Addison-Wesley; pp. 160–63.

Mathews, F., Honess, P., Wolfensohn, S. (2001). Refinements in wildlife anaesthesia. *Veterinary Record* 150, 785–87.

McKenzie, A.A. (ed.) (1993). *The Capture and Care Manual: Capture, Care, Accommodation and Transportation of Wild African Animals.* Wildlife Decision Support Services CC and The South African Veterinary Foundation, South Africa.

Osofsky, S.A. and Hirsch, K.J. (2000) Chemical restraint of endangered mammals for conservation purposes: a practical primer. *Oryx* 34, 27–33.

RCVS Legislation Affecting the Veterinary Profession in the UK.

Redfern, C. (2001). *The Ringers Manual*. BTO, Thetford.

*Management and Welfare of Farm Animals* (1994). UFAW, London.

Vogel, P. (1980). Metabolic levels and biological strategies in shrews. In *Comparative Physiology, Primitive Mammals* (eds. K. Schmidt-Nielsen, L. Bolis and C.R. Taylor). Cambridge, Cambridge University Press; pp. 170–80.

Summary of Legislation Relation to Animal Welfare at Levels of the European Community and the Council of Europe. Brussels, Eurogroup for Animal Welfare.

## WEBSITES

Guidelines for the Capture, Handling and Care of Mammals as approved by the American Society of Mammologists: http://www.mammalsociety.org/committees/index.asp

The Mammal Society: http://www.abdn.ac.uk/mammal/

The British Trust for Ornithology: http://www.bto.org/

CITES: www.cites.org

Association for the Study of Animal Behaviour: http://www.societies.ncl.ac.uk/asab/

English Nature: www.english-nature.org.uk

# Glossary

**Acidosis**  A reduction in the pH of the blood, commonly due to an increase in blood carbon dioxide level.

**Adjuvant**  An added substance which assists or increases the effect of the main ingredient.

**Akinesia**  Absence or loss of voluntary movement.

**Alar**  Related to the wing.

**Alopecia**  Hair loss.

**Anaphylaxis**  Increased susceptibility to hypersensitivity or infection on second exposure to a substance characterised by a very rapid reaction.

**Anorexic**  Not eating.

**Anterior**  An anatomical term meaning towards the front (usually head) end.

**Apnoea**  Respiratory arrest.

**Arrhythmia**  Irregularity of the heart beat.

**Ataxia**  Loss of muscular coordination.

**Atopy**  A form of hypersensitivity where there is a familial tendency to develop conditions such as hay fever, asthma and eczema.

**Axenic**  Animals, which are free from detectable micro-organisms.

**Barbering**  The chewing and nibbling of whiskers and fur by one rodent to exert dominance over another.

**Cardiac tamponade**  Effusion of blood or fluid into the pericardium which prevents the heart from being able to fill effectively, thereby causing circulatory failure.

**Caudal**  An anatomical term meaning towards the tail.

**Cloned animal**  An animal produced by inserting nuclear material from one cell into another by nucleus transfer.

**Coprophagy**  The eating of faeces carried out by rodents and lagomorphs to allow nutrients released during microbial digestion in the hindgut to be absorbed.

**Cranial**  An anatomical term meaning towards the head.

**Crepuscular**  Active at dawn and dusk.

**Cyanosis**  Bluish colouration of the skin and mucous membranes due to poor blood oxygenation.

**Cystocentesis**  A method of sampling urine by passing a needle through the abdominal wall into the lumen of the bladder (under aseptic conditions).

**Decerebration**  Removal or separation of the cerebral cortex, leaving the brain stem intact. Such animals are considered to be insentient but are still alive.

**Diuretic**   Promoting the excretion of urine.

**Dorsal**   An anatomical term meaning towards the back.

**Dyscrasia**   Any disease causing abnormalities in the cellular constituents of blood.

**Dystocia**   Difficulty in giving birth.

**Dysuria**   Difficulty or pain on urination.

**Effusion**   Escape of fluid from blood vessels or lymphatics into a body cavity.

**Embolism**   The passage of a blood clot or other particulate matter in the blood-stream to a site distant from the site of origin, causing blockage of a vessel.

**Emesis**   Vomiting.

**Endotoxaemia**   The presence of endotoxin (bacterial products) in the blood, which frequently results in shock, due to vasodilation.

**Epidemic**   A disease affecting a large proportion of individuals in a colony simultaneously.

**Exudate**   The extravasation of fluid and/or cells from the blood into the tissues, any body cavity or the surface, usually due to inflammation.

**Genetically altered animal**   An animal in which the heritable DNA has been manipulated intentionally. This includes genetically modified animals and harmful mutants.

**Genetically modified animal**   An animal in which there has been insertion or deletion of DNA in a way that does not occur naturally.

**Genotype**   The genetic makeup of an animal.

**Gnotobiotic**   Animals that harbour known micro-organisms.

**Haemolysis**   The splitting or disintegration of red blood cells resulting in the release of haemoglobin.

**Harmful mutant**   An animal in which the genome has been altered by point mutation or chromosomal changes, without insertion or deletion of DNA, with resulting potential for harm.

**Hepatotoxin**   A compound which is toxic to the liver.

**Hypercapnia**   A high level of carbon dioxide in the blood.

**Hypertonic**   One of two solutions, which has the higher osmotic pressure.

**Hypnotic**   As narcotic. A drug, which induces sleep.

**Hypoglycaemia**   A low blood glucose level.

**Hypotonic**   One of two solutions, which has the lower osmotic pressure.

**Hypoxia**   A low blood oxygen level.

**Iatrogenic**   Caused through medical intervention.

**Infarction**   Necrosis of part of an organ or tissue due to blockage of its arterial supply, by a thrombus or embolus in the end arteriole.

**Isotonic**   Two solutions having equal osmotic pressure.

**Laparoscopy**   Examination of the abdominal cavity usually via the passage of an endoscope through a keyhole incision, for diagnosis or to perform surgical procedures.

**Laparotomy**   A surgical procedure involving incision into the abdominal cavity.

**Lordosis**   A position adopted by female animals in oestrus to facilitate copulation, with the back arched and the tail held to one side.

**Meconium**   The first intestinal discharge from a neonate.

**Morbidity**   The proportion of a colony infected by a disease.

**Mortality**   The proportion of individuals affected by a disease, which die from it.

**Mutagenesis**   Exposing animals to chemicals, viruses or radiation in order to increase the rate of mutation of genes.

**Narcotic**   A substance which induces sleep.

**Nephrotoxin**   A substance which is toxic to the kidney.

**Nystagmus**   A repetitive movement of the eyeballs, consisting of a slow movement in one direction followed by a rapid return.

**Phenotype**   The physical characteristics of an animal.

**Pheromone**   Hormone-like substance secreted by one animal, which causes behavioural, physiological, or endocrine changes in another.

**Phlebitis**   Inflammation of a vein.

**Posterior**   An anatomical term meaning towards the rear.

**Pyrexia**   Fever.

**Rostral**   An anatomical term meaning towards the nose or beak, used for describing structures on the head.

**Ruminal tympani**   Distension of the forestomach (rumen) with gas.

**Sedative**   A drug which produces a calming effect and drowsiness.

**Sentient**   Capable of feeling, perceiving sensations.

**Skin tenting**   A phenomenon, usually caused by dehydration, in which a fold of skin remains raised for several seconds after being pinched.

**Specific pathogen free**   Animals free from particular (named) micro-organisms.

**Stereotypy**   The performance of unusual motor acts, repeatedly and often invariably, which serve no apparent purpose. Often indicative of an inadequate environment.

**Subclinical**   A period prior to the appearance of manifest symptoms in the development of a disease.

**Syncope**   A sudden fall in blood pressure or heart failure leading to cerebral anaemia and loss of consciousness.

**Tachycardia**   Rapid heart beat.

**Teratogenesis**   The production of abnormalities in a fetus, due to exposure of the dam to physical or chemical insult.

**Therapeutic index**   The ratio between the lethal dose of a drug and its effective clinical dose.

**Thrombosis**   The inappropriate formation of a blood clot.

**Tranquiliser**   A drug which produces a calming effect without drowsiness.

**Transgenic**   An animal in which additional genes have been inserted.

**Transudate**   The passage of fluid into the tissues or a body cavity, usually passively without inflammation.

**Urticaria**   Nettle rash.

**Ventilation**   A term used to describe forced breathing, by the application of positive pressure to the airways (intermittent positive pressure ventilation).

**Ventral**   An anatomical term meaning towards the belly.

**Xiphisternum**   Cartilaginous process on the caudal end of the sternum.

**Zoonosis**   A disease communicable from animals to man.

# Index